[redacted]

FORTY FIFTH EDITION

MODELL'S DRUGS IN CURRENT USE AND NEW DRUGS

1999

Elizabeth A. Duthie, RN, MA
Editor

SPRINGER PUBLISHING COMPANY
New York

[redacted]

ORDER YOUR 2000 EDITION

Prepublication price: $28.95 10 or more copies, 10% discount

The $28.95 price and quantity discount will be retained for all orders mailed before **December 1, 1999.** The final price for the 2000 edition will be higher.

To receive your Modell's DRUGS IN CURRENT USE AND NEW DRUGS 2000 upon its publication in January 2000, send your order with payment to:

Springer Publishing Co., Inc.
536 Broadway
New York, N. Y. 10012

Please send ________ copies of MODELL'S DRUGS IN CURRENT USE AND NEW DRUGS 2000. Enclosed is $28.95 plus $4.50 for postage for first copy, $1.50 for each additional copy. New York State residents add sales tax.

Name ____

Institution ____

Street address _______________________________________

City ________________ State __________ Zip _______________

Telephone ________________

If you wish to charge it:

Charge to: ❑ Visa ❑ Mastercard ❑ Amex

Card no: _________________________ Exp. date _________________

MODELL'S DRUGS IN CURRENT USE AND NEW DRUGS

1999

536 Broadway New York, New York 10012

Library of Congress Catalog Card Number: 72-622-911
International Standard Book Number: 0-8261-7657-7
International Standard Serial Number: 1044-0704
Printed in U.S.A.

The Editor and Publisher have made every attempt to check dosages and nursing content for accuracy. Because the science of pharmacology is continually advancing, our knowledge base continues to expand. Therefore we recommend that the reader always check product information for changes in dosage or administration before administering any medication. This is particularly important with new or rarely used drugs.

The Publisher shall not be liable for any special, consequential, or exemplary damages resulting, in whole or in part, from the readers' use of, or reliance on, the information contained in this book.

ABOUT THE EDITOR

Elizabeth A. Duthie, RN, MA, attended St. Vincent's Hospital School of Nursing in New York City and received her BSN from Seton Hall University in South Orange, NJ and her MA in Nursing Education from New York University. She is currently matriculated at New York University in the Ph.D. program in nursing research. Ms. Duthie is employed at New York University Medical Center as the Director of Nursing for Education and Patient Care Systems. She taught Pharmacotherapeutics to undergraduate nursing students at New York University for 10 years and Advanced Pharmacology to graduate-level nursing students in the Nurse Practitioner Program. Ms. Duthie is a member of the Pharmacology & Therapeutics Committee of the medical board at the hospital and chairs a multidisciplinary committee that assesses practices surrounding medication administration and implements procedures to facilitate safe delivery of drugs. Ms. Duthie writes procedures to guide nursing practice in the administration of drugs at the hospital and collaborates with the pharmacy staff in developing nursing guidelines for the administration of investigational agents. An area of primary interest for Ms. Duthie is in error prevention in the administration of medications.

CONTENTS

Preface ix

PART I **Drugs in Current Use (an alphabetical listing)** 1

PART II **New Drugs** 255

Actonel® 284
Aggrastat® 289
Alatrofloxacin 293
Amerge® 280
Amlexanox 5% 257
Anzemet® 267
Aphthasol® 257
Ardeparin 258
Avapro® 275
Baycol® 264
Becaplermin 264
Bromfenac 260
Budesonide 261
Capecitabine 262
Carvedilol 263
Cerivastatin 264
Clopidogrel 265
Coreg® 263
Danaparoid Sodium 266
Detrol® 291
Dolasetron Mesylate 267
Duract® 260
Eptifibatide 269
Evista® 282
Fareston® 292
Femara® 277
Fenofibrate 270
Finasteride 271
Flomax® 287
Gabitril® 288
Grepafloxacin 272
Hydroquinone 273
Integrilin® 269
Interferon Alfacon-1 274
Intergen® 274
Irbesartan 275
Lepirudan 276

Letrozole 277
Lustra® 273
Meridia® 285
Mometasone Furoate 278
Montelukast 279
Naratriptan 280
Nasonex® 278
Normiflo® 258
Orgaran® 266
Plavix® 265
Prandin® 283
Propecia® 271
Pulmicort Turbuhaler® 261
Quetiapine 281
Raloxifene HCL 282
Raxar® 272
Refludan® 276
Regranex® 259
Repaglinide 283
Risedronate 284
Seroquel® 281
Sibutramine Hydrochloride 285
Sildenafil Citrate 286
Singulair® 279
Tamsulosin Hydrochloride 287
Tasmar® 290
Tiagabine Hydrochloride 288
Tirofiban® 289
Tolcapone 290
Tolterodine Tartrate 291
Toremifene 292
Tricor® 270
Trovafloxacin 293
Trovan® 293
Viagra® 286
Xeloda® 262
Zolmitriptan 294
Zomig® 294

PREFACE

The publication of the forty-fifth edition continues a longstanding commitment to provide timely information regarding the newest therapeutic agents, as well as useful and concise information concerning other drugs in current use. The general format that has been used in recent editions has been continued in this new edition. Part I consists of an alphabetical listing of drugs currently in use. Part II gives special attention to the drugs that have been recently introduced (most within the past year) in the United States. The addition of new drugs in this edition reflects a very productive period of new drug introductions. Although some of the new agents are used very infrequently for very specific indications, other new drugs are already widely prescribed. The new drugs are considered in greater detail because many of them are not yet considered in other references, and it is often difficult to obtain information about them.

The purpose of Part I is to provide useful and concise information concerning drugs in current use. The primary trade names, uses, and preparations are provided for each of the medications included in this section. More detailed information, including precautionary statements regarding important adverse reactions and serious drug interactions, is included for those agents that are most frequently used in current therapy, as well as for the relatively new drugs that have been introduced during the last several years, but prior to the introduction of the agents included in Part II.

The drugs included in both Parts I and II are listed alphabetically by their generic names. Common trade names and synonyms are included, but the listing of the trade names of many of the medications available from multiple companies is not complete. Trade names are followed by the symbol®.

Although the emphasis of *Drugs in Current Use* continues to be on the properties and use of individual therapeutic agents, a number of combination products are also listed. The combination products selected for inclusion are those that are most frequently used and about which questions are most frequently asked of health professionals.

The formulations in which drugs are available may contain a particular salt or ester of those drugs and, when this is the case, the salt or ester is usually designated. In some situations several salts and/or esters of a drug are used in available formulations of a particular drug. The different salts and/or esters are usually identified when this is an important consideration with respect to the use or route of administration of the drug; however, the properties of the drug may be discussed just once in the consideration of the primary drug. The potency of available formulations of drugs that are available in a salt or ester form may be expressed in terms of the primary drug or its salt/ester. The potencies noted in this reference are the ones in common usage and may not always distinguish between the quantity of drug and its salt or ester.

Dosage information is provided for the new drugs listed in Part II. However, in view of the many factors that will influence dosage determinations for a particular patient, this information is not provided for the agents included in Part I, and the product labeling or other more comprehensive references should be consulted.

The focus of *Drugs in Current Use* is on those agents used for therapeutic purposes. Thus, most agents used for diagnostic purposes, biological products such as vaccines, and ingredients in pharmaceutical formulations that are not pharmacologically active have not been included.

This reference is designed to provide rapid access to what is considered to be the most pertinent information regarding the drugs used in current therapy. However, such a publication cannot be all-inclusive, and the product literature and/or more comprehensive references should be consulted for prescribing purposes or when additional information is needed.

ELIZABETH A. DUTHIE, RN, MA

Note to the reader: We try to keep the information on the new drugs in Part II as up-to-date as possible, but there is an inevitable lag between our publisher's deadline for copy and publication of the book. In addition, new drugs are often approved near the end of a calendar year, so it is not always possible to include all the drugs that were introduced toward the end of the preceding year.

PART I

Drugs in Current Use

A

A-200 PYRINATE®, see Pyrethrins

ABBOKINASE®, see Urokinase

ABCIXIMAB—ReoPro®

Platelet aggregation inhibitor.

Actions and Uses: Inhibits platelet aggregation by preventing binding of fibrinogen and other adhesive molecules to receptor sites on activated platelets. Indicated as an adjunct to percutaneous transluminal coronary angioplasty (PTCA) or arthrectomy for the prevention of acute cardiac ischemic complications in patients at high risk for abrupt closure of the treated coronary vessel. Is used in conjunction with heparin and aspirin.

Warnings: Contraindicated in situations in which a significant risk of bleeding complications exists, when intravenous dextran is used before or during PTCA and in individuals with known hypersensitivity to any component of the product or to murine proteins.

Administration: Intravenous. An intravenous bolus of 0.25 mg/kg is administered 10–60 minutes before the start of PTCA followed by 10ug/minute for 12 hours.

Preparations: Vials (5 ml) 2 mg/ml. Vials should be stored in refrigerator; but not frozen. Do not shake vials.

ABELCET®—Amphotericin B lipid complex

ACARBOSE—Precose®

Oral antidiabetic agent (alpha-glucosidase inhibitor).

Actions and Uses: Reduces blood sugar by inhibiting alpha glucosidase enzymes in the GI tract resulting in delayed glucose absorption. Indicated as an adjunct to diet in non-insulin-dependent diabetes mellitus (NIDDM). Administered alone or with sulfonylurea oral hypoglycemic agents.

Warnings: Risk of hypogyclemia is increased when used with oral hypoglycemic agents. Treat mild-to-moderate hypoglycemia with oral glucose (e.g., glucose tablets). Adverse reactions include flatulence, diarrhea, and abdominal pain. Contraindicated in ketoacidosis, cirrhosis, inflammatory bowel disease, chronic ulceration, partial or predisposition to intestinal obstruction, chronic intestinal disease with marked disorders of digestion or absorbency, and in conditions that may deteriorate from increased intestinal gas formation.

Administration: Oral. Take with first bite of each main meal.

Preparation: Scored tablets, 25, 50 and 100 mg.

ACCOLATE®, see Zafirlukast

ACCUPRIL®, see Quinapril

ACCUTANE®, see Isotretinoin

ACEBUTOLOL HYDROCHLORIDE—Sectral®

Antihypertensive and antiarrhythmic agent.

Actions and Uses: A cardioselective beta-adrenergic blocking agent possessing mild intrinsic sympathomimetic activity. Indicated for the treatment of hypertension, and may be used alone or in combination with other agents, usually a thiazide diuretic. Is also indicated in the management of ventricular premature beats.

Warnings: Contraindicated in patients with persistently severe bradycardia, second- and third-degree heart block in the absence of a functioning artificial pacemaker, overt cardiac failure, and cardiogenic shock. Adverse reactions include fatigue, dizziness, headache, nausea, dyspepsia, arthralgias, and myalgias. Use is best avoided in patients with bronchospastic diseases and therapy in diabetic patients must be closely monitored.

Administration: Oral. Patients should be cautioned about the interruption or discontinuation of therapy.

Preparations: Capsules, 200 and 400 mg.

ACETAMINOPHEN—Panadol®, Tempra®, Tylenol®

Analgesic/antipyretic.

Actions and Uses: Used in the treatment of mild to moderate pain, and fever.

Warnings: Overdosage may result in hepatotoxicity; acetylcysteine is the antidote.

Administration: Oral and rectal.

Preparations: tablets/capsules/caplets, 80, 160, 325, 500, and 650 mg. Controlled-release caplets, 650 mg. Chewable tablets, 80 mg. Granules, 80 mg. Liquid, 160 mg/5 ml, 500 mg/15 ml, and 100 mg/ml. Drops, 100 mg/ml. Suppositories, 120, 325, and 650 mg.

ACETAZOLAMIDE—Diamox®

Carbonic anhydrase inhibitor indicated in the treatment of glaucoma, edema, certain convulsive disorders, and for the prevention or relief of symptoms associated with acute mountain sickness.

Preparations: tablets, 125 and 250 mg. Controlled release capsules, 500 mg. Vials (sodium salt), 500 mg.

ACETIC ACID—VoSol®

Anti-infective agent used as a bladder irrigant, for otic infections, and certain dermatologic conditions.

Preparations: Solution (bladder irrigation), 0.25%. Otic solution (VoSol®), 2%.

ACETOHEXAMIDE—Dymelor®

First-generation sulfonylurea hypoglycemic agent indicated in the treatment of non-insulin-dependent diabetes mellitus.

Preparations: tablets, 250 and 500 mg.

ACETOHYDROXAMIC ACID—Lithostat®

Adjunctive therapy in certain urinary tract infections. Inhibits the bacterial enzyme urease, thereby inhibiting the hydrolysis of urea and production of ammonia in urine infected with urea-splitting organisms.

Preparation: tablets, 250 mg.

ACETOPHENAZINE MALEATE—Tindal®

Phenothiazine antipsychotic agent indicated for psychotic disorders.

Preparations: tablets, 20 mg.

ACETYLCARBROMAL—Paxarel®

Central nervous system depressant used as a sedative and hypnotic.

Preparation: tablets, 250 mg.

ACETYLCYSTEINE—Mucomyst®

Mucolytic agent indicated as adjunctive therapy in patients with abnormal or viscid mucous secretions in various pulmonary disorders. Also indicated in the management of acetaminophen overdosage.

Preparations: Vials (solution of sodium salt), 10% and 20%. Administered by nebulization or direct instillation, or enterally. Usually administered via nasogastric tube as noxious taste causes regurgitation.

ACETYLSALICYLIC ACID, see Aspirin

ACHROMYCIN V®, see Tetracycline

ACLOVATE®, see Alclometasone

ACRIVASTINE/PSEUDOEPHEDRINE HYDROCHLORIDE—Semprex-D®

Antihistamine/decongestant combination.

Actions and Uses: Indicated for the relief of symptoms associated with seasonal allergic rhinitis.

Warnings: Contraindicated in patients with severe hypertension or severe coronary artery disease, and in patients taking a monoamine oxidase inhibitor. Adverse reactions preclude driving and operating machinery until response is ascertained. Avoid CNS-acting drugs including alcohol. Patients should be advised against the concurrent use with nonprescription antihistamines and/or decongestants.

Administration: Oral.

Preparation: Capsules, 8 mg of acrivastine and 60 mg of pseudophedrine hydrochloride.

ACTH, see Corticotropin

ACTHAR®, see Corticotropin

ACTIGALL®, see Ursodiol

ACTIMMUNE®, see Interferon gamma-1b

ACTINEX®, see Masoprocol

ACTISITE®, see Tetracycline hydrochloride

ACTIVASE®, see Alteplase, recombinant

ACTRON®, see Ketoprofen

ACULAR®, see Ketorolac

ACUTRIM®, see Phenylpropanolamine

ACYCLOVIR—Zovirax®

Antiviral agent indicated in the treatment of genital herpes infections, varicella (chickenpox) infections, varicella zoster (shingles) infections, herpes simplex encephalitis, and mucosal and cutaneous herpes simplex (HSV-1 and HSV-2) infections in immunocompromised patients.

Preparations: Capsules, 200 mg. tablets, 800 mg. Suspension, 200 mg/5ml. Ointment, 5%. Vials (sodium salt), 500 and 1000 mg (administered by IV infusion).

ADAGEN®, see Pegademase bovine

ADALAT®, see Nifedipine

ADALAT CC®, see Nifedipine

ADAPALENE—Differin®

A synthetic analogue, alcohol-free topical gel indicated in the treatment of acne vulgaris.

Warning: Do not use on cuts, abrasions, or broken eczematous or sunburned skin. Avoid contact with eyes, lips, angles of the nose, and mucous membranes. Minimize exposure to sun and UV light. Increased irritation may occur in extreme weather (e.g., wind, cold). Reduce frequency or discontinue if prolonged or severe irritation occurs. Do not use concomitantly with other topical irritants. Adverse reactions include erythema, scaling, dryness, pruritis, burning, and acne flares.

Administration: Apply a thin film to affected areas once daily at bedtime after washing.

Preparation: 0.1%. gel, topical (alcohol free), 15, 45 g.

ADENOCARD®, see Adenosine

ADENOSINE—Adenocard®

Antiarrhythmic agent.

Actions and Uses: Slows conduction through the AV node of the heart and reestablishes normal heart rhythm. Has a rapid onset of action and a very short duration of action. Indicated for the conversion to sinus rhythm of paroxysmal supraventricular tachycardia (PSVT), including that associated with accessory bypass tracts (Wolff-Parkinson-White syndrome).

Warnings: Contraindicated in second- or third-degree AV block (except in patients with a functioning artificial pacemaker), sick sinus syndrome (except in patients with a functioning artificial pacemaker), atrial flutter, atrial fibrillation, and ventricular tachycardia. Adverse reactions include myocardial conduction abnormalities, facial flushing, headache, shortness of breath/dyspnea, chest pressure, lightheadedness, and nausea. Action may be potentiated by dipyridamole. Caution must be exercised in patients receiving carbamazepine concurrently because a higher degree of heart block may be produced. Actions of adenosine may be competitively antagonized by methylxanthines such as theophylline and caffeine.

Administration: Administered as a rapid bolus IV injection over a one-to-two-second period. To be certain the solution reaches the systemic circulation, it should be administered either directly into a vein or, if given into an IV line, it should be given as proximal as possible and followed by a rapid saline flush.

Preparations: Vials, 6 mg/2ml. The product should not be refrigerated as crystallization may occur.

ADIPEX®, see Phentermine

ADRENALIN®, see Epinephrine

ADRIAMYCIN PFS®, see Doxorubicin

ADRIAMYCIN RDF®, see Doxorubicin

ADRUCIL®, see Fluorouracil

ADVIL®, see Ibuprofen

AEROBID®, see Flunisolide

AEROSPORIN®, see Polymyxin B

AFRIN®, see Oxymetazoline

AFRINOL®, see Pseudoephedrine

AGRYLIN®, see Anagrelide

AKINETON®, see Biperiden

AKNE-MYCIN®, see Erythromycin base (topical)

ALBAMYCIN®, see Novobiocin

ALBENZA®, see Albendazole

ALBENDAZOLE—Albenza®

Actions and Uses: Anthelmintic indicated for treatment of cystic hydatid disease of the liver, lung, and peritoneum caused by the larval form of the dog tapeworm, (Echonococcus granulosus) and for parenchymal neurocysticercosis from active lesions caused by larval forms of the pork tapeworm (Taenia solium). Also indicated in the treatment of ascariasis, hookworm, strongyloidiasis, giardiasis, and microsporidiosis in patients with HIV.

Warnings: In treating neurocysticercosis during the 1st week of therapy administer steroid and anticonvulsant therapy concurrently to prevent cerebral hypertension. The most common adverse drug reactions are alterations in LFTs, abdominal pain, and nausea and vomiting. Monitor LFT's prior and during therapy. If enzymes significantly increase, discontinue the albendazole. Therapy can be reinstituted when enzymes have returned to pretreatment levels. Monitor white blood cells (WBC) as reversible reductions in total WBC's have been noted.

Administration:

- Hydatid disease: 800–1200 mg/day, in divided doses for 28 days.
- Neurocysticercosis: 15 mg/kg for 8–30 days.
- Roundworm, pinworm, hookworm: 400 mg, as a single dose.
- Giardiasis, strongyloidiasis, and tapeworm: 400 mg/day for 3 days.

Preparation: Tablets, 200 mg.

ALBUMIN (HUMAN)—Albuminar®, Buminate®, Plasbumin®

Plasma protein fraction indicated as supportive treatment in patients in shock, or patients with burns, hepatic cirrhosis, nephrosis, and certain other conditions.

Preparations: Vials, 5% and 25%, administered by IV infusion.

ALBUMINAR®, see Albumin

ALBUTEROL—Proventil®, Proventil HFA Inhaler®, Ventolin®, Volmax®

Bronchodilator.

Actions and Uses: Stimulates beta 2-adrenergic receptors. Indicated for the relief of bronchospasm in patients with reversible obstructive airway disease and for the prevention of exercise-induced bronchospasm.

Warnings: Adverse reactions include nervousness, tremor, headache, tachycardia, and palpitations. Should be used cautiously in patients with cardiovascular disorders. Concurrent use with other adrenergic (sympathomimetic) agents will have additive adrenergic effects. Must be used with caution in patients being treated with a tricyclic antidepressant or monoamine oxidase inhibitor because the action of albuterol may be increased. Beta-adrenergic blocking agents and albuterol may inhibit the effect of each other.

Administration: Oral and oral inhalation.

Preparations: tablets, 2 and 4 mg. Controlled-release tablets, 4 and 8 mg. Capsules for inhalation, 200 ug. Syrup, 2 mg/5 ml. Metered-dose inhaler. (HFA inhaler is chlorofluro-carbon free). Solution for inhalation.

ALCLOMETASONE DIPROPIONATE—Aclovate®

Topical corticosteroid.

Actions and Uses: Indicated for relief of the inflammatory and pruritic manifestations of corticosteroid-responsive dermatoses.

Warnings: Adverse reactions include itching, burning, erythema, dryness, irritation, and papular rashes. Children may absorb proportionally larger amounts of the drug and thus be more susceptible to the development of systemic effects.

Administration: Topical.

Preparations: Cream and ointment, 0.05%.

ALCOHOL—Ethyl alcohol

Antiseptic, astringent, and solvent when applied topically. Also used intravenously as a source of calories.

Preparations: Solution (topical), 70%. Bottles (intravenous), 5% and 10% with 5% dextrose in water.

ALDACTONE®, see Spironolactone

ALDARA®, see Imiquimod

ALDESLEUKIN—Proleukin®

Antineoplastic agent.

Actions and Uses: A human recombinant interleukin-2 product (rIL-2) produced by recombinant DNA technology using a genetically engineered *E. coli* strain containing an analog of the human interleukin-2 gene. Indicated for the treatment of adults (18 years of age and older) with metastatic renal cell carcinoma.

Warnings: Contraindicated in patients with organ allografts and in patients who do not have normal cardiac and pulmonary functions as defined by thallium stress testing and formal pulmonary function testing. Many adverse reactions are associated with capillary leak syndrome which results in hypotension and reduced organ perfusion. Pressor agents may be necessary to sustain blood pressure and the use of dopamine to help maintain organ perfusion. Other adverse reactions include renal dysfunction with oliguria/ anuria, pulmonary congestion, dyspnea, respiratory failure, mental status changes, seizure, myocardial ischemia, myocarditis, gastrointestinal bleeding, intestinal perforation/ileus, sinus tachycardia, nausea, vomiting, diarrhea, anemia, thrombocytopenia, pruritus, erythema, fever and/or chills, pain, fatigue, and edema. Treatment should be monitored closely and hematologic tests (including CBC, differential and platelet counts), blood chemistries (including electrolytes, renal and hepatic function tests), and chest X-rays should be conducted prior to beginning treatment and then daily during drug administration. Use is associated with an increased risk of disseminated infection, including sepsis and bacterial endocarditis; therefore, preexisting infections should be adequately treated prior to starting therapy. Patients with indwelling central lines should be evaluated for antibiotic prophylaxis against *Staphylococcus aureus.*

Administration: Intravenous. Each course of treatment consists of two 5-day treatment cycles separated by a rest period of 9 days.

Preparations: Vials, 22 million units (1.3 mg).

ALDOMET®, see Methyldopa

ALDORIL®, Combination of methyldopa and hydrochlorothiazide

ALENDRONATE SODIUM—Fosamax®

Bone resorption inhibitor.

Actions and Uses: Inhibits resorption of bone by inhibiting osteoclast activity. Indicated in the prevention and treatment of osteoporosis in postmenopausal women and treatment of Paget's disease of the bone.

Warnings: Should not be used in patients whose creatinine clearance is less than 35 ml/minute, or during pregnancy and lactation. Adverse reactions include headache, GI symptoms, rash, and musculoskeletal pain.

Administration: Oral. Administer first thing in the morning with 6–8 oz. of plain water 30 minutes prior to other medication, beverages, or food. (Must also avoid lying down for at least 30 minutes after the dose is administered.)

Preparation: tablets, 10 mg.

ALESSE®—Levonorgestrel

10 mg ethinyl estradiol, 20 ug Low dose combination oral contraceptive.

ALEVE®, see Naproxen sodium

ALFENTA®, see Alfentanil

ALFENTANIL HYDROCHLORIDE—Alfenta®

Opioid analgesic/anesthetic.

Actions and Uses: Indicated (1) as an analgesic adjunct given in incremental doses in the maintenance of anesthesia with barbiturate/nitrous oxide/oxygen, (2) as an analgesic administered by continuous infusion with nitrous oxide/oxygen in the maintenance of general anesthesia, and (3) as a primary anesthetic agent for the induction of anesthesia in patients undergoing general surgery in which endotracheal intubation and mechanical ventilation are required. Has an almost immediate onset of action and a short duration of action.

Warnings: Skeletal muscle rigidity of the chest wall, trunk, and extremities is one of the most common adverse reactions; the incidence may be reduced by the appropriate use of a neuromuscular blocking agent. Respiratory depression including delayed respiratory depression and respiratory arrest have been reported, and the monitoring of the patient must be continued well after surgery; caution must be exercised in patients with pulmonary disease or those with potentially compromised respiration. Other adverse reactions include cardiovascular effects (e.g., bradycardia, hypotension, arrhythmias), nausea, vomiting, and dizziness. When administered with other central nervous system depressants the dose of one or both agents should be reduced. It can produce dependence and has the potential for being abused; is included in Schedule II under the provisions of the Controlled Substances Act.

Administration: Intravenous.

Preparations: Ampules (2, 5, 10, and 20 ml) containing the equivalent of 500 μg. of alfentanil base in each ml.

ALFERON N®, see Interferon alfa-n3

ALGLUCERASE—Ceredase®

Agent for Gaucher disease.

Actions and Uses: Is a modified form of the enzyme glucocerebrosidase. Indicated for use as long-term enzyme replacement therapy for patients with a confirmed diagnosis of Type 1 Gaucher disease who exhibit signs and symptoms that are severe enough to result in one or more of the following conditions: moderate to severe anemia; thrombocytopenia with bleeding tendency; bone disease; significant hepatomegaly or splenomegaly.

Warnings: Adverse reactions include fever, chills, abdominal discomfort, nausea, vomiting, and discomfort, burning, and swelling at the site of venipuncture.

Administration: Intravenous. Is administered by IV infusion over 1–2 hours. Dosage should be individualized for each patient.

Preparations: Vials, 10 units/ml and 80 units/ml.

ALKERAN®, see Melphalan

ALLEGRA®, see Fexofenadine Hydrochloride

ALLEGRA®—Combination agent Fexotenadine hydrochloride and psuedoephedrine hydrochloride (Antighistrmine and sympothomimetic)

ALLOPURINOL—Lopurin®, Zyloprim®

Agent for gout.

Actions and Uses: A xanthine oxidase inhibitor indicated in the management of (1) gout; (2) patients with leukemia, lymphoma, and malignancies who are receiving cancer therapy that causes elevations of serum and urinary uric acid levels; and (3) patients with recurrent calcium oxalate calculi.

Warnings: Adverse reactions include hypersensitivity reactions, and therapy should be discontinued at the first appearance of rash or other signs of an allergic response. Will increase the action of azathioprine and mercaptopurine, and the dosage of these agents should be reduced to one-third to one-quarter the usual dose when allopurinol is administered concomitantly.

Administration: Oral.

Preparations: tablets, 100 and 300 mg.

ALOMIDE®, see Lodoxamide tromethamine

ALORA®, see Estradio

ALPHAGAN®, see Brimonidine Tartrate

ALPHA1-ANTITRYPSIN, see Alpha$_1$-Proteinase Inhibitor

ALPHA1-PROTEINASE INHIBITOR (HUMAN)—Prolastin®

Agent for alpha1-proteinase inhibitor deficiency.

Actions and Uses: Also known as alpha$_1$-antitrypsin, it is indicated for chronic replacement therapy in individuals having congenitial deficiency of alpha$_1$-proteinase inhibitor with clinically demonstrable panacinar emphysema.

Warnings: Preparation is purified from large pools of fresh human plasma obtained from many donors, and the presence of hepatitis viruses in such pools must be assumed. It is, therefore recommended that patients be immunized against hepatitis B.

Administration: Intravenous.

Preparation: Vials, with the activity, in milligrams, stated on the label of each vial.

ALPRAZOLAM—Xanax®

Benzodiazepine antianxiety agent.

Actions and Uses: A CNS depressant indicated for the management of anxiety disorders or the short-term relief of the symptoms of anxiety. Anxiety associated with depression is also responsive. Also indicated in the treatment of panic disorder.

Warnings: Contraindicated in patients with acute narrow-angle glaucoma. Adverse reactions include drowsiness and other CNS effects; patients should be cautioned regarding activities such as driving and operating machinery, as well as interactions with other CNS-acting drugs including alcohol. Can cause dependence and is included in Schedule IV.

Administration: Oral.

Preparations: tablets, 0.25, 0.5, 1, and 2 mg.

ALPROSTADIL—Caverject®, Edex®, Prostin VR Pediatric®, Prostaglandin E_1, PGE_1

Prostaglandin indicated (Prostin VR Pediatric®) for palliative therapy to temporarily maintain the patency of the ductus arteriosus until corrective or palliative surgery can be performed in neonates who have congenital heart defects and who depend upon the patent ductus for survival. Also indicated (Caverject®) for the diagnosis and treatment of male erectile dysfunction due to neurologic, vascular, psychological, or mixed causes.

Administration: Intravenous infusion (Prostin VR Pediatric®) and into an area along the shaft of the penis known as the corpus cavernosum (Caverject®).

Preparations: Ampules, 500 µg (Prostin VR Pediatric®). Vials, 5, 10, 20, and 40 µg (Caverject®).

ALREX®, see Loteprednol Etabonate

ALTACE®, see Ramipril

ALTEPLASE, RECOMBINANT—Activase®

Fibrinolytic agent.

Actions and Uses: Is a form of the body's natural tissue plasminogen activator (TPA) that promotes the conversion of plasminogen to plasmin, which is fibrinolytic. Indicated for the management of acute myocardial infarction in adults for the lysis of thrombi obstructing coronary arteries, the improvement of ventricular function, and reduction of the incidence of congestive heart failure. Also indicated for the management of acute massive pulmonary embolism and acute ischemic stroke.

Warnings: Contraindicated in patients with active bleeding, history of cerebrovascular accident, recent (within 2 months) intracranial or intraspinal surgery or trauma, intracranial neoplasm, arteriovenous malformation or aneurysm, known bleeding diathesis, or severe uncontrolled hypertension. Serious bleeding reactions (i.e., internal and/or surface bleeding) may occur and appropriate precautions must be taken. Intramuscular injections should be avoided. Intracranial bleeding has occurred in some patients. The coronary thrombolysis produced by the drug may result in arrhythmias associated with reperfusion.

Administration: Intravenous infusion.

Preparations: Vials, 20 mg (11.6 million IU) and 50 mg (29 million IU).

ALternaGEL®, see Aluminum hydroxide gel

ALTRETAMINE—Hexalen®

Antineoplastic agent.

Actions and Uses: A synthetic cytotoxic agent that must be me TABolized for its cytotoxic effect to develop. Indicated for use as a single agent in the palliative treatment of patients with persistent or recurrent ovarian cancer following first-line therapy with a cisplatin and/or alkylating agent-based combination.

Warnings: Should not be used in patients with preexisting severe bone marrow depression or severe neurologic toxicity. Adverse reactions include nausea, vomiting, peripheral neuropathy, and CNS symptoms (e.g., mood disorders, ataxia, dizziness, vertigo). Neurologic examinations should be performed regularly. May cause myelosuppression (e.g., leukopenia, thrombocytopenia) and peripheral blood counts should be monitored at least monthly, prior to the initiation of each course of the drug. May cause fetal damage if administered during pregnancy. If a nursing mother is to be treated with the drug it is recommended that breast-feeding be discontinued. Concurrent use with a monoamine oxidase inhibitor may cause severe orthostatic hypotension. Activity may be increased by the concurrent use of cimetidine.

Administration: Oral. The total daily dose should be given as 4 divided doses after meals and at bedtime.

Preparations: Capsules, 50 mg.

ALUDROX®, see Aluminum and magnesium hydroxides

ALUMINUM ACETATE

Astringent used as a wet dressing (e.g., Burow's solution) for relief of inflammatory conditions of the skin.

Preparation: Solution.

ALUMINUM AND MAGNESIUM HYDROXIDES—Aludrox®, Maalox®

Antacid indicated for hyperacidity associated with ulcers and other GI conditions.

Preparations: Liquid and tablets.

ALUMINUM CARBONATE GEL, BASIC—Basaljel®

Antacid indicated for hyperacidity associated with ulcers and other GI conditions. Also indicated for the management of hyperphosphatemia or for use with a low phosphate diet to prevent formation of phosphate urinary stones.

Preparations: Capsules, tablets, and suspension.

ALUMINUM HYDROXIDE GEL—Amphojel®, ALternaGEL®

Antacid indicated for hyperacidity associated with ulcers and other GI conditions.

Preparation: Capsules, tablets, suspension.

ALUMINUM PHOSPHATE GEL—Phosphaljel®

Indicated to reduce fecal excretion of phosphates.

Preparation: Suspension.

ALUPENT®, see Metaproterenol

ALURATE®, see Aprobarbital

AMANTADINE HYDROCHLORIDE—Symmetrel®

Antiviral agent and antiparkinson agent.

Actions and Uses: Indicated in the prevention and treatment of respiratory tract illness caused by influenza A virus strains. Also indicated for parkinsonism and drug-induced extrapyramidal reactions.

Warnings: Adverse reactions include orthostatic hypotensive episodes, urinary retention, depression, psychosis, and congestive heart failure.

Administration: Oral.

Preparations: Capsules, 100 mg. Syrup, 50 mg/5 ml.

AMARYL, see Glimepiride

AMBENONIUM CHLORIDE—Mytelase®

Anticholinesterase indicated for the treatment of myasthenia gravis.

Preparation: tablets, 10 mg.

AMBIEN®, see Zolpidem tartrate

AMCINONIDE—Cyclocort®

Corticosteroid indicated in the topical treatment of corticosteroid-responsive dermatoses.

Preparations: Cream, ointment, and lotion, 0.1%.

AMICAR®, see Aminocaproic acid

AMIDATE®, see Etomidate

AMIFOSTINE—Ethyol

Cytoprotective agent (for cisplatin).

Actions and Uses: Reduces renal toxicity due to cumulative effects of cisplatin in patients being treated for ovarian cancer or non-small-cell lung cancer.

Warnings: Should not be used in patients with hypotension or dehydration. Adverse effects most commonly seen are hypotension, nausea, and vomiting.

Administration: Intravenous.

Preparation: Powder for injection, 500 mg/vial (with 500 mg mannitol).

AMIKACIN SULFATE—Amikin®

Aminoglycoside antibiotic.

Actions and Uses: Indicated in the treatment of serious infections caused by gram-negative bacteria including *Pseudomonas aeruginosa.* Is also effective in the treatment of staphylococcal infections.

Warnings: May cause nephrotoxicity, ototoxicity, and neurotoxicity, and the concurrent or serial use of other nephrotoxic or ototoxic agents should be avoided.

Administration: Intravenous and intramuscular. Clinical response and dosage should be closely monitored.

Preparations: Vials, 100 and 500 mg, and 1 g. Syringes, 500 mg.

AMIKIN®, see Amikacin

AMILORIDE HYDROCHLORIDE—Midamor®

Diuretic (potassium-sparing) indicated as adjunctive treatment with thiazide or other potassium-depleting diuretics in patients with congestive heart failure or hypertension. Should be administered with food.

Preparation: tablets, 5 mg.

AMINOACETIC ACID—Glycine

Anti-infective for urological irrigation. Has also been used in conjunction with antacids.

Preparations: Solutions (for irrigation), 1.5%.

AMINOCAPROIC ACID—Amicar®

Coagulant that inhibits fibrinolysis. Useful in enhancing hemostasis when fibrinolysis contributes to bleeding.

Preparations: tablets, 500 mg. Syrup, 250 mg/ml. Vials (for IV use) 250 mg/ml.

AMINOPHYLLINE—Theophylline ethylenediamine, Phyllocontin®

Bronchodilator indicated for the management of bronchial asthma, chronic bronchitis, and emphysema. Has been used as a diuretic and in certain cardiovascular disorders.

Preparations: tablets, 100 and 200 mg. Controlled-release tablets, 225 mg. Liquid, 105 mg/5 ml. Suppositories, 250 and 500 mg. Ampules and vials, 250 mg.

AMINOSALICYLATE SODIUM—Para-aminosalicylate sodium, PAS sodium

Antitubercular agent indicated for tuberculosis in combination with other antitubercular agents.

Preparations: tablets, 500 mg. Powder.

AMINOSALICYLIC ACID, see Aminosalicylate sodium

AMIODARONE HYDROCHLORIDE—Cordarone®

Antiarrhythmic agent.

Actions and Uses: A class III antiarrhythmic agent indicated for documented, life-threatening recurrent ventricular fibrillation, and for recurrent, hemodynamically unstable ventricular tachycardia, when these conditions have not responded to treatment with other antiarrhythmic agents or when alternative drugs were not tolerated. Is often effective in patients with serious ventricular arrhythmias that are refractory to other agents.

Warnings: Contraindicated in patients with severe sinus-node dysfunction, causing marked sinus bradycardia; second- and third-degree AV block, and when episodes of bradycardia have caused syncope (except when used in conjunction with a pacemaker). Adverse reactions include pulmonary toxicity that may be fatal, proarrhythmic events, GI effects, neurologic effects (e.g., fatigue, tremor), ocular effects (e.g., visual halos, blurred vision), hepatic dysfunction, and dermatologic effects (e.g., photosensitivity reactions). May interact with and increase the activity of digoxin, warfarin, diltiazem, and other antiarrhythmic agents. Orally has variable absorption. Slow onset of action and long duration of action make dosing and monitoring of therapy difficult. IV administration results in complete bioavailability.

Administration: Oral/IV.

Preparation: tablets, 200 mg. Injection, 50 mg/ml in 3 ml ampules.

AMITRIPTYLINE HYDROCHLORIDE—Elavil®, Endep®

Tricyclic antidepressant.

Actions and Uses: Indicated for the relief of symptoms of depression.

Warnings: Should not be given concomitantly with a monoamine oxidase inhibitor. Is not recommended for use during the acute recovery phase following myocardial infarction. Adverse reactions include CNS effects, and patients should be cautioned regarding activities such as driving and operating machinery, as well as interactions with other CNS-acting drugs including alcohol. Other adverse reactions include anticholinergic effects (e.g., dry mouth, blurred vision), GI effects (e.g., nausea, vomiting), and cardiovascular effects (e.g., orthostatic hypotension). Caution should be exercised in patients with cardiovascular disorders. May reduce the action of guanethidine and guanadrel.

Administration: Oral and intramuscular.

Preparations: tablets, 10, 25, 50, 75, 100, and 150 mg. Vials, 10 mg/ml.

AMLODIPINE BESYLATE—Norvasc®

Antihypertensive and antianginal agent.

Actions and Uses: Is a calcium channel blocking agent that causes a reduction in peripheral vascular resistance and a lowering in blood pressure. Indicated for the treatment of hypertension. Also indicated for the treatment of chronic s@TABle angina and vasospastic angina (Prinzmetal's or variant angina).

Warnings: Adverse reactions include edema, flushing, palpitation, dizziness, fatigue, somnolence, nausea, and abdominal pain.

Administration: Oral.

Preparations: tablets, 2.5, 5, and 10 mg.

AMMONIA, AROMATIC SPIRIT—Aromatic ammonia spirit

Respiratory stimulant used by inhalation to treat or prevent fainting.

Preparations: Inhalant and solution.

AMMONIATED MERCURY

Anti-infective agent used for the topical treatment of certain skin infections and conditions such as psoriasis.

Preparations: Ointment, 5% and 10%.

AMMONIUM CARBONATE

Respiratory stimulant used in the preparation of aromatic ammonia spirit and as a source of ammonia in smelling salts.

AMMONIUM CHLORIDE

Expectorant, diuretic, and acidifying agent. Used orally as an expectorant, diuretic, and to acidify the urine, and intravenously in the treatment of certain hypochloremic states and metabolic alkalosis.

Preparations: tablets, 500 mg and 1 g. Vials and bottles, 0.4 mEq/ml and 5 mEq/ml.

AMMONIUM LACTATE—Lac-Hydrin®

Actions and Uses: Emollient indicated in treatment of dry skin and ichthyosis vulgaris. Transient stinging or burning, erythema, peeling, eczema, petechiae, dryness, and hyperpigmentation may occur.

Administration: Apply and rub into affected areas twice daily.

Preparations: Lotion and cream, 12%.

AMOBARBITAL SODIUM—Amytal sodium®

Barbiturate sedative-hypnotic indicated for the treatment of anxiety and convulsive disorders, for preanesthetic sedation, and in narcoanalysis and narcotherapy.

Preparations: Vials, 250 and 500 mg.

AMOXAPINE—Asendin®

Antidepressant (dibenzoxazepine) indicated for the relief of symptoms of depression, and for depression accompanied by anxiety or agitation.

Preparations: tablets, 25, 50, 100, and 150 mg.

AMOXICILLIN—Amoxil®, Polymox®, Trimox®

Penicillin antibiotic.

Actions and Uses: Is bactericidal and exhibits activity that is most similar to that of ampicillin. Indicated for the treatment of infections caused by susceptible strains of *Escherichia coli, Haemophilus influenzae, Proteus mirabilis, Neisseria gonorrhoeae,* streptococci, and non-penicillinase-producing staph-ylococci. Is commonly used in the treatment of respiratory tract infections, otitis media, urinary tract infections, and uncomplicated gonorrhea.

Warnings: Contraindicated in patients with a history of allergic reaction to any of the penicillins. Adverse reactions include hypersensitivity reactions, rash, urticaria, nausea, vomiting, and diarrhea.

Administration: Oral. May be administered without regard to meals.

Preparations: Capsules, 250 and 500 mg. Chewable tablets, 125 and 250 mg. Powder for oral suspension, 125 and 250 mg/5 ml when reconstituted.

AMOXICILLIN/CLAVULANATE POTASSIUM—Augmentin®

Penicillin antibiotic with beta-lactamase inhibitor.

Actions and Uses: Clavulanic acid inhibits beta-lactamase enzymes and protects amoxicillin from degradation by these enzymes; the spectrum of action of amoxicillin is extended to include many gram-positive and gram-negative bacteria, including *Moraxella catarrhalis.* Indicated for the treatment of lower respiratory infections, otitis media, sinusitis, skin and skin-structure infections, and urinary tract infections.

Warnings: Contraindicated in patients with a history of allergic reaction to any of the penicillins. Adverse reactions include hypersensitivity reactions, rash, urticaria, nausea, vomiting, and diarrhea. Incidence of GI effects is higher than when amoxicillin is administered alone. Due to clavulanic acid component, 2 Augmentin 250 mg are not equivalent to 1 Augmentin 500 mg.

Administration: Oral. May be administered without regard to meals.

Preparations: Tablets, 250, 500, and 875 mg with 125 mg potassium clavulanate. Chewable tablets, 125 mg amoxicillin with 31.25 mg of clavulanic acid, 200 mg amoxicillin, with 28.5 mg clavulanic acid, 250 mg amoxicillin with 62.5 mg of clavulanic acid, and 400 mg amoxicillin with 57 mg of clavulonic acid. Powder for oral suspension, 125 mg amoxicillin with 31.25 mg clavulonic acid/5 ml; 200 mg amoxicillin with 28.5 mg clavulanic acid/5ml; and 400 amoxicillin with 57 mg clavulanic acid.

AMPHETAMINE SULFATE

Central nervous system stimulant indicated in the treatment of narcolepsy, attention deficit disorder in children, and exogenous obesity.

Preparations: tablets, 5 and 10 mg.

AMPHOJEL®, see Aluminum hydroxide gel

AMPHOTEC®—Amphotericin B cholesteryl sulfate, also, Ambisome®—Amphotericin B liposome for injection

Administration: Intravenous. An intravenous bolus of 0.25 mg/kg is administered 10–60 minutes.

Antifungal.

Uses: Indicated in patients with aspergillosis who are intolerant or refractory to conventional dosage form of Amphotericin B. Empiric treatment of persumed fungal infections in febrile neutropenic patients.

Administration: Intravenous infusion after dilution.

Preparations: Vials, 100 mg with single-use filter needle.

AMPHOTERICIN B—Fungizone®

Antifungal agent indicated for the intravenous treatment of systemic fungal infections, topical treatment of cutaneous candidal infections and oral suspension for oral candidiasis.

Warnings: Be fully familiar with the use of this product. Administer under close supervision; cardiopulmonary resuscitation facilities should be available. Monitor serum creatinine, liver function, serum electrolytes (esp. magnesium and potassium), and CBC.

Preparations: Vials, 50 mg. Oral suspension, 100 mg/mL. Cream, ointment, and lotion, 3%.

AMPICILLIN—Omnipen®, Polycillin®, Principen®, Totacillin®
AMPICILLIN SODIUM

Penicillin antibiotic.

Actions and Uses: Is bactericidal. Indicated for the treatment of infections caused by susceptible strains of *Escherichia coli, Haemophilus influenzae, Neisseria gonorrhoeae, Neisseria meningitidis, Proteus mirabilis, Salmonella* species, *Shigella,* streptococci, and nonpenicillinase-producing staphylococci. Is used in the treatment of urinary tract infections, respiratory tract infections, and uncomplicated gonorrhea. Used intravenously in the treatment of meningitis and septicemia caused by susceptible organisms.

Warnings: Contraindicated in patients with a history of allergic reaction to any of the penicillins. Adverse reactions include hypersensitivity reactions, rash, urticaria, nausea, vomiting, and diarrhea.

Administration: Oral, intravenous, and intramuscular. When administered orally, it is best administered apart from meals.

Preparations: Capsules, 250 and 500 mg. Powder for oral suspension, 125, 250, and 500 mg/5 ml (when reconstituted). Vials, ampicillin sodium equivalent to 125, 500 mg, 1, 2, and 10 g of ampicillin per vial.

AMPICILLIN SODIUM/SULBACTAM SODIUM—Unasyn®

Penicillin antibiotic with beta-lactamase inhibitor.

Actions and Uses: A combination of ampicillin and a beta-lactamase inhibitor, sulbactam. By irreversibly binding to beta-lactamase enzymes that are produced by certain bacteria, sulbactam protects ampicillin against inactivation by these enzymes, thereby extending the spectrum of ampicillin to include many bacteria that are resistant to it when it is given alone. Indicated for intra-abdominal, gynecological, and skin structure infections caused by susceptible bacteria. Among the bacteria that are susceptible are beta-lactamase producing strains of *Acinetobacter calcoaceticus, Bacteroides* species (including *B. fragilis*), *Enterobacter* species, *Escherichia coli, Klebsiella* species (including *K. pneumoniae*), *Proteus mirabilis,* and *Staphylococcus aureus.*

Warnings: Contraindicated in patients with a known hypersensitivity to any of the penicillins. Adverse reactions include diarrhea, rash, pain at the intramuscular and intravenous injection sites, and thrombophlebitis. Should not be used in patients with mononucleosis because of the likelihood of a nonallergic skin rash developing.

Administration: Intravenous and intramuscular. The coadministration of lidocaine significantly decreases the incidence of local pain following intramus- cular injection.

Preparations: Vials and piggyback bottles containing 1.5 g (1 g ampicillin sodium plus 0.5 g sulbactam sodium) and 3 g (2 g ampicillin sodium plus 1 g sulbactam sodium).

AMRINONE—Inocor®
Inotropic agent.

Actions and Uses: Increases myocardial contractility and decreases preload and afterload by a direct dilating effect on vascular smooth muscle. Indicated for short-term treatment of congestive heart failure unresponsive to glycosides, diuretics, and vasodilators.

Warnings: Contraindicated in idiopathic hypertrophic subaortic stenosis (IHSS). Correct fluid and electrolytes associated with previous aggressive diuretic therapy prior to initiating amrinone. Adverse reactions include arrhythmias, hypotension, thrombocytopenia, and tachyphylaxis. Initiate in monitored environment.

Administration: Intravenous.

Preparation: Injection, 5 mg/ml.

AMYL NITRITE

Antianginal agent administered by inhalation for the relief of acute angina pectoris.

Preparations: Inhalant, 0.18 and 0.3 ml.

AMYTAL®, see Amobarbital

ANADROL-50®, see Oxymetholone

ANAFRANIL®, see Clomipramine hydrochloride

ANAGRELIDE—Agrylin®

Actions and Uses: Indicated in the treatment of essential thrombocythemia. Reduces platelet counts at therapeutic doses and at higher doses inhibits platelet aggregation as well. Does not affect WBC counts or coagulation parameters at therapeutic doses although it may have clinically insignificant effect on RBC parameters.

Warnings: Use cautiously in cardiovascular disease, hepatic or renal dysfunction. Adverse reactions include headache, palpitations, tachycardia, anorexia, edema, pain, dizziness, dyspnea, rash, paresthesia, tachycardia, anorexia, CHF, MI, malaise, cardiomyopathy, cardiomegaly, complete heart block, atrial fibrillation, CVA, pericarditis, pulmonary infiltrates/fibrosis, hypertension, pancreatitis, ulcer, and seizures. Instruct patients to report signs/symptoms of hepatic, renal, or cardiac dysfunction.

Administration: 0.5 mg 4 times daily or 1 mg twice daily for at least 1 week. Then adjust to the lowest effective dosage required to reduce and maintain platelet count < 600,000/mcl.

Preparation: Capsules, 0.5 and 1 mg.

ANAPROX®, see Naproxen sodium

ANAPROX DS®, see Naproxen sodium

ANASPAZ, see Hyoscyamine

ANASTROZOLE—Arimidex®

Antiestrogen.

Action and Uses: Exerts antineoplastic effect and is indicated in advanced breast cancer in post-menopausal women with disease progression after tamoxifen therapy.

Warnings: Contraindicated in pregnancy. Asthenia, GI disturbances, headache, hot flashes, pain, dyspnea, rash, dry mouth, peripheral edema, depression, parenthesia, and vaginal bleeding may occur.

Administration: Oral, 1 mg once daily.

Preparation: Tablets, 1 mg.

ANCEF®, see Cefazolin

ANCOBON®, see Flucytosine

ANDRODERM®, see Testosterone

ANECTINE®, see Succinylcholine

ANISINDIONE—Miradon®

Anticoagulant (indandione) indicated for the prophylaxis and treatment of conditions such as venous thrombosis and pulmonary embolism.

Preparation: tablets, 50 mg.

ANISOTROPINE METHYLBROMIDE

Anticholinergic agent indicated as adjunctive therapy in the management of peptic ulcer.

Preparation: tablets, 50 mg.

ANISTREPLASE—Eminase®

Thrombolytic agent.

Actions and Uses: Also known as anisoylated plasminogen streptokinase activator complex (APSAC). Promotes the conversion of plasminogen to plasmin, which is fibrinolytic. Indicated for acute management of coronary thrombosis (myocardial infarction). Treatment should be initiated as soon as possible after the onset of AMI symptoms.

Warnings: Contraindicated in patients who are hypersensitive to the drug or to streptokinase. Is also contraindicated in patients with active internal bleeding, history of cerebrovascular accident, recent intracranial or intraspinal surgery or trauma, intracranial neoplasm, arteriovenous malformation, or aneurysm, known bleeding diathesis, or severe, uncontrolled hypertension. Serious bleeding reactions (e. g., internal bleeding and/or superficial or surface bleeding) may occur and appropriate precautions must be taken. Con- current use of heparin anticoagulation may contribute to the bleeding. Warfarin, aspirin, and dipyridamole may increase the risk of bleeding if administered prior to anistreplase therapy. Intramuscular injections should be avoided during treatment with anistreplase. Other adverse reactions include hypotension and allergic-type reactions.

Administration: Intravenous.

Preparations: Vials, 30 units.

ANSAID®, see Flurbiprofen

ANSPOR®, see Cephradine

ANTABUSE®, see Disulfiram

ANTEPAR®, see Piperazine citrate

ANTHRA-DERM®, see Anthralin

ANTHRALIN—Anthra-Derm®, Dithranol

Used in the topical management of psoriasis and certain other dermatologic disorders.

Preparations: Cream and ointment, 0.1%, 0.2%, 0.25%, 0.4%, 0.5%, and 1%.

ANTILIRIUM®, see Physostigmine

ANTIMINTH®, see Pyrantel pamoate

ANTISPAS®, see Dicyclomine

ANTITHROMBIN III (HUMAN)—ATnativ®

Coagulation inhibitor.

Actions and Uses: Is identical with heparin cofactor I, a factor that is necessary for heparin to exert its anticoagulant effect. Inactivates thrombin and the activated forms of Factors IX, X, XI, and XII. Indicated for the treatment of patients with hereditary antithrombin III deficiency in connection with surgical or obstetrical procedures or when they suffer from thromboembolism.

Warnings: The anticoagulant effect of heparin is increased by concurrent treatment with antithrombin III and the dosage of heparin should be reduced.

Administration. Intravenous. Plasma antithrombin III levels should be measured preceding and 30 minutes after the dose until the patient is stabilized, and thereafter measured once a day immediately before the next infusion.

Preparations: Infusion bottles, 500 international units.

ANTIVERT®, see Meclizine

ANTURANE®, see Sulfinpyrazone

A.P.L.®, see Chorionic gonadotropin

APRACLONIDINE HYDROCHLORIDE—Iopidine®

Ocular laser surgical agent.

Actions and Uses: An alpha adrenergic agonist which, when instilled into the eye, reduces intraocular pressure. Indicated (1% solution) to control or prevent postsurgical elevations in intraocular pressure that occur in patients after argon laser trabeculoplasty or argon laser iridotomy. Also indicated (0.5% solution) for short-term adjunctive therapy in patients on maximally tolerated medical therapy who require additional intraocular pressure reduction.

Warnings: Adverse reactions include upper lid elevation, conjunctival blanching, and mydriasis.

Administration: Ophthalmic.

Preparation: Ophthalmic solution, containing the equivalent of 0.5% and 1% apraclonidine base.

APRESOLINE®, see Hydralazine

APROBARBITAL—Alurate®

Barbiturate sedative-hypnotic indicated for the treatment of anxiety and insomnia.

Preparation: Elixir, 40 mg/5 ml.

APROTININ—Trasylol®

Antifibrinolytic agent.

Actions and Uses: Is a natural protease inhibitor that inhibits fibrinolysis and decreases bleeding, and reduces the need for donor blood or blood products. Indicated for prophylactic use to reduce perioperative blood loss and the need for blood transfusion in patients undergoing cardiopulmonary bypass in the course of repeat coronary artery bypass graft (CABG) surgery. Is also indicated in selected cases of primary CABG surgery where the risk of bleeding is especially high or where transfusion is unavailable or unacceptable.

Warnings: Adverse reactions include anaphylactic reactions, renal dysfunction, and abnormal liver function tests. All patients should first receive a test dose to assess the potential for allergic reactions. Patients who experience any allergic reaction to the test dose should not receive further administration of the drug. Particular caution is necessary when administering aprotinin (even test doses) to patients who have received the drug in the past. In re-exposure cases, an antihistamine should be administered intravenously shortly before the loading dose. May inhibit the effects of fibrinolytic agents. May be administered concurrently with heparin; however, aprotinin prolongs the activated clotting time (ACT) and some patients may require additional heparin, even in the presence of ACT levels that appear to represent adequate anticoagulation.

Administration: Intravenous. Is administered through a central line and other drugs should not be administered using the same line. A 1 ml (10,000 Kallikrein Inhibitor Units [KIU]) test dose should be administered at least 10 minutes before the loading dose. The loading dose is given slowly over 20–30 minutes after induction of anesthesia but prior to sternotomy. When the loading dose is complete, it is followed by the constant infusion dose, which is continued until surgery is complete and the patient leaves the operating room. A "pump prime" dose is added to the priming fluid of the cardiopulmonary bypass circuit, by replacement of an aliquot of the priming fluid, prior to the institution of the cardiopulmonary bypass.

Preparations: Vials 1,000,000 and 2,000,000 Kallikrein Inhibitor Units (KIU). One million units represents 140 mg of the drug.

AQUA MEPHYTON®, see Phytonadione

AQUACARE®, see Urea

AQUASOL A®, see Vitamin A

AQUASOL E®, see Vitamin E

ARA-C, see Cytarabine

ARALEN®, see Chloroquine

ARAMINE®, see Metaraminol

ARDUAN®, see Pipecuronium bromide

AREDIA®, see Pamidronate disodium

ARGININE HYDROCHLORIDE—R-Gene®

Diagnostic agent administered intravenously in the evaluation of pituitary function.

Preparation: Solution, 10%.

ARICEPT®, see Triamcino

ARISTOCORT®, see Donepezil Hydrochloride

ARIMIDEX, see Anastrozole

ARISTOSPAN®, see Triamcinolone hexacetonide

AROMATIC SPIRIT OF AMMONIA, see Ammonia, aromatic spirit

ARTANE®, see Trihexyphenidyl

ARTHROPAN®, see Choline salicylate

ARTHROTEC®—Combination agent diclotenac sodium and misoprostol

ASA, see Aspirin

ASACOL®, see Mesalamine

ASCORBIC ACID, see Vitamin C

ASENDIN®, see Amoxapine

A-SPAS®, see Dicyclomine

ASPARAGINASE—Elspar®

Antineoplastic agent indicated in the treatment of acute lymphocytic leukemia.

Preparation: Vials, 10,000 IU.

ASPERCREME®, see Trolamine salicylate

ASPIRIN—Acetylsalicylic acid, ASA, Bayer aspirin®, Easprin®, Ecotrin®, Empirin®, ZORprin®

Analgesic/antipyretic and anti-inflammatory agent.

Actions and Uses: A salicylate used in the treatment of mild to moderate pain, fever, and arthritic and other disorders associated with inflammation. Also indicated for reducing the risk of stroke in male patients with recurrent ischemic attacks, and to reduce the risk of death and/or nonfatal myocardial infarction in patients with a previous infarction or unstable angina pectoris.

Warnings: Contraindicated in patients known to be hypersensitive to salicylates or in individuals with the syndrome of nasal polyps, angioedema, and bronchospastic reactivity to aspirin. May cause GI effects, and use should be avoided in patients with active GI tract disease and closely supervised in patients with a previous history of such disorders. Other adverse reactions include rash, tinnitus, interference with hemostasis, aspirin intolerance, and salicylism. May interact with and increase the effect of anticoagulants, hypoglycemic agents, and methotrexate. May reduce the effect of probenecid and sulfinpyrazone. Discontinue the drug 7–10 days before elective surgical procedures. Use in children or teenagers with influenza or chickenpox may be associated with the development of Reye's syndrome. Use during pregnancy is best avoided, especially in the third trimester.

Administration: Oral and rectal. Enteric-coated and controlled-release formulations should be swallowed intact.

Preparations: tablets, 81, 325, and 500 mg. Enteric-coated tablets/capsules, 325, 500, 650, and 975 mg. Controlled-release tablets, 650, and 800 mg. Suppositories, 60, 130, 200, 325, and 650 mg.

ASTELIN®, see Azelastine Hydrochloride

ASTEMIZOLE—Hismanal®

Antihistamine.

Actions and Uses: Has a long duration of action which permits once-daily dosing but also has a slow onset of action. Is not likely to cause sedation and is often designated as a nonsedating antihistamine. Indicated for the relief of symptoms associated with seasonal allergic rhinitis (e.g., sneezing, runny nose, pruritus) and in the management of chronic idiopathic urticaria.

Warnings: Adverse reactions include increased appetite and weight gain. Elevated drug plasma concentrations have been associated with electrocardiographic QT prolongation, cardiac arrest, torsades de pointes, and other ventricular arrhythmias. Use is contraindicated in patients with severe hepabic dysfunction or concurrent use of erythromycin, ketoconazole, itraconazole, fluvoxamine, or nefazoclone and in severe hepatic dysfunction.

Administration: Oral. Absorption may be reduced by as much as 60% when the medication is taken with meals; therefore, it should be taken on an empty stomach (e.g., at least 2 hours after a meal) and no additional food should be taken for at least 1 hour post-dosing.

Preparation: tablets, 10 mg.

ASTRAMORPH PF®, see Morphine.

ATARAX®, see Hydroxyzine

ATENOLOL—Tenormin®

Antihypertensive and antianginal agent.

Actions and Uses: A cardioselective beta-adrenergic blocking agent indicated in the management of hypertension, angina pectoris, and myocardial infarction.

Warnings: Contraindicated in patients with sinus bradycardia, heart block greater than first degree, cardiogenic shock, and overt cardiac failure. Adverse reactions include dizziness, fatigue, bradycardia, postural hypotension, and nausea. Use is best avoided in patients with bronchospastic diseases, and therapy in diabetic patients must be closely monitored.

Administration: Oral and intravenous. Patients should be cautioned about the interruption or discontinuation of therapy; exacerbation of angina pectoris has occurred following the abrupt cessation of therapy and, when therapy is to be discontinued, the dosage should be gradually reduced over a period of 1 to 2 weeks.

Preparations: tablets, 25, 50, and 100 mg. Ampules, 5 mg/10 ml.

ATIVAN®, see Lorazepam

ATnativ®, see Antithrombin III (Human)

ATOVAQUONE—Mepron®

Antiprotozoal agent.

Actions and Uses: Indicated for the treatment of mild to moderate *Pneumocystis carinii* pneumonia (PCP) in patients who are intolerant to trimethoprim-sulfamethoxazole.

Warnings: Adverse reactions include rash, nausea, vomiting, diarrhea, headache, fever, insomnia, and elevations of liver enzymes.

Administration: Oral. Should be taken with meals. Patients should be advised of the importance of administering the drug with meals.

Preparations: Suspension, 750 mg/ 5 ml.

ATRACURIUM BESYLATE—Tracrium®

Nondepolarizing skeletal muscle relaxant administered intravenously as an adjunct to general anesthesia, to facilitate endotracheal intubation, and to provide skeletal muscle relaxation during surgery or mechanical ventilation.

Preparations: Ampules and vials, 10 mg/ml.

ATROMID-S®, see Clofibrate

ATROPINE SULFATE

Anticholinergic, mydriatic, and cycloplegic agent used parenterally in a number of conditions including peptic ulcer, biliary and ureteral colic, bronchial spasm, and parkinsonism, to lessen the degree of AV heart block, to restore cardiac rate and arterial pressure during anesthesia in certain situations, and as preanesthetic medication. Used via ophthalmic administration for cycloplegic refraction, or for pupil dilation in certain acute ocular inflammatory conditions.

Preparations: Ampules, vials, and syringes, 0.05, 0.1, 0.3, 0.4, 0.5, 0.8, 1, and 1.2 mg/ml. tablets 0.4 mg. Hypodermic tablets, 0.3, 0.4, and 0.6 mg. Ophthalmic solution, 0.5%, 1%, 2%, and 3%. Ophthalmic ointment, 0.5%, and 1%.

ATORVASTATIN—Lipitor®

Actions and Uses: An HMG-CoA reductase inhibitor indicated as an adjunct to diet for the reduction of elevated total and LDL-cholesterol levels in patients with primary hypercholesterolemia and mixed dyslipidemia.

Warnings: Contraindicated in active liver disease, unexplained peristent elevated serum transaminases, and pregnancy. Monitor liver function before and during therapy. Reduce or discontinue dose if serum transaminase levels > 3 times the upper limit of normal persist. Use cautiously in patients with chronic alcohol ingestion. Discontinue if myopathy or elevated CPK levels occur. Suspend therapy if predisposition to development of renal failure secondary to rhabdomyolysis develops. Adverse reactions include constipation, flatulence, dyspepsia, abdominal pain, headache, myalgia, arthralgia, rash, asthenia, and elevated serum transaminases.

Administration: Initially 10 mg once daily. Range 10–80 mg once daily.

Preparation: Tablets, 10, 20, and 40 mg.

ATROVENT®, see Ipratropium

AUGMENTIN®, see Amoxicillin/clavulanate potassium

AURANOFIN—Ridaura®

Antiarthritic Agent.

Actions and Uses: An orally administered gold-containing formulation indicated in the management of rheumatoid arthritis in adult patients who have had an insufficient therapeutic response to one or more nonsteroidal anti-inflammatory drugs or who are intolerant of such drugs.

Warnings: Adverse reactions include loose stools or diarrhea, abdominal pain, nausea, vomiting, rash, pruritus, stomatitis, proteinuria. A complete blood count (CBC) with differential and platelet count, urinalysis, and physical examination of the mouth and skin should be done at least monthly during therapy.

Administration: Oral.

Preparation: Capsules, 3 mg.

AUREOMYCIN®, see Chlortetracycline

AUROTHIOGLUCOSE—Solganal®

Gold formulation administered intramuscularly in the treatment of rheumatoid arthritis.

Preparation: Vials, 50 mg/ml.

AVC®, see Sulfanilamide

AVENTYL®, see Nortriptyline

AVITA®, see Tretinoin

AVLOSULFON®, see Dapsone

AVONEX®, see Interferon beta-1A

AXID®, see Nizatidine

AZACTAM®, see Aztreonam

AZATADINE MALEATE—Optimine®

Antihistamine indicated for the treatment of perennial and seasonal allergic rhinitis and chronic urticaria.

Preparation: tablets, 1 mg.

AZATHIOPRINE—Imuran®

Immunosuppressant indicated as an adjunct for the prevention of rejection in renal homotransplantation, and in the management of severe rheumatoid arthritis that has not responded satisfactorily to other agents.

Preparations: tablets, 50 mg. Vials (sodium salt), 100 mg.

AZELAIC ACID—Azelex®

Topical antibacterial.

Action and Uses: Exerts antibacterial and keratolytic activity when applied topically. Indicated for treatment of mild to moderate inflammatory acne vulgaris.

Warnings: Not recommended for use in children. Monitor patients with dark complexion for hypopigmentation. Discontinue if sensitivity or severe irritation develops. Pruritis, burning, stinging, tingling, exacerbation of acne, hypopigmentation, contact dermatitis, vitiligo, depigmentation, and hypertrichosis may occur.

Administration: Massage thin film on clean, dry affected areas twice daily. Wash hands after application. If persistent irritation occurs may decrease to once daily.

Preparations: 20% topical cream.

AZELASTINE HYDROCHLORIDE—Astelin®

Antihistamine indicated in the treatment of seasonal allergic rhinitis symptoms including rhinorrhea. A nasal spray formulation of an H_1 antagonist.

Warnings: Avoid contact with eyes. May potentiate CNS depression of other drugs or alcohol. Adverse reactions include bitter taste, somnolence, headache, weight increase, myalgia, nasal burning, sneezing, and nausea.

Administration: Two sprays in each nostril twice daily.

Preparation: Aqueous nasal spray 137 μg/actuation.

AZELEX®, see Azelaic Acid

AZITHROMYCIN—Zithromax®, Z-Pak®

Azalide antibiotic.

Actions and Uses: Inhibits protein synthesis and usually exhibits a bacteriostatic action against gram-positive and gram-negative bacteria. Indicated for upper respiratory tract infections, lower respiratory tract infections, and uncomplicated skin and skin structure infections caused by susceptible organisms. Also indicated for nongonococcal urethritis and cervicitis caused by *Chlamydia trachomatis.* Used to treat acute otitis media.

Warnings: Contraindicated in patients with a known hypersensitivity to any of the macrolide antibiotics. Adverse reactions include diarrhea/loose stools, nausea, vomiting, abdominal pain, and vaginitis. Aluminum- and magnesium-containing antacids may reduce the rate of absorption, and the two agents should not be administered at the same time.

Administration: Oral (should be administered at least one hour before or 2 hours after a meal) and intravenous.

Preparation: Tablets 250 (scored) and 650 mg. Oral suspension 100 mg/5ml, and200 mg/5ml. Single-dose packets for oral suspension, 1 g. Vials for IV infusion after reconstitution, 500 mg/vial.

AZMACORT®, see Triamcinolone acetonide

AZO-STANDARD®, see Phenazopyridine hydrochloride

AZT, see Zidovudine

AZTREONAM—Azactam®

Monobactam antibiotic.

Actions and Uses: Indicated for urinary tract infections, lower respiratory tract infections, septicemia, skin and skin-structure infections, intra-abdominal infections, and gynecologic infections caused by susceptible gram-negative bacteria. Among the organisms that are susceptible to the drug are *Pseudomonas aeruginosa, Haemophilus influenzae, Escherichia coli, Klebsiella pneumoniae, Proteus mirabilis, Serratia* species, *Enterobacter* species, and *Citrobacter* species. It is also indicated as adjunctive therapy to surgery in the management of infections caused by susceptible organisms.

Warnings: It has only a weak potential to cause hypersensitivity reactions or to demonstrate cross-reactivity with the penicillins and cephalosporins. Adverse reactions include diarrhea, nausea and/or vomiting, rash, phlebitis/thrombophlebitis following intravenous administration, discomfort at the injection site following intramuscular administration, and superinfection with gram-positive bacteria such as enterococci.

Administration: Intravenous and intramuscular.

Preparations: Vials, 500 mg, 1 and 2 g. Intravenous infusion bottles, 500 mg, 1 and 2 g.

B

BACAMPICILLIN HYDROCHLORIDE —Spectrobid®

Penicillin antibiotic. Is a prodrug which is hydrolyzed to ampicillin following administration. Indicated in the treatment of respiratory tract, urinary tract, and dermatologic infections caused by susceptible bacteria, and also in the management of gonorrhea. tablets may be given without regard to meals but the suspension should be administered apart from meals.

Preparations: tablets, 400 mg. Powder for oral suspension, 125 mg/5 ml when reconstituted.

BACITRACIN

Anti-infective agent that is primarily active against gram-positive bacteria such as staphylococci. Most often used topically.

Preparations: Ointment and ophthalmic ointment, 500 units/g. Vials (for parenteral administration), 10,000 and 50,000 units.

BACLOFEN—Lioresal®

Muscle relaxant and antispastic agent indicated for the alleviation of signs and symptoms of spasticity resulting from multiple sclerosis, and also in the management of certain spinal cord injuries and diseases.

Preparations: tablets, 10 and 20 mg.

Ampules (for intrathecal use), 10 mg/5 ml and 10 mg/20 ml.

BACTRIM®, see Trimethoprim-sulfamethoxazole

BACTROBAN®, see Mupirocin

BAKING SODA, see Sodium bicarbonate

BAL, see Dimercaprol

BARIUM SULFATE

Diagnostic agent used in the x-ray examination of the gastrointestinal tract.

BASALJEL®, see Aluminum carbonate gel, basic

BAYER ASPIRIN®, see Aspirin

BECLOMETHASONE DIPROPIONATE—Beclovent®, Vanceril®, Beconase®, Beconase AQ®, Vancenase®, Vancenase AQ®, Double Strength®, Vanceril®, Double strength

Corticosteroid administered by oral inhalation (Beclovent®, Vanceril®) or nasal spray in patients who require chronic treatment with corticosteroids to control the symptoms of bronchial asthma. Also administered by nasal inhalation for the relief of symptoms of seasonal or perennial rhinitis.

Preparation: Aerosol, 42 and 84 µg per actuation. Nasal spray (Beconase AQ®, Vancenase AQ®), 84 µg/spray.

BECLOVENT®, see Beclomethasone dipropionate

BECONASE®, see Beclomethasone dipropionate

BECONASE AQ®, see Beclometha- sone dipropionate

BEEPEN VK®, see Penicillin V potassium

BELLADONNA

Anticholinergic. Contains atropine, hyoscyamine and scopolamine alkaloids and has been used in the treatment of gastrointestinal disorders and parkinsonism.

Preparation: Tincture of belladonna.

BENADRYL®, see Diphenhydramine

BENAZEPRIL HYDROCHLORIDE—Lotensin®

Antihypertensive agent.

Actions and Uses: An angiotensin-converting enzyme (ACE) inhibitor that is a prodrug. Following oral administration, is converted to its active metabolite, benazeprilat. Indicated for the treatment of hypertension and may be used alone or in combination with a thiazide diuretic.

Warnings: Adverse reactions include headache, dizziness, fatigue, cough, and nausea. May cause an elevation in serum potassium levels; the risk of hyperkalemia is increased in patients also taking a potassium-sparing diuretic, a potassium supplement, and/ or a potassium-containing salt substitute. May cause symptomatic postural hypotension. There have been infrequent reports of angioedema of the face, extremities, lips, tongue, glottis, and larynx, especially following the first dose. Patients should be told to report immediately any symptoms suggesting angioedema and to stop taking the drug. When used during the second and third trimesters of pregnancy, ACE inhibitors have been reported to be associated with the development of neonatal hypertension, renal failure, and skull hypoplasia; use during pregnancy should be avoided. May increase serum lithium levels and concurrent therapy should be closely monitored.

Administration: Oral.

Preparations: tablets, 5, 10, 20, and 40 mg.

BENDROFLUMETHIAZIDE—Naturetin®

Thiazide diuretic indicated as adjunctive therapy in the treatment of edema and in the management of hypertension.

Preparations: tablets, 2.5, 5, and 10 mg.

BENEMID®, see Probenecid

BENOQUIN®, see Monobenzone

BENOXINATE HYDROCHLORIDE

Local anesthetic sometimes employed to provide anesthesia in certain ophthalmic procedures.

BENTYL®, see Dicyclomine

BENYLIN COUGH®, see Diphenhydramine hydrochloride

BENYLIN DM®, see Dextromethorphan

BENZALKONIUM CHLORIDE—Zephiran®

Anti-infective agent used topically as an antiseptic, in the irrigation of certain tissues, and in the preoperative preparation of the skin. Also used as a preservative (e.g., in ophthalmic solutions) and in the sterile storage of instruments.

Preparations: Solution and tincture, 1:750. Concentrate (to be diluted), 17%.

BENZATHINE PENICILLIN G—Bicillin®, Permapen®

Penicillin antibiotic that has a long duration of action following intramuscular administration. Indicated in infections caused by highly susceptible organisms such as streptococci. Also used in the prevention of recurrent rheumatic fever and in the treatment of syphilis.

Preparations: Vials, 300,000 units/ml. Syringes, 600,000, 1,200,000, and 2,400,000 units.

BENZEDREX®, see Propylhexedrine

BENZOCAINE—Ethyl aminobenzoate, Zilabrace®, Ziladent®

Local anesthetic administered topically in dermatologic disorders, locally to provide oral and mucosal anesthesia, and orally as an adjunct in a weight reduction regimen.

Preparations: Cream, ointment, solution, and lotion, 0.5% to 20%. Gel, 6% and 10%. Candy and gum (in weight-reduction regimen), 6 mg.

BENZOIC ACID

Anti-infective agent used topically in the treatment of fungal infections, usually in combination with salicylic acid in an ointment formulation known as Whitfield's ointment (6% benzoic acid and 3% salicylic acid).

BENZOIN

Protectant used topically to protect the skin against irritants and to coat sores. Tincture and compound benzoin tincture have sometimes been placed in boiling water as steam inhalants to provide an expectorant and soothing action in certain respiratory conditions.

Preparation: Tincture.

BENZONATATE—Tessalon®

Antitussive indicated for the symptomatic relief of cough.

Preparation: Capsules, 100 mg.

BENZPHETAMINE HYDROCHLORIDE—Didrex®

Anorexiant indicated in the management of exogenous obesity as a short-term adjunct in a regimen of weight reduction based on caloric restriction.

Preparation: tablets, 25 and 50 mg.

BENZTHIAZIDE—Exna®

Thiazide diuretic indicated in the treatment of edema in the management of hypertension.

Preparation: tablets, 50 mg.

BENZTROPINE MESYLATE—Cogentin®

Antiparkinson agent.

Actions and Uses: Exhibits anticholinergic activity, and is indicated for the treatment of parkinsonism and the control of drug-induced extrapyramidal reactions.

Warnings: Adverse reactions include dry mouth, nausea, vomiting, blurred vision, tachycardia, confusion, nervousness, and urinary retention.

Administration: Oral, intravenous and intramuscular.

Preparations: Tablets, 0.5, 1, and 2 mg. Ampules, 1 mg/ml.

BEPRIDIL HYDROCHLORIDE—Vascor®

Antianginal agent.

Actions and Uses: A calcium channel blocking agent that is indicated for the treatment of chronic stable angina (classic effort-associated angina) in patients who have failed to respond optimally to, or are intolerant of, other antianginal medications. May be used alone or in combination with beta-blockers and/or nitrates.

Warnings: Contraindicated in patients with a history of serious ventricular arrhythmias, sick sinus syndrome or second- or third-degree AV block except in the presence of a functioning ventricular pacemaker, hypotension, uncompensated cardiac insufficiency, congenital QT interval prolongation, and in patients taking other drugs that prolong QT interval. May cause proarrhythmic effects including serious ventricular arrhythmias. May prolong the QT interval and the QTc interval which has been associated with the development of torsades-de-pointes-type ventricular tachycardia. The risk of this reaction is increased by the presence of antecedent bradycardia, hypokalemia, and the use of potassium-depleting diuretics. If the concurrent use of a diuretic is needed, a potassium-sparing diuretic should be used if possible. Any potassium deficiency should be corrected before bepridil therapy is initiated and serum potassium levels should be monitored periodically. Other adverse reactions include nausea, diarrhea, dyspepsia, GI distress, dizziness, asthenia, and nervousness. Agranulocytosis has been reported rarely. Other agents that may prolong the QT interval (e.g., quinidine, procainamide, tricyclic antidepressants) should not be used concurrently because of a greater potential for ventricular arrhythmias. Concurrent use with digoxin may result in an increase in serum digoxin levels and therapy should be closely monitored.

Administration. Oral.

Preparations: Tablets, 200, 300, and 400 g.

BERACTANT—Survanta®

Agent for respiratory distress syndrome.

Actions and Uses: A pulmonary surfactant of bovine origin that contains phospholipids, neutral lipids, fatty acids, and surfactant-associated proteins, to which colfosceril palmitate, palmitic acid, and tripalmitin are added to standardize the composition and to mimic the surface tension lowering properties of natural lung surfactant. Replenishes surfactant and restores surface activity to the lungs. Indicated for the prevention and treatment of respiratory distress syndrome in premature infants.

Warnings: Adverse reactions include bradycardia and oxygen desaturation. May rapidly affect oxygenation and lung compliance.

Administration: Intratracheal. If settling has occurred during storage, swirl the vial gently (do not shake) to redisperse. Is stored refrigerated and, before administration, should be warmed by standing at room temperature for at least 20 minutes or warmed in the hand for at least 8 minutes. Is administered intratracheally by instillation through a 5 French end-hole catheter inserted into the infant's endotracheal tube. Each dose is divided into four quarter-doses and each quarter-dose is administered with the infant in a different position.

Preparations: Vials, 200 mg phospholipids/8ml.

BETADINE®, see Povidone-Iodine

BETAGAN®, see Levobunolol

BETAMETHASONE, BETAMETHASONE SODIUM PHOSPHATE, BETAMETHASONE ACETATE—Celestone®

Corticosteroid.

Actions and Uses: Indicated in a wide range of endocrine, rheumatic, allergic, dermatologic, respiratory, hematologic, neoplastic, and other disorders.

Preparations: Tablets, 0.6 mg. Syrup, 0.6 mg/5 ml. Vials (solution), 4 mg as the sodium phosphate per ml. Vials (suspension), 6 mg as the sodium phosphate and acetate per ml.

BETAMETHASONE BENZOATE—Uticort®

Topical corticosteroid.

Preparations: Cream, lotion, and gel, 0.025%.

BETAMETHASONE DIPROPIONATE—Diprosone®, Maxivate®

Topical corticosteroid.

Preparations: Cream, ointment, and lotion, 0.05%.

Topical aerosol, 0.1%.

BETAMETHASONE DIPROPIONATE AUGMENTED—Diprolene®, Diprolene AF®

Topical corticosteroid.

Actions and Uses: Specially formulated vehicle increases penetration and potency. Indicated for the short-term treatment of the inflammatory and pruritic manifestations of moderate to severe corticosteroid-responsive dermatoses.

Warnings: Is highly potent and is more likely than less potent analogs to cause systemic effects including suppression of the hypothalamic-pituitary-adrenal (HPA) axis. Treatment period should be limited to 2 weeks and the total dosage should not exceed 45 g per week. Occlusive dressings should not be used.

Administration: Topical.

Preparations: Cream, ointment, and lotion, 0.05%.

BETAMETHASONE VALERATE—Valisone®

Topical corticosteroid.

Actions and Uses: Indicated for relief of the inflammatory and pruritic manifestations of corticosteroid-responsive dermatoses.

Warnings: Adverse reactions include burning, itching, irritation, dryness, and a potential for systemic effect.

Administration: Topical.

Preparations: Cream, ointment, and lotion, 0.1%.

Reduced-strength cream 0.01%.

BETAPACE®, see Sotalol hydrochloride

BETAPEN VK®, see Penicillin V potassium

BETASERON®, see Interferon beta-1b

BETAXOLOL HYDROCHLORIDE—Betoptic®, Betoptic S®, Kerlone®

Antihypertensive agent and agent for glaucoma.

Actions and Uses: A cardioselective beta-adrenergic blocking agent indicated in the treatment of hypertension, and for ophthalmic administration in the treatment of chronic open-angle glaucoma and ocular hypertension.

Warnings: Contraindicated in patients with sinus bradycardia, second- and third-degree AV block in the absence of a functioning artificial pacemaker, overt cardiac failure, or cardiogenic shock. Adverse reactions include fatigue, dizziness, and bradycardia, and, when administered in the ophthalmic dosage forms, transient stinging during instillation. Use is best avoided in patients with bronchospastic diseases, and therapy in diabetic patients must be closely monitored.

Administration: Oral and ophthalmic. Patients should be cautioned about the interruption or discontinuation of oral therapy; exacerbation of angina pectoris has occurred following the abrupt cessation of therapy and when therapy is to be discontinued, the dosage should be gradually reduced over a period of 2 weeks.

Preparations: Tablets (Kerlone), 10 and 20 mg. Ophthalmic suspension (Betoptic S), 0.25%. Ophthalmic solution (Betoptic), 0.5%.

BETHANECHOL CHLORIDE—Urecholine®

Cholinergic agent indicated for the treatment of acute postoperative and postpartum nonobstructive urinary retention, and for neurogenic atony of the urinary bladder with retention.

Preparations: Tablets, 5, 10, 25, and 50 mg. Vials, 5 mg/ml.

BETIMOL®, see Timolol

BETOPTIC®, see Betaxolol

BIAXIN®, see Clarithromycin

BICALUTAMIDE—Casodex®

Antineoplastic, antiandrogen hormone.

Uses and Actions: Antagonizes the effects of androgen (action is usually against a more potent androgen) at the cellular level. Indicated in the treatment of metastatic prostate carcinoma in conjunction with luteinizing hormone releasing hormone (LHRH) analogs (goserelin, leuprolide).

Warnings: May cause moderate to severe hepatic impairment. Monitor hepatic function and prostate specific antigen (PSA). Adverse reactions include weakness, constipation, nausea, diarrhea, back pain, pelvic pain, hot flashes, and generalized pain.

Administration: Oral, 50 mg once daily (must be given concurrently with LHRH analog).

Preparation: Tablets, 50 mg.

BICILLIN®, see Benzathine penicillin G

BICITRA®, see Sodium citrate

BICNU®, see Carmustine

BILTRICIDE®, see Praziquantel

BIPERIDEN—Akineton®

Antiparkinson agent indicated for the treatment of parkinsonism and the control of extrapyramidal disorders secondary to neuroleptic drug therapy.

Preparations: Tablets (as the hydrochloride), 2 mg. Ampules (as the lactate), 5 mg.

BISACODYL—Dulcolax®

Laxative indicated for acute constipation, chronic constipation, preparation for x-rays, preoperative preparation, and other situations.

Preparations: Tablets, 5 mg. Suppositories, 5 and 10 mg.

BISMUTH SUBCARBONATE

Antacid included in some combination formulations.

BISMUTH SUBSALICYLATE—PeptoBismol®

Antidiarrheal/antacid and analgesic used in the management of nausea, gas pains, abdominal cramps, and diarrhea. Has been used in the prevention and treatment of traveler's diarrhea. Also indicated in regimens for the treatment of gastrointestinal disorders caused by Helicobacter pylori.

Preparations: Chewable tablets, 262 mg. Suspension, 262 mg/15 ml and 524 mg/15 ml.

BISOPROLOL FUMARATE—Zebeta®

Antihypertensive agent.

Actions and Uses: Is a cardioselective beta-adrenergic blocking agent that is indicated for the treatment of hypertension.

Warnings: Contraindicated in patients in cardiogenic shock, or with overt cardiac failure, second- and third-degree heart block, or marked sinus bradycardia. Adverse reactions include headache, fatigue, dizziness, diarrhea, and cold extremities. Use is best avoided in patients with bronchospastic diseases and therapy in diabetic patients must be closely monitored.

Administration: Oral. When therapy is to be discontinued, the dosage should be gradually reduced over a period of one week.

Preparations: Tablets, 5 and 10 mg. Also available in combination formulations (Ziac) with hydrochlorothiazide that contain 2.5, 5, and 10 mg of bisoprolol fumarate with 6.25 mg of the diuretic.

BITOLTEROL MESYLATE—Tornalate®

Bronchodilator used by oral inhalation for prophylactic and therapeutic use for bronchial asthma and for reversible bronchospasm.

Preparations: Metered dose inhaler, 0.37 mg per actuation. Inhalation solution, 0.2%

BLENOXANE®, see Bleomycin

BLEOMYCIN SULFATE—
Blenoxane®

Antineoplastic agent indicated for parenteral use as a palliative treatment in the management of squamous cell carcinomas, lymphomas, and testicular carcinoma.

Preparation: Vials, 15 units.

BLOCADREN®, see Timolol

BONINE®, see Meclizine

BONTRIL®, see Phendimetrazine

BORIC ACID

Antiseptic used topically for conditions associated with irritation of the skin, and for the treatment of irritated and inflamed eyelids.

Preparations: Ointment and ophthalmic ointment, 5% and 10%.

BOTOX®, see Botulinum toxin type A

BOTULINUM TOXIN TYPE A—
Botox®

Agent for muscle disorders.

Actions and Uses: Is produced from a culture of *Clostridium botulinum* and, following injection into eye muscles, inhibits the release of acetylcholine resulting in a localized reversible muscle paralysis. Indicated for the treatment of strabismus and blepharospasm associated with dystonia, including benign essential blepharospasm or seventh cranial nerve disorders. Is also being evaluated in a number of other muscle disorders.

Warnings: Adverse reactions when used in the treatment of strabismus include spatial disorientation, double vision, ptosis, vertical deviation, and retrobulbar hemorrhages resulting from needle penetrations into the orbit. Adverse reactions when used in the treatment of blepharospasm include ptosis, irritatioon/tearing, ecchymosis, rash,and local swelling of the eyelid skin.

Administration: Ocular injection. In the treatment of strabismus the drug is injected using electromyographic guidance to facilitate placement within the target muscle. Paralysis of the injected muscles lasts for 2 to 6 weeks. In the treatment of blepharospasm the drug is injected into the orbicularis oculi without electromyographic guidance. Each treatment lasts approximately 3 months.

Preparations: Vials, 100 units.

BRETHAIRE®, see Terbutaline

BRETHINE®, see Terbutaline

BRETYLIUM TOSYLATE—
Bretylol®

Antiarrhythmic agent indicated for parenteral use in the prophylaxis and treatment of ventricular fibrillation and also in the treatment of life-threatening ventricular arrhythmias that have not responded to other agents.

Preparations: Ampules, vials, and syringes, 500 mg.

BRETYLOL®, see Bretylium

BREVIBLOC®, see Esmolol

BREVITAL®, see Methohexital

BRICANYL®, see Terbutaline

BRIMONIDINE TARTRATE—Alphagan®

Antiglaucoma agent used to lower intraocular pressure in patients with open-angle Glaucoma or Ocular Hypertension.

Warning: Use cautiously in severe cardiovascular diseases, hepatic or renal impairment, depression, cerebral disease, Raynaud's phenomenon, orthostatic hypertension, and thromboangiitis obliterans. Contraindicated with concomitant MAOI use. Adverse reactions include xerostomia, ocular hyperemia, burning/stinging, headache, blurred vision, foreign body sensation, fatigue/drowsiness, conjunctival follicles, ocular allergic reactions, ocular pruritis, corneal staining/erosion, photophobia, eyelid erythema, ocular ache/pain/dryness, tearing, upper respiratory symptoms, eyelid edema, conjunctival blanching, abnormal vision, and muscular pain.

Administration: One drop in affected eye(s) every 8 hours. Remove soft contact lenses before instillation and for 15 minutes after dose administration.

Preparation: 0.2% ophthalmic solution.

BROMOCRIPTINE MESYLATE—Parlodel®

Dopamine receptor agonist indicated for the treatment of dysfunctions associated with hyperprolactinemia (e.g., amenorrhea, infertility), acromegaly, and parkinsonism. Is an ergot derivative.

Preparations: Tablets, 2.5 mg. Capsules, 5 mg.

BROMODIPHENHYDRAMINE HYDROCHLORIDE

Antihistamine included in some combination formulations.

BROMPHENIRAMINE MALEATE—Dimetane®

Antihistamine indicated for the management of allergic disorders.

Preparations: Tablets, 4 mg. Controlled-release tablets, 8 and 12 mg. Elixir, 2 mg/5 ml. Vials, 10 mg/ml.

BRONKAID MIST, see Epinephrine

BRONKEPHRINE®, see Isoetharine

BRONKOMETER®, see Isoetharine

BRONKOSOL®, see Isoetharine

BUCLADIN-S®, see Buclizine

BUCLIZINE HYDROCHLORIDE—Bucladin-S®

Antiemetic indicated in the management of nausea, vomiting, and dizziness associated with motion sickness.

Preparation: Tablets, 50 mg.

BUDESONIDE—Rhinocort®

Corticosteroid.

Actions and Uses: Indicated for use by nasal inhalation for the treatment of symptoms of seasonal or perennial allergic rhinitis in adults and children, and nonallergic perennial rhinitis in adults.

Warnings: Adverse reactions include nasal irritation, pharyngitis, increased cough, and epistaxis. Caution must be exercised when transferring a patient from systemic corticosteroid therapy to budesonide therapy.

Administration: Nasal inhalation.

Preparation: Metered-dose inhaler, 32 ug per actuation.

BUMETANIDE—Bumex®

Diuretic.

Actions and Uses: Is a loop diuretic indicated for the treatment of edema associated with congestive heart failure, hepatic disease, and renal disease, including the nephrotic syndrome.

Warnings: Is contraindicated in anuria, and in patients in hepatic coma or in states of severe electrolyte depletion until the condition is improved or corrected. May cause volume and electrolyte depletion. Potential for hypokalemia warrants periodic measurement of serum potassium levels. Concurrent use with lithium is best avoided because of an increased risk of lithium toxicity. Parenteral administration is best avoided in patients receiving aminoglycoside antibiotics because of an increased risk of ototoxicity.

Administration: Oral, intravenous, and intramuscular.

Preparations: Tablets, 0.5, 1, and 2 mg. Ampules and vials, 0.25 mg/ml.

BUMEX®, see Bumetanide

BUMINATE®, see Albumin

BUPIVACAINE HYDROCHLORIDE —Marcaine®

Local anesthetic administered by injection for the production of local or regional anesthesia or analgesia for surgery, dental and oral surgery procedures, diagnostic and therapeutic procedures, and for obstetrical procedures. A formulation is also available for the production of subarachnoid block (spinal anesthesia).

Preparations: Ampules and vials, 0.25%, 0.5%, and 0.75%, and in combination with epinephrine. Ampules for spinal anesthesia, 15 mg.

BUPRENEX®, see Buprenorphine

BUPRENORPHINE HYDROCHLORIDE—Buprenex®

Analgesic.

Actions and Uses: Demonstrates both opiate agonist and antagonist actions, and is indicated for the relief of moderate to severe pain.

Warnings: Adverse reactions include sedation, dizziness, and vertigo; caution should be exercised in patients also receiving other CNS depressants. Is less likely than many other potent analgesics to cause dependence and is included in Schedule V. May precipitate withdrawal symptoms in patients who are physically dependent on other opiates. Respiratory depression produced by buprenorphine is only partially reversed by naloxone and doxapram may be used.

Administration: Intravenous and intramuscular.

Preparation: Ampules, 0.3 mg.

BUPROPION HYDROCHLORIDE —Wellbutrin®, 2 g bar®

Antidepressant.

Actions and Uses: Indicated for the treatment of depression and as an aid to smoking cessation treatment.

Warnings: Contraindicated in patients with seizure disorders, and also in patients with a current or prior diagnosis of bulimia or anorexia nervosa because of a higher incidence of seizures noted in such patients when treated with bupropion. Concurrent use with a monoamine oxidase inhibitor is contraindicated and at least 14 days should elapse between discontinuation of a MAO inhibitor and initiation of treatment with bupropion. Adverse reactions most commonly encountered include nausea/vomiting, constipation, dry mouth, agitation, insomnia, headache/migraine, and tremor. Some patients experience weight loss. Patients should be cautioned regarding activities such as driving and operating machinery, as well as interactions with other CNS-acting drugs including alcohol. Extreme caution should be exercised in patients with a history of seizures or other predisposition toward seizure, and in patients treated with other medications (e.g., antipsychotics) that may lower seizure threshold. Is extensively metabolized and its activity may be changed by other medications known to affect hepatic enzyme systems (e.g., phenobarbital, cimetidine).

Administration: Oral. Because of a greater risk of seizures, no single dose should exceed 150 mg and the total daily dosage should not exceed 450 mg. Consecutive 150 mg doses should be separated by an interval of at least 6 hours, and consecutive 100 mg doses by an interval of at least 4 hours. For smoking cessation, treat for 7–12 week; avoid bedtime dosing. Patients should aim to stop smoking within 1–2 weeks after starting bupropion. May be used with transdermal nicotine (quit smoking when starting nicotine).

Preparations: Tablets, 75 and 100 mg. Sustained release tabs, 100 and 150 mg.

BUROW'S SOLUTION, see Aluminum acetate

BuSpar®, see Buspirone

BUSPIRONE HYDROCHLORIDE—BuSpar®

Antianxiety agent.

Actions and Uses: Indicated for the management of anxiety disorders or the short-term relief of the symptoms of anxiety.

Warnings: Adverse reactions include dizziness, headache, nervousness, lightheadedness, excitement, and nausea. Buspirone is less likely than other antianxiety agents to cause effects such as sedation; however, because its CNS effects in any individual patient are usually not predictable, patients should be cautioned about engaging in activities such as operating an automobile or machinery. The concurrent use with other CNS-active drugs should be closely monitored, and the consumption of alcoholic beverages is best avoided. The drug should not be used concomitantly with a monoamine oxidase inhibitor because of the possibility of blood pressure elevations.

Administration: Oral.

Preparations: Tablets, 5, 10 and 15 mg.

BUSULFAN—Myleran®

Antineoplastic agent indicated for the palliative treatment of chronic myelogenous leukemia.

Preparation: Tablets, 2 mg.

BUTABARBITAL SODIUM—Butisol sodium®

Barbiturate sedative-hypnotic indicated for the treatment of anxiety and insomnia.

Preparations: Tablets, 15, 30, 50, and 100 mg. Elixir, 30 mg/5 ml.

BUTALBITAL

Barbiturate sedative used in combination with analgesics in the management of muscle-contraction headaches.

BUTAMBEN PICRATE—Butesin picrate®

Local anesthetic indicated for the temporary relief of pain due to minor burns.

Preparation: Ointment, 1%.

BUTENAFINE HYDROCHLORIDE—Mentax®

Anitfungal agent indicated in the treatment of tinea corporis, tinea cruris, and interdigital tinea pedis.

Warnings: Avoid eyes, nose, mouth,

and mucous membranes. Do not occlude area of application. Discontinue if irritation develops and confirm diagnosis. Use cautiously in patients with hypersensitivity to allylamines. Adverse reactions include burning/stinging, worsening of condition and other local irritation.

Administration: Apply to affected area and immediately surrounding area according to the following guidelines:

Tinea pedis: once daily for 4 weeks.

Tinea corporis, cruris once daily for 2 weeks.

If no improvement within 4 weeks reconfirm diagnosis.

Preparation: 1% cream.

BUTESIN PICRATE®, see Butamben picrate

BUTISOL®, see Butabarbital

BUTOCONAZOLE NITRATE—Femstat®

Imidazole antifungal agent.

Actions and Uses: Indicated for the treatment of vulvovaginal mycotic infections caused by *Candida* species.

Warnings: Use during the first trimester of pregnancy should be avoided. Adverse reactions include vulvar/vaginal burning and/or vulvar itching.

Administration: Vaginal.

Preparation: Vaginal cream, 2%.

BUTORPHANOL TARTRATE—Stadol®, Stadol NS®

Analgesic also possessing narcotic antagonist activity. Indicated for parenteral use in the relief of moderate to severe pain, for preoperative or preanesthetic medication, as a supplement to balanced anesthesia, and for the relief of prepartum pain. Also indicated for nasal use in the management of pain (including postoperative analgesia).

Preparations: Vials and syringes, 1 mg/ml and 2 mg/ml. Nasal spray, 10 mg/ml.

BUTYL METHOXYDIBENZOYLMETHANE/PADIMATE O—Photoplex®

Sunscreen.

Actions and Uses: A combination of padimate O, which is highly protective against short-wave ultraviolet radiation [UVB (290-320 nm)], and butyl methoxydibenzoylmethane, which protects against long-wave ultraviolet radiation [UVA (320-400 nm)]. The combination of the two agents has been designated as a "broad" or "full" spectrum sunscreen. Indicated to provide protection against the acute (e.g., sunburn) and long-term (e.g. photoaging, skin cancer) risks associated with UVA and UVB light exposure.

Warnings: Contraindicated in patients with a history of allergy to paraaminobenzoic acid, sulfonamides, benzocaine, or aniline dyes. The formulation may stain some fabrics.

Administration: Topical.

Preparation: Lotion containing butyl methoxydibenzoylmethane in a 3% concentration and padimate O in a 7% concentration.

C

CABERGOLINE—Dostinex®

Dopamine agonist indicated in treatment of hyperprolactinemic disorders, either idiopathic or due to pituitary tumors.

Warnings: Not for pregnancy-induced hypertension or postpartum lactation inhibition or suppression. Use cautiously in hepatic dysfunction. Contraindicated in uncontrolled hypertension and previous sensitivity to ergot alkaloids. Monitor prolactin levels monthly, until normalized.

Administration: Initially 0.25 mg twice weekly. Dose may be increased at 4-week intervals by 0.25 mg twice weekly. Maximum dose is 1 mg twice weekly.

Preparations: Scored tablets, 0.5 mg.

CAFERGOT®, Combination of ergotamine tartrate and caffeine

CAFFEINE—NoDoz®

Central nervous system stimulant used as an aid in staying awake and as an adjunct to analgesics in the management of pain.

Preparations: Tablets, 100 and 200 mg. Controlled-release capsules, 200 and 250 mg.

CAFFEINE AND SODIUM BENZOATE

Central nervous system stimulant that has been administered parenterally as a diuretic, as a stimulant in acute circulatory failure, in the treatment of poisoning, and to alleviate headaches following spinal puncture.

Preparation: Ampules, 250 mg/ml (equal parts caffeine and sodium benzoate).

CALAMINE

Protectant applied topically in the treatment of dermatologic conditions associated with itching, pain, and irritation.

Preparation: Lotion, 8% with 8% zinc oxide.

CALAN®, see Verapamil

CALAN SR®, see Verapamil

CALCIFEDIOL—Calderol®

Vitamin D derivative indicated in the management of metabolic bone disease or hypocalcemia associated with chronic renal failure in patients undergoing renal dialysis.

Preparations: Capsules, 20 and 50 μg.

CALCIBIND®, see Sodium cellulose phosphate

CALCIJEX®, see Calcitriol

CALCIMAR®, see Calcitonin—Salmon

CALCIPOTRIENE—Dovonex®

Agent for psoriasis.

Actions and Uses: Is a synthetic analog of vitamin D_3 that is indicated for the topical treatment of moderate plaque psoriasis.

Warnings: Contraindicated in patients with demonstrated hypercalcemia or evidence of vitamin D toxicity. Is also contraindicated for use on the face. Adverse reactions include burning, itching, skin irritation, and hypercalcemia. If an elevation in serum calcium outside the normal range should occur, treatment should be discontinued until normal calcium levels are restored.

Administration: Topical.

Preparation: Cream, ointment, scalp solution, 0.005%.

CALCITONIN—SALMON—Calcimar®, Miacalcin©

Hormone indicated for the parenteral treatment of symptomatic Paget's disease of bone, hypercalcemia, and postmenopausal osteoporosis.

Preparation: Vials, 200 IU/ml. Nasal spray, 200 units/spray.

CALCITRIOL—Calcijex®, Rocaltrol®

Vitamin D derivative indicated in the management of hypocalcemia and the resultant metabolic bone disease in patients undergoing chronic renal dialysis. Is also indicated in the management of hypocalcemia in patients with hypoparathyroidism.

Preparations: Capsules, 0.25 and 0.5 µg. Ampules, 1 µg/ml and 2 µg/ml.

CALCIUM ACETATE—PhosLo®

Phosphate binding agent indicated for the control of hyperphosphatemia in end stage renal failure.

Preparations: Tablets, 667 mg.

CALCIUM CARBONATE—Caltrate®, Os-Cal®, Tums®

Antacid and source of calcium used in the treatment of gastrointestinal conditions, and in the treatment of hypocalcemic disorders and in situations in which calcium intake is inadequate.

Preparations: Chewable tablets, 350, 500, 750, and 850 mg. Tablets, 1.25 and 1.5 g.

CALCIUM CHLORIDE

Source of calcium and is administered intravenously in the treatment of hypocalcemic disorders. Also used IV in the treatment of magnesium intoxication, certain hyperkalemic conditions, and cardiac resuscitation.

Preparations: Ampules, vials, and syringes, 10%.

CALCIUM DISODIUM VERSENATE®, see Edetate calcium disodium

CALCIUM GLUCEPTATE

Source of calcium and is administered parenterally in the treatment of hypocalcemic disorders and certain other conditions.

Preparations: Ampules and vials, 1.1 g/5 ml.

CALCIUM GLUCONATE

Source of calcium and is administered orally and intravenously in the treatment of hypocalcemic disorders and in situations in which calcium intake is inadequate.

Preparations: Tablets, 500 and 650 mg, 1 g. Ampules and vials, 10%.

CALCIUM LACTATE

Source of calcium used in the treatment of hypocalcemic disorders and in situations in which calcium intake is inadequate.

Preparations: Tablets, 325 and 650 mg.

CALCIUM PHOSPHATE, TRIBASIC—Tricalcium phosphate, Posture®

Source of calcium used in the treatment of hypocalcemic disorders and in situations in which calcium intake is inadequate.

Preparations: Tablets, 300 and 600 mg.

CALCIUM UNDECYLENATE—Caldesene®

Antifungal agent applied topically in the management of dermatologic fungal infections.

Preparation: Powder, 10%.

CALDEROL®, see Calcifediol

CALDESENE®, see Calcium undecylenate

CALTRATE®, see Calcium carbonate

CAMPHOR

Analgesic and antipruritic. Is used in topically applied formulations used in the management of various dermatologic conditions.

CAMPHORATED OPIUM TINCTURE, see Paregoric

CANTIL®, see Mepenzolate

CAPASTAT®, see Capreomycin

CAPOTEN®, see Captopril

CAPOZIDE®, Combination of captopril and hydrochlorothiazide

CAPREOMYCIN SULFATE—Capastat®

Antitubercular agent used for the intramuscular treatment of tuberculosis, in conjunction with other antitubercular agents.

Preparation: Vials, 1 g.

CAPSAICIN—Zostrix®, Zostrix-HP®

Topical analgesic indicated for the relief of neuralgias that may accompany herpes zoster infections, diabetic neuropathy, or follow surgery.

Preparations: Cream, 0.025% and 0.075%.

CAPTOPRIL—Capoten®

Antihypertensive agent and agent for treatment of heart failure.

Actions and Uses: Is an angiotensin-converting enzyme (ACE) inhibitor. Indicated for the treatment of hypertension, and in patients with congestive heart failure who have not responded adequately to treatment with diuretics and digitalis. Also indicated to improve survival following myocardial infarction in clinically stable patients with left ventricular dysfunction. Also indicated for the treatment of diabetic nephropathy.

Warnings: Adverse reactions include cough, rash, pruritus, dysgeusia, hypotension, hyperkalemia, proteinuria, and nephrotic syndrome. Neutropenia and agranulocytosis have occurred, and patients should be advised to report promptly any indication of infection (e.g., sore throat, fever) that may be a sign of neutropenia. Use during pregnancy should be avoided.

Administration: Oral. Food reduces absorption and the drug should be given one hour before meals.

Preparations: Tablets, 12.5, 25, 50, and 100 mg.

CARAFATE®, see Sucralfate

CARBACHOL—Isopto Carbachol®, Miostat®

Cholinergic and miotic agent indicated for ophthalmic administration (Isopto Carbachol®) to lower intraocular pressure in the treatment of glaucoma, and for intraocular administration (Miostat®) to provide miosis during surgery.

Preparations: Ophthalmic solution (Isopto-Carbachol®, 0.75%, 1.5%, 2.25%, and 3%. Solution for intraocular administration (Miostat®), 0.01%.

CARBAMAZEPINE—Carbatrol®, Tegretol®

Anticonvulsant and agent for trigeminal neuralgia.

Actions and Uses: Indicated in the following conditions in patients who have not responded satisfactorily to treatment with other agents such as phenytoin, phenobarbital, or primidone: (1) partial seizures with complex symptomatology, (2) generalized tonic-clonic seizures (grand mal), and (3) mixed seizure patterns that include the above, or other partial or generalized seizures. Also indicated in the treatment of pain associated with trigeminal neuralgia and glossopharyngeal neuralgia.

Warnings: Is structurally related to the

tricyclic antidepressants and should not be used in patients with a history of hypersensitivity to any of these agents. May cause serious hematologic reactions and should not be used in patients with a history of serious bone marrow depression. Patients should be advised to report immediately signs and symptoms of a potential hemattologic problem, such as sorethroat, fever, ulcers in the mouth, and easy brusing. Other adverse reactions include dizziness, drowsiness, nausea, vomiting, and dermatologic effects. Concurrent use with a monoamine oxidase inhibitor is not recommended.

Administration: Oral.

Preparations: Tablets, 200 mg. Extended release 100, 200, 300, and 400 mg. Chewable tablets, 100 mg. Suspension, 100 mg/5 ml.

CARBAMIDE PEROXIDE—Urea peroxide, Debrox®, Gly-Oxide®

Antiseptic and cleansing agent administered in the mouth for the treatment and prevention of minor oral inflammation such as canker sores, and in the ear to soften and remove earwax.

Preparations: Solution, 6.5% (otic use) and 10% (oral use).

CARBATROL®, see Carbamazepine

CARBENICILLIN INDANYL SODIUM—Geocillin®

Penicillin antibiotic indicated in the oral treatment of urinary tract and prostatic infections caused by susceptible bacteria.

Preparation: Tablets, equivalent to 382 mg of carbenicillin.

CARBIDOPA—Lodosyn®

Inhibits the peripheral decarboxylation of levodopa and is used in combination with that agent in the treatment of parkinsonism.

Preparation: Tablets, 25 mg.

CARBINOXAMINE MALEATE

Antihistamine used in combination with other medications.

CARBOCAINE®, see Mepivacaine

CARBOL-FUCHSIN SOLUTION—Castellani paint

Antifungal formulation used topically in the management of dermatologic fungal infections. Fuchsin is a dye and causes staining.

Preparation: Solution containing phenol and resorcinol in addition to fuchsin.

CARBOLIC ACID, see Phenol

CARBON DIOXIDE

Respiratory stimulant used by inhalation in conjunction with oxygen.

Preparation: Gas, available in mixtures with oxygen.

CARBOPLATIN—Paraplatin®

Antineoplastic agent.

Actions and Uses: A platinum compound related to cisplatin. Indicated for the palliative treatment of patients with ovarian carcinoma recurrent after prior chemotherapy, including patients who have been previously treated with cisplatin. Also indicated for the initial treatment of advanced ovarian carcinoma.

Warnings: Should not be used in patients with severe bone marrow depression or significant bleeding. Thrombocytopenia, neutropenia, leukopenia, and anemia are often experienced and therapy must be closely monitored. Serious allergic reactions may occur. Other adverse reactions include nausea, vomiting, abdominal pain, diarrhea, constipation, peripheral neuropathies, abnormal hepatic and renal function tests, electrolyte changes, alopecia, and cardiovascular, respiratory, genitourinary, and mucosal effects. Concomitant treatment with aminoglycosides has resulted in increased renal and/or audiologic toxicity. The drug may cause fetal harm when administered during pregnancy.

Administration: Intravenous infusion (lasting 15 minutes or longer). Carboplatin reacts with aluminum, causing precipitate formation and loss of potency; therefore, needles or intravenous sets containing aluminum parts that may come in contact with the drug must not be used for the preparation or administration of carboplatin.

Preparations: Vials, 50, 150, and 450 mg.

CARBOPROST TROMETHAMINE—Hemabate®

Abortifacient administered intramuscularly for the termination of pregnancy during the period from 13 to 20 gestational weeks. Also indicated for the treatment of postpartum hemorrhage due to uterine atony that has not responded to conventional management.

Preparation: Ampules, 250 μg carboprost and 83 μg tromethamine per ml.

CARBOWAX®, see Polyethylene glycol

CARDENE®, see Nicardipine

CARDENE IV®, see Nicardipine

CARDILATE®, see Erythrityl tetranitrate

CARDIOQUIN®, see Quinidine polygalacturonate

CARDIZEM®, see Diltiazem

CARDIZEM CD®, see Diltiazem

CARDIZEM SR®, see Diltiazem

CARDURA®, see Doxazosin mesylate

CARISOPRODOL—Rela®, Soma®

Skeletal muscle relaxant indicated as an adjunct to rest, physical therapy, and other measures for the relief of discomfort associated with acute, painful musculoskeletal conditions.

Preparation: Tablets, 350 mg.

CARMUSTINE—BiCNU®

Antineoplastic agent administered intravenously as palliative therapy for brain tumors, multiple myeloma, Hodgkin's disease, and non-Hodgkin's lymphomas.

Preparation: Vials, 100 mg.

L-CARNITINE—Carnitor®, Vitacarn®

Agent for carnitine deficiency.

Actions and Uses: Indicated in the treatment of primary systemic carnitine deficiency.

Warnings: Adverse reactions include nausea, vomiting, abdominal cramps, diarrhea, and patient body odor. Reducing the dosage often decreases or eliminates the GI effects or drug-related odor.

Administration: Oral.

Preparations: Tablets, 330 mg. Enteral liquid, 100 mg/ml.

CARNITOR®, see L-Carnitine

CARTEOLOL HYDROCHLORIDE—Cartrol®, Ocupress®

Antihypertensive agent and agent for glaucoma.

Actions and Uses: A nonselective beta-adrenergic blocking agent with intrinsic sympathomimetic activity. Indicated in the treatment of hypertension, and for ophthalmic administration in the treatment of chronic open-angle glaucoma and intraocular hypertension.

Warnings: Contraindicated in patients with bronchial asthma, cardiogenic shock, severe bradycardia, and second and third degree atrioventricular conduction block in the absence of a functioning artificial pacemaker. Adverse reactions include weakness, tiredness, fatigue, and muscle cramps. Use is best avoided in patients with bronchospastic diseases and therapy in diabetic patients must be closely monitored.

Administration: Oral and ophthalmic. Patients should be cautioned about the interruption or discontinuation of therapy; exacerbation of angina pectoris has occurred following the abrupt cessation of therapy and, when therapy is to be discontinued, the dosage should be gradually reduced over a period of 1 to 2 weeks.

Preparations: Tablets (Cartrol), 2.5 and 5 mg. Ophthalmic solution (Ocupress), 1%.

CARTROL®, see Carteolol

CASANTHRANOL

Laxative included in combination formulations indicated for constipation.

CASCARA SAGRADA

Laxative used in the treatment of constipation.

Preparations: Tablets, 325 mg. Aromatic fluid extract.

CASODEX®, see Bicalutamide

CASTELLANI PAINT, see Carbolfuchsin solution.

CASTOR OIL

Laxative indicated for the treatment of constipation and preparation of the colon for x-ray and endoscopic examination.

Preparations: Liquid. Emulsions, 36%, 60%, 67%, and 95%.

CATAPRES®, see Clonidine

CATAPRES-TTS®, see Clonidine

CAVERJECT®, see Alprostadil

CCNU®, see Lomustine

CECLOR®, see Cefaclor

CEDAX®, see Ceftibuten

CeeNU®, see Lomustine

CEFACLOR—Ceclor®

Second-generation cephalosporin antibiotic.

Actions and Uses: Spectrum of action includes many gram-positive and gram-negative bacteria. Indicated in upper and lower respiratory infections, otitis media, urinary tract infections, and skin and skin-structure infections caused by susceptible organisms.

Warnings: Must be used cautiously in penicillin-sensitive patients and use should be avoided in patients with a history of immediate and/or severe reactions to penicillin.

Administration: Oral. May be administered without regard to meals.

Preparations: Capsules, 250 and 500 mg. Extended release tablets, 375 and 500 mg. Powder for oral suspension,

125, 187, 250, and 375 mg/5 ml when reconstituted.

CEFADROXIL—Duricef®, Ultracef®

First-generation cephalosporin antibiotic.

Actions and Uses: Spectrum of action includes many gram-positive and gram-negative bacteria. Indicated in pharyngitis and tonsillitis, urinary tract infections, and skin and skin-structure infections caused by susceptible organisms.

Warnings: Must be used cautiously in penicillin-sensitive patients and use should be avoided in patients with a history of immediate and/or severe reactions to penicillin.

Administration: Oral. May be administered without regard to meals.

Preparations: Capsules, 500 mg. Tablets, 1 g. Powder for oral suspension, 125, 250, and 500 mg/5 ml when reconstituted.

CEFADYL®, see Cephapirin

CEFAMANDOLE NAFTATE—Mandol®

Second-generation cephalosporin antibiotic.

Actions and Uses: Active against many gram-positive and gram-negative bacteria. Indicated for lower respiratory infections, urinary tract infections, peritonitis, septicemia, skin and skin-structure infections, and bone and joint infections caused by susceptible organisms. May also be used for surgical prophylaxis.

Warnings: Must be used cautiously, if at all, in penicillin-sensitive patients and use should be avoided in patients with a history of immediate and/or severe reactions to penicillin. Therapy in patients at risk of bleeding reactions must be closely monitored. Disulfiram-like reactions may occcur following the consumption of alcoholic beverages.

Administration: Intravenous and intramuscular.

Preparations: Vials, 500 mg, 1, 2, and 10 g of cefamandole activity.

CEFANEX®, see Cephalexin

CEFAZOLIN SODIUM—Ancef®, Kefzol®, Zolicef®

First-generation cephalosporin antibiotic.

Actions and Uses: Active against many gram-positive and gram-negative bacteria. Indicated for respiratory tract infections, genitourinary tract infections, skin and skin-structure infections, biliary tract infections, bone and joint infections, septicemia, and endocarditis caused by susceptible organisms. Is often used for surgical prophylaxis.

Warnings: Must be used cautiously, if at all, in penicillin-sensitive patients and use should be avoided in patients with a history of immediate and/or severe reactions to penicillins.

Administration: Intravenous and intramuscular.

Preparations: Vials, 250 and 500 mg, 1, 5, and 10 g of cefazolin.

CEFEPIME—Maxipime®

Fourth generation cephalosporin indicated in treatment of susceptible uncomplicated or complicated urinary tract infections, uncomplicated skin and skin structure infections, and moderate to severe pneumonia.

Warnings: Use cautiously in patients with compromised renal or hepatic function, poor nutritional state, elderly or debilitated, and history of GI disease (esp. colitis). Monitor prothrombin time. Contraindicated in patients allergic to cephalasporins. Adverse reactions include local reactions to IV infusion (e.g., pain, phlebitis, inflammation), rash, pseudomembranous colitis, and superinfection.

Administration: IV infusion over 30 minutes or IM every 12 hours for 7–10 days.

Preparation: Powder for reconstitution, 500 mg , 1 and 2 g.

CEFIXIME—Suprax®

Antibiotic.

Actions and Uses: An orally-administered, third-generation cephalosporin antibiotic that is especially active against gram-negative bacteria. Indicated in the treatment of otitis media, pharyngitis and tonsillitis, acute bronchitis and acute exacerbations of chronic bronchitis, uncomplicated gonorrhea, and uncomplicated urinary tract infections caused by susceptible bacteria. Among the bacteria that are susceptible are *Branhamella (Moraxella) catarrhalis, Escherichia coli, Haemophilus influenzae, Neisseria gonorrhoeae, Proteus mirabilis, Streptococcus pneumoniae, and Streptococcus pyogenes.*

Warnings: Must be used cautiously in penicillin-sensitive patients and use should be avoided in patients with a history of immediate and/or severe reactions to penicillin. Adverse reactions include diarrhea, loose or frequent stools, abdominal pain, nausea, dyspepsia, flatulence, headache, dizziness, pruritus, and rash.

Administration: Oral. The suspension formulation should be used in the treatment of otitis media. Because the suspension formulation provides higher peak blood levels than the tablet when administered at the same dose, patients should not be switched from the suspension to the tablets. May be administered without regard to meals.

Preparations: Tablets, 200 and 400 mg. Powder for oral suspension, 100mg/5ml when reconstituted.

CEFIZOX®, see Ceftizoxime

CEFMETAZOLE SODIUM—Zefazone®

Second-generation cephalosporin antibiotic.

Actions and Uses: Active against many aerobic and anaerobic gram-positive and gram-negative bacteria; spectrum of action includes *Bacteroides fragilis.* Indicated in the treatment of urinary tract, lower respiratory tract, skin and skin structure, and intraabdominal infections caused by susceptible bacteria. Is also indicated for surgical prophylaxis.

Warnings: Must be used cautiously, if at all, in penicillin-sensitive patients and use should be avoided in patients with a history of immediate and/or severe reactions to penicillin. Adverse reactions include diarrhea, nausea, epigastric pain, bleeding, allergic reactions, rash, pruritus, superinfection, pain and/or swelling at the injection site, thrombophlebitis, and prolonged prothrombin time. Prothrombin time should be monitored for patients at risk. Disulfiram-like reactions may occur when alcohol is ingested within 24 hours of cefmetazole administration.

Administration: Intravenous.

Preparations: Vials, 1 and 2 grams.

CEFOBID®, see Cefoperazone

CEFONICID SODIUM—Monocid®

Second-generation cephalosporin antibitic.

Actions and Uses: Active against many gram-positive and gram-negative bacteria. Indicated for lower respiratory tract infections, urinary tract infections, septicemia, and bone and joint infections caused by susceptible organisms. May also be used for surgical prophylaxis.

Warnings: Must be used cautiously, if at all, in penicillin-sensitive patients and use should be avoided in patients with a history of immediate and/or severe reactions to penicillin.

Administration: Intravenous and intramuscular. Long duration of action permits once-daily dosing in many infections.

Preparations: Vials, 500 mg, 1 and 10 g of cefonicid.

CEFOPERAZONE SODIUM—
Cefobid®

Third-generation cephalosporin antibiotic.

Actions and Uses: Highly active against many gram-negative bacteria and also effective against some gram-positive bacteria; spectrum of action includes *Pseudomonas aeruginosa.* Indicated for respiratory tract infections, peritonitis and other intra-abdominal infections, septicemia, skin and skin-structure infections, urinary tract infections, and pelvic inflammatory disease and other female genital tract infections caused by susceptible organisms.

Warnings: Must be used cautiously, if at all, in penicillin-sensitive patients and use should be avoided in patients with a history of immediate and/or severe reactions to penicillin. Therapy in patients at risk of bleeding reactions must be closely monitored. Is excreted via biliary mechanisms to a greater extent than are other cephalosporins and use is associated with a higher incidence of diarrhea. Disulfiram-like reactions may occur following the consumption of alcoholic beverages.

Administration: Intravenous and intramuscular.

Preparations: Vials, 1, 2, and 10 g of cefoperazone.

CEFOTAN®, see Cefotetan

CEFOTAXIME SODIUM—
Claforan®

Third-generation cephalosporin antibiotic.

Actions and Uses: Highly active against many gram-negative bacteria and also effective against some gram-positive bacteria. Indicated for lower respiratory tract infections, bacteremia/septicemia, skin and skin-structure infections, intra-abdominal infections, bone and/or joint infections, and central nervous system infections caused by susceptible organisms. May also be used for surgical prophylaxis.

Warnings: Must be used cautiously, if at all, in penicillin-sensitive patients and use should be avoided in patients with a history of immediate and/or severe reactions to penicillins.

Administration: Intravenous and intramuscular.

Preparations: Vials, 1, 2, and 10 g of cefotaxime.

CEFOTETAN DISODIUM—
Cefotan®

Second-generation cephalosporin antibiotic.

Actions and Uses: Active against many gram-positive and gram-negative bacteria; spectrum of action includes *Bacteroides fragilis.* Indicated for urinary tract infections, lower respiratory tract infections, skin and skin-structure infections, gynecologic infections, intra-abdominal infections, and bone and joint infections caused by susceptible organisms. May also be used for surgical prophylaxis.

Warnings: Must be used cautiously, if at all, in penicillin-sensitive patients and use should be avoided in patients with a history of immediate and/or severe reactions to penicillin. Disulfiram-like reactions may occur when alcohol is ingested within 72 hours of cefotetan administration. Prothrombin times should be monitored in patients at risk of bleeding reactions.

Administration: Intravenous and intramuscular.

Preparations: Vials, 1, 2, and 10 g of cefotetan activity.

CEFOXITIN SODIUM—Mefoxin®

Second-generation cephalosporin antibiotic.

Actions and Uses: Active against many gram-positive and gram-negative bacteria; spectrum of action includes *Bacteroides fragilis.* Indicated for lower respiratory tract infections, genitourinary infections, intra-abdominal infections, gynecological infections, septicemia, bone and joint infections, and skin and skin-structure infections caused by susceptible organisms. May also be used for surgical prophylaxis.

Warnings: Must be used cautiously, if at all, in penicillin-sensitive patients and use should be avoided in patients with a history of immediate and/or severe reactions to penicillins.

Administration: Intravenous and intramuscular.

Preparations: Vials, 1, 2, and 10 g of cefoxitin.

CEFPODOXIME PROXETIL—Vantin®

Third-generation cephalosporin antibiotic.

Actions and Uses: Is a prodrug that is converted to its active metabolite, cefpodoxime. Inhibits bacterial cell wall synthesis and exhibits a bactericidal action against many gram-positive and gram-negative bacteria. Indicated for upper respiratory tract infections, lower respiratory tract infections, uncomplicated skin and skin structure infections, and uncomplicated urinary tract infections (cystitis) caused by susceptible organisms. Also indicated for acute, uncomplicated urethral and cervical gonorrhea, and acute, uncomplicated ano-rectal infections in women due to *Neisseria gonorrhoeae.*

Warnings: Must be used cautiously in penicillin-sensitive patients and use should be avoided in patients with a history of immediate and/or severe reactions to penicillins. Adverse reactions include diarrhea, nausea, abdominal pain, vomiting, vaginal fungal infections, rash, and headache. Absorption may be reduced by the concomitant administration of an antacid or histamine H_2-receptor antagonist.

Administration: Oral. Tablet formulation should be administered with food.

Preparations: Tablets, 100 and 200 mg. Powder for oral suspension, 50 mg/5 ml and 100 mg/5 ml.

CEFPROZIL—Cefzil®

Second-generation cephalosporin antibiotic.

Actions and Uses: Inhibits bacterial cell wall synthesis and exhibits a bactericidal action against many gram-positive and gram-negative bacteria. Indicated for upper respiratory tract infections (including pharyngitis and tonsilitis), lower respiratory tract infections, and uncomplicated skin and skin structure infections caused by susceptible organisms.

Warnings: Must be used cautiously in penicillin-sensitive patients and use should be avoided in patients with a history of immediate and/or severe reactions to penicillins. Adverse reactions include diarrhea, nausea, vomiting, abdominal pain, rash, eosinophilia, vaginitis, and superinfection.

Administration: Oral.

Preparations: Tablets, 250 and 500 mg. Powder for

oral suspension, 125 mg/5 ml and 250 mg/5 ml.

CEFTAZIDIME—Ceptaz®, Fortaz®, Tazicef®, Tazidime®

Third-generation cephalosporin antibiotic.

Actions and Uses: Highly active against many gram-negative bacteria and also effective against some gram-positive bacteria; spectrum of action includes *Pseudomonas aeruginosa.* Indicated for lower respiratory tract infections, skin and skin-structure infections, urinary tract infections, bacterial septicemia, bone and joint infections, gynecological infections, intra-abdominal infections, and central nervous system infections caused by susceptible organisms.

Warnings: Must be used cautiously, if at all, in penicillin-sensitive patients and use should be avoided in patients with a history of immediate and/or severe reactions to penicillin.

Administration: Intravenous and intramuscular.

Preparations: Vials, 500 mg, 1, 2, and 6 g. Ceptaz formulation contains L-arginine instead of sodium carbonate, and does not release carbon dioxide following reconstitution as the other formulations do.

CEFTIBUTEN—Cedax®

Third-generation cephalosporin.

Actions and Uses: Indicated in susceptible mild to moderate acute bacterial exacerbations of chronic bronchitis, acute bacterial otitis media, and pharyngitis /tonsillitis.

Warnings: May cause GI upset, headache, dizziness. Adjust dosing in renal impairment. Must be used cautiously in penicillin sensitive patients and use should be avoided in patients with a history of immediate and/or severe reactions to penicillin.

Administration: Oral. Suspension should be taken on an empty stomach. Capsules may be taken regardless of food intake.

Preparations: Capsules, 400 mg. Suspension, 90 mg/5 ml.

CEFTIN®, see Cefuroxime axetil

CEFTIZOXIME SODIUM—Cefizox®

Third-generation cephalosporin antibiotic.

Actions and Uses: Highly active against many gram-negative bacteria and also effective against some gram-positive bacteria. Indicated for lower respiratory tract infections, urinary tract infections, gonorrhea, pelvic inflammatory disease, intra-abdominal infections, septicemia, skin and skin-structure infections, bone and joint infections, and meningitis caused by susceptible organisms.

Warnings: Must be used cautiously, if at all, in penicillin-sensitive patients and use should be avoided in patients with a history of immediate and/or severe reactions to penicillins.

Administration: Intravenous and intramuscular.

Preparations: Vials, 1, 2, and 10 g of ceftizoxime.

CEFTRIAXONE SODIUM—Rocephin®

Third-generation cephalosporin antibiotic.

Actions and Uses: Highly active against many gram-negative bacteria and also effective against some gram-positive bacteria. Indicated for lower respiratory tract infections, skin and skin-structure infections, urinary tract infections, gonorrhea, including pharyngeal gonorrhea, pelvic inflammatory disease, septicemia, bone and joint infections, intra-abdominal infections, and meningitis caused by susceptible organisms. May also be used for surgical prophylaxis.

Warnings: Must be used cautiously, if at all, in penicillin-sensitive patients and use should be avoided in patients with a history of immediate and/or severe reactions to penicillins.

Administration: Intravenous and intramuscular. Long duration of action permits once-daily dosing in most infections.

Preparations: Vials, 250 and 500 mg, 1, 2, and 10 g of ceftriaxone.

CEFUROXIME AXETIL—Ceftin®

Second-generation cephalosporin antibiotic.

Actions and Uses: Spectrum of action includes many gram-positive and gram-negative bacteria. Indicated in pharyngitis and tonsillitis, otitis media, lower respiratory tract infections, urinary tract infections, gonorrhea, and skin and skin-structure infections caused by susceptible organisms.

Warnings: Must be used cautiously in penicillin-sensitive patients and use should be avoided in patients with a history of immediate and/or severe reactions to penicillin.

Administration: Oral. Tablets may be administered without regard to meals but the suspension should be administered with food.

Preparations: Tablets, 125, 250, and 500 mg. Powder for oral suspension, 125mg/5ml and 250mg/5ml.

CEFUROXIME SODIUM—Kefurox®, Zinacef®

Second-generation cephalosporin antibiotic.

Actions and Uses: Active against many gram-positive and gram-negative bacteria. Indicated for lower respiratory tract infections, urinary tract infections, skin and skin-structure infections, septicemia, bone and joint infections, meningitis, and gonorrhea caused by susceptible organisms. May also be used for surgical prophylaxis.

Warnings: Must be used cautiously, if at all, in penicillin-sensitive patients and use should be avoided in patients with a history of immediate and/or severe reactions to penicillins.

Administration: Intravenous and intramuscular.

Preparations: Vials, 750 mg, 1.5 and 7.5 g of cefuroxime.

CEFZIL®, see Cefprozil

CELESTONE®, see Betamethasone

CELLCEPT®, see Mycophenolate mofetil.

CELONTIN®, see Methsuximide

CENTRAX®, see Prazepam

CEPACOL®, see Cetylpyridinium

CEPHALEXIN—Cefanex®, Keflex®

CEPHALEXIN HYDROCHLORIDE—Keftab®

First-generation cephalosporin antibiotic.

Actions and Uses: Spectrum of action includes many gram-positive and gram-negative bacteria. Indicated in respiratory tract infections, otitis media, skin and skin-structure infections, bone infections, and genitourinary tract infections caused by susceptible organisms.

Warnings: Must be used cautiously in penicillin-sensitive patients and use should be avoided in patients with a history of immediate and/or severe reactions to penicillin.

Administration: Oral. May be administered without regard to meals.

Preparations: Capsules and tablets, 250 and 500 mg, 1 g. Powder for oral suspension, 125 and 250 mg/5 ml when reconstituted, and formulation for pediatric use, 100 mg/ml when reconstituted.

CEPHALOTHIN SODIUM—Keflin®

First-generation cephalosporin antibiotic indicated for the parenteral treatment of infections caused by susceptible organisms.

Preparations: Vials, 1, 2, 4 and 20 g.

CEPHAPIRIN SODIUM—Cefadyl®

First-generation cephalosporin antibiotic indicated for the parenteral treatment of infections caused by susceptible organisms.

Preparations: Vials, 500 mg, 1, 2, 4, and 20 g.

CEPHRADINE—Anspor®, Velosef®

First-generation cephalosporin antibiotic.

Actions and Uses: Active against many gram-positive and gram-negative bacteria. Indicated for the oral treatment of respiratory tract infections, otitis media, skin and skin-structure infections, and urinary tract infections caused by susceptible organisms. May also be administered parenterally for these infections as well as for bone infections and septicemia caused by susceptible organisms. May be used parenterally for surgical prophylaxis.

Warnings: Must be used cautiously, if at all, in penicillin-sensitive patients and use should be avoided in patients with a history of immediate and/or severe reactions to penicillins.

Administration: Oral, intravenous, and intramuscular. May be administered orally without regard to meals.

Preparations: Capsules, 250 and 500 mg. Powder for oral suspension, 125 and 250 mg/5 ml when reconstituted. Vials, 250 and 500 mg, 1, 2, and 4 g.

CEPHULAC®, see Lactulose

CEPTAZ®, see Ceftazidime

CEREBYX®, see Fosphenytoin

CEREDASE®, see Alglucerase

CEREZYME®, see Imiglucerase

CERUBIDINE®, see Daunorubicin

CETIRIZINE HYDROCHLORIDE—Zyrtec®

Actions and Uses: Antihistamine indicated in the treatment of seasonal rhinitis, perennial allergic rhinitis, and chronic idiopathic urticaria.

Warnings: Contraindicated in hydroxyzine sensitivity. Use cautiously in hepatic or renal dysfunction. Use in nursing mothers and children not recommended. Potentiates CNS depression with alcohol and other CNS depressants. Adverse reactions include somnolence, fatigue, dry mouth, and dizziness.

Administration: Oral. Adjust dose in hepatic or renal impairment.

Preparations: Tablets, 5 and 10 mg, syrup 1 mg/mL

CETYLPYRIDINIUM CHLORIDE—Cepacol®

Antiseptic included in formulations used in minor sore throat and in conditions in which there is minor irritation of the mouth or throat.

Preparations: Lozenges, 0.07%. Mouthwash, 0.05%.

CHARCOAL, ACTIVATED

Adsorbent used for relief of intestinal gas, diarrhea, and GI distress. Also used as an antidote in the treatment of poisoning by many drugs and chemicals.

Preparations: Capsules, 260 mg. Liquid. Powder.

CHEMET®, see Succimer

CHIBROXIN®, see Norfloxacin

CHILDREN'S ADVIL®—see Ibuprofen

CHILDREN'S MOTRIN®—see Ibuprofen

CHLORAL HYDRATE

Sedative-hypnotic used in the treatment of insomnia and as an anesthetic adjunct for reduction of anxiety preoperatively.

Preparations: Capsules, 250 and 500 mg. Syrup, 500 mg/5ml. Suppositories, 324, 500, and 648 mg.

CHLORAMBUCIL—Leukeran®

Antineoplastic agent indicated in the treatment of chronic lymphocytic leukemia, malignant lymphomas including lymphosarcoma, giant follicular lymphoma, and Hodgkin's disease.

Preparation: Tablets, 2 mg.

CHLORAMPHENICOL—Chloromycetin®

Antibiotic with a broad spectrum of activity that has been used in the treatment of systemic, dermatologic, ophthalmic, and otic infections. Is of greatest value in systemic infections caused by *Salmonella typhi, Haemophilus influenzae* (e.g., meningitis), and rickettsial organisms.

Preparations: Vials (as the sodium succinate), 1 g. Ophthalmic solution (0.5%) and ointment (1%). Otic solution, 0.5%.

CHLORDIAZEPOXIDE—Librium®, Libritabs®

Benzodiazepine antianxiety agent.

Actions and Uses: A CNS depressant indicated for the management of anxiety disorders or for the short-term relief of symptoms of anxiety, withdrawal symptoms of acute alcoholism, and preoperative apprehension and anxiety.

Warnings: Adverse reactions include drowsiness and other CNS effects; patients should be cautioned regarding activities such as driving and operating machinery, as well as interactions with other CNS-acting drugs including alcohol. Can cause dependence and is included in Schedule IV.

Administration: Oral, intravenous, and intramuscular.

Preparations: Capsules (as the hydrochloride) and tablets, 5, 10, and 25 mg. Ampules (as the hydrochloride), 100 mg.

CHLORESIUM®, see Chlorophyll

CHLORHEXIDINE GLUCONATE—Hibiclens®, Hibistat®, Peridex®

Antiseptic and cleanser indicated for topical use as a skin wound cleanser and general skin cleanser, as a surgical scrub, for patient preoperative showering and bathing, as a patient preoperative skin preparation, and as a health-care personnel handwash or germicidal hand rise. Also used as an oral rinse (Peridex®) for the treatment of gingivitis.

Preparations: Skin cleanser, 4%. Germicidal hand rinse, 0.5%. Oral rinse, 0.12%.

CHLORMEZANONE—Trancopal®

Antianxiety agent indicated for the treatment of mild anxiety and tension states.

Preparations: Tablets, 100 and 200 mg.

CHLOROMYCETIN®, see Chloramphenicol

CHLOROPHYLL-Chloresium®, Derifil®

Deodorizing agent used topically to reduce malodors in wounds, burns, and other dermatologic conditions, and orally for the control of fecal and urinary odor associated with incontinence and ostomy conditions, body odors, and odor of surface lesions.

Preparations: Solution, 0.2%. Ointment, 0.5%. Tablets, 100 mg.

CHLOROPROCAINE HYDROCHLORIDE—Nesacaine®, Nesacaine-CE®

Local anesthetic indicated for the production of local anesthesia by infiltration and peripheral nerve block. Formulation without preservatives (Nesacaine-CE®) may also be used by central nerve block, including lumbar and caudal epidural blocks.

Preparations: Vials, 1% and 2%. Vials (Nesacaine-CE), 2% and 3%.

CHLOROQUINE—Aralen®

Antimalarial agent and amebicide. Indicated for acute attacks of malaria and prophylaxis against malaria. Also indicated for the treatment of extraintestinal amebiasis.

Preparations: Tablets (as the phosphate), 500 mg. Vials (as the dihydrochloride), 50 mg/ml.

CHLOROTHIAZIDE—Diuril®

Thiazide diuretic indicated as adjunctive therapy in edema and in the management of hypertension.

Preparations: Tablets, 250 and 500 mg. *Suspension,* 250 mg/5 ml.

CHLOROTRIANISENE—Tace®

Estrogen indicated for the treatment of postpartum breast engorgement, moderate to severe vasomotor symptoms associated with the menopause, atrophic vaginitis, kraurosis vulvae, and female hypogonadism. Also used as palliative therapy of advanced prostatic carcinoma.

Preparations: Capsules, 12, 25, and 72 mg.

CHLORPHENESIN CARBAMATE—Maolate®

Skeletal muscle relaxant indicated as an adjunct to rest, physical therapy, and other measures for relief of discomfort associated with acute, painful musculoskeletal conditions.

Preparation: Tablets, 400 mg.

CHLORPHENIRAMINE MALEATE—Chlor-Trimeton®, Teldrin®

Antihistamine.

Actions and Uses: Indicated in the treatment of various allergic disorders.

Warnings: Adverse effects include drowsiness and other CNS effects; patients should be cautioned regarding activities such as driving and operating machinery, as well as interactions with other CNS-acting drugs including alcohol.

Administration: Oral, intravenous, intramuscular, and subcutaneous.

Preparations: Tablets, 2 and 4 mg. Controlled-release tablets and capsules, 8 and 12 mg. Syrup, 2 mg/5 ml. Vials, 10 mg/ml.

CHLORPROMAZINE—Thorazine®

Phenothiazine antipsychotic and antiemetic agent. Indicated in the management of psychotic disorders, to control nausea and vomiting, as a preoperative medication, as an adjunct in the treatment of tetanus, for relief of intractable hiccups, to control the manifestations of the manic type of manic-depressive illness, and for acute intermittent porphyria. Also indicated for the treatment of certain severe behavioral problems in children, and in the short-term treatment of certain hyperactive children.

Preparations: Tablets, 10, 25, 50, 100, and 200 mg. Controlled-release capsules, 30, 75, 150, 200 and 300 mg. Syrup (as the hydrochloride), 10 mg/5 ml., Oral concentrate (as the hydrochloride), 30 and 100 mg/ml. Suppositories, 25 and 100 mg. Ampules and vials (as the hydrochloride) 25 mg/ml.

CHLORPROPAMIDE—Diabinese®

Sulfonylurea hypoglycemic agent.

Actions and Uses: Indicated as an adjunct to diet to lower the blood glucose in patients with non-insulin-dependent diabetes mellitus whose hyperglycemia cannot be controlled by diet alone.

Warnings: May cause hypoglycemia and patients should be advised to contact their physician if symptoms of hypoglycemia develop. Adverse reactions include nausea, vomiting, diarrhea, pruritus, and rash. Oral hypoglycemic agents have been suggested to be associated with increased cardiovascular mortality as compared with treatment by diet alone or diet plus insulin. May cause disulfiram-like reactions following the consumption of alcoholic beverages. Therapy in patients also receiving a beta-adrenergic blocking agent should be monitored closely.

Administration: Oral.

Preparations: Tablets, 100 and 250 mg.

CHLORPROTHIXENE

Antipsychotic agent indicated for the management of manifestations of psychotic disorders.

Preparations: Tablets, 10, 25, 50 and 100 mg. Oral concentrate (as the lactate and hydrochloride), 100 mg chlorprothixene/5 ml. Ampules (as the hydrochloride), 25 mg chlorprothixene/2 ml.

CHLORTETRACYCLINE—Aureomycin®

Tetracycline antibiotic used in the treatment of dermatologic and ocular infections.

Preparations: Ointment, 3%.

CHLORTHALIDONE—Hygroton®

Diuretic and antihypertensive agent.

Actions and Uses: Action is similar to that of the thiazide diuretics. Indicated in the management of hypertension, and as adjunctive therapy in edema associated with congestive heart failure, hepatic cirrhosis, and corticosteroid and estrogen therapy. Is also useful in edema due to various forms of renal dysfunction such as nephrotic syndrome.

Warnings: May cause hypokalemia and serum potassium levels should be determined periodically. Concurrent use with lithium is best avoided because of an increased risk of lithium toxicity. May cause hyperglycemia and hyperuricemia, and therapy in patients having diabetes or gout should be closely monitored.

Administration: Oral.

Preparations: Tablets, 25, 50, and 100 mg.

CHLOR-TRIMETON®, see Chlorpheniramine

CHLORZOXAZONE—Paraflex®, Parafon Forte DSC®

Skeletal muscle relaxant indicated as an adjunct to rest, physical therapy, and other measures for the relief of discomfort associated with acute, painful skeletal muscle conditions.

Preparation: Tablets, 250 mg.

CHOLECALCIFEROL—Vitamin D_3

A form of Vitamin D used as a supplement to treat or prevent Vitamin D deficiency.

Preparations: Tablets 400 and 1000 IU.

CHOLEDYL®, see Oxtriphylline

CHOLESTYRAMINE—Questran®, Questran Light®

Antihyperlipidemic agent indicated as adjunctive therapy to diet for the reduction of elevated serum cholesterol in patients with primary hypercholesterolemia. Also indicated for the relief of pruritus associated with partial biliary obstruction.

Preparations: Powder and packets, 4 g/9 g of powder. (Questran). Powder and packets, 4g/5g of powder (Questran Light with aspartame). Chewable bar, 4g.

CHOLINE MAGNESIUM TRISALICYLATE—Trilisate®

Salicylate analgesic/anti-inflammatory agent indicated in the treatment of rheumatoid arthritis, osteoarthritis, and acute painful shoulder.

Preparations: Tablets, 500 and 750 mg., 1 gram of salicylate. Liquid, 500 mg salicylate/5 ml.

CHOLINE SALICYLATE—Arthropan®

Salicylate analgesic/anti-inflammatory agent used in the treatment of conditions associated with mild to moderate pain and/or inflammation.

Preparation: Liquid, 870 mg/5 ml.

CHOLINE THEOPHYLLINATE, see Oxtriphylline

CHOLOXIN®, see Dextrothyroxine

CHORIONIC GONADOTROPIN—A.P.L.®, Follutein®

Hormone indicated for intramuscular use for cryptorchidism not due to anatomic obstruction, selected cases of male hypogonadism secondary to pituitary failure, and induction of ovulation and pregnancy in the anovulatory, infertile woman in selected situations.

Preparations: Vials, 5,000, 10,000, and 20,000 units.

CHYMODIACTIN®, see Chymopapain

CHYMOPAPAIN—Chymodiactin®

Proteolytic enzyme indicated for intradiscal injection for the treatment of documented herniated lumbar intervertebral discs in patients whose symptoms and signs have not responded to adequate periods of conservative therapy.

Preparations: Vials, 4,000 units.

CICLOPIROX OLAMINE—Loprox®

Antifungal agent indicated for the topical treatment of tinea pedis, tinea cruris, tinea corporis, candidiasis, and tinea versicolor.

Preparation: Cream and lotion, 1%.

CIDOFOVIR—Vistide®

Nucleoside analogue indicated in the treatment of cytomegalovirus (CMV) retinitis in patients with AIDS.

Warnings: Not recommended for use in patients with CrCl of < 55 ml/min. Do not exceed recommended dose as this may increase the risk of nephrotoxicity. Women should use effective contraception during and 1 month after therapy. Men should use barrier contraception during and 3 months after therapy. Monitor serum creatinine, urine protein, WBC, with differential before each dose; monitor intraocular pressure, visual acuity, and ocular symptoms periodically. Use cautiously in the elderly. Adverse reactions include elevated serum creatinine, proteinuria, neutropenia, ocular hypotony, metabolic acidosis, GI disturbances, fever, asthenia, rash, headache, alopecia, infection, chills, and dyspnea. Contraindicated in severe probenecid or other sulfa allergy. Not for intraocular injection.

Administration: Give as an IV infusion over 1 hr. Pretreat with oral probenecid and hydrate with Normal Saline as per manufacturer's guidelines. Induction is 5 mg/kg once weekly for 2 consecutive weeks.

Maintenance is 5 mg/kg once every 2 weeks. Adjust dosing for preexisting renal dysfunction or if function deteriorates during treatment as per manufacturer's recommendations.

Preparation: Solution for IV infusion after dilution, 75 mg/5ml.

CILOXAN®, see Ciprofloxacin

CIMETIDINE—Tagamet®, Tagamet HB®

Antiulcer agent.

Actions and Uses: A histamine H2 receptor antagonist that inhibits gastric acid secretion. Indicated in (1) short-term treatment of active duodenal ulcer, (2) maintenance therapy for duodenal ulcer patients at reduced dosage after healing of active ulcer, (3) short-term treatment of active benign gastric ulcer, (4) the treatment of erosive gastroesophageal reflux disease, (5) the treatment of pathological hypersecretory conditions (e.g., Zollinger-Ellison syndrome), and (6) the prevention of upper gastrointestiinal bleeding in critically ill patients. Available without a prescription (Tagamet HB®) to relieve heartburn and acid indigestion.

Warnings: Adverse reactions include diarrhea, rash, dizziness, somnolence, and confusional states. Has a weak antiandrogenic effect and has caused gynecomastia and impotence, particularly when used in high doses and/or for long periods.

Administration: Oral, intravenous, and intramuscular.

Preparations: Tablets, 100 (Tagamet HB®) 200, 300, 400, and 800 mg. Liquid (as the hydrochloride), 300 mg/5 ml. Vials and syringes (as the hydrochloride), 300mg/2 ml. Plastic containers, 300 mg/50 ml.

CIPRO®, see Ciprofloxacin

CIPRO HC Otic®—Combination agent ciprofloxacin and hydrocortisone (quinolone antibiotic and steroid)

CIPRO IV®, see Ciprofloxacin

CIPROFLOXACIN HYDROCHLORIDE—Ciloxan®, Cipro®, Cipro IV®

Anti-infective agent.

Actions and Uses: A fluoroquinolone antibacterial agent with a broad spectrum of action. Indicated for lower respiratory tract, urinary tract, skin and skin structure, and bone and joint infections, urethral/cervical gonococcal infections, typhoid fever, infectious diarrhea, complicated intra-abdominal infections (used with metranidazole), and ocular infections caused by susceptible bacteria.

Warnings: Contraindicated in patients with a known hypersensitivity to the drug and is also best avoided in patients with a history of hypersensitivity to other fluoroquinolone/quinolone derivatives. It should not be used in children or pregnant women because it and related drugs have been shown to cause arthropathy and damage to the weight-bearing joints in immature animals. Adverse reactions include nausea, vomiting, diarrhea, abdominal discomfort, headache, dizziness, restlessness, and rash. Because the drug may cause CNS effects, patients should be cautioned about engaging in activities that require mental alertness and coordination, and the drug should be used cautiously in patients with epilepsy or other CNS disorders. Concurrent use of ciprofloxacin and theophylline has resulted in elevated plasma concentrations of theophylline and a corresponding increase in the risk of adverse effects with this agent.

Administration: Oral, intravenous, and ophthalmic.

Preparations: Tablets, 250, 500, and 750 mg. Oral suspension, 5% (250 mg/5ml) and 10% (500 mg/5 ml) microcapsules for suspension after reconsitution in strawberry flavor. Vials, 200 and 400 mg. Ophthalmic solution, 0.3% (Ciloxan).

CISAPRIDE—Propulsid®

Gastrointestinal prokinetic agent.

Actions and Uses: Increases gastrointestinal motility through a cholinergically-mediated mechanism. Indicated for the symptomatic treatment of patients with nocturnal heartburn due to gastroesophageal reflux disease.

Warnings: Contraindicated in patients in whom an increase in gastrointestinal motility could be harmful (e.g., in the presence of gastrointestinal hemorrhage, mechanical obstruction, or perforation). Concurrent use with ketoconazole, itraconazole, miconazole (intravenously), or troleandomycin is contraindicated. Adverse reactions include headache, diarrhea, constipation, abdominal pain, dyspepsia, and rhinitis.

Administration: Oral. Should be administered at least 15 minutes before meals and at bedtime. Suspension, 1 mg/ml.

Preparations: Tablets, 10 and 20 mg.

CISPLATIN—Platinol®

Antineoplastic agent indicated for intravenous use as palliative therapy for metastatic testicular tumors, metastatic ovarian tumors, and advanced bladder cancer.

Preparations: Vials, 10 and 50 mg.

CITANEST®, see Prilocaine

CITRATE OF MAGNESIA, see Magnesium citrate

CITROVORUM FACTOR, see Leucovorin calcium.

CITRUCEL®, see Methylcellulose

CLADRIBINE—Leustatin®

Antineoplastic agent.

Actions and Uses: Also known as 2-chlorodeoxyadenosine or 2-CdA, it crosses lymphocyte cell membranes and is metabolized to a triphosphate derivative that disrupts cell metabolism and is cytotoxic to both actively dividing and resting cells. Indicated for the treatment of active hairy cell leukemia.

Warnings: May cause myelosuppression (neutropenia, thrombocytopenia, anemia) and peripheral blood counts should be performed, particularly during the first 4 to 8 weeks following initiation of therapy. Caution should be exercised if cladribine is to be administered in conjunction with or following other drugs known to cause myelosuppression. Fever is often experienced (most often in neutropenic patients) and infection may develop; empiric antibiotic therapy should be initiated as necessary. Other adverse reactions include nausea, decreased appetite, vomiting, diarrhea, abnormal breath sounds, cough, fatigue, headache, injection site reactions, purpura, and rash. Women of childbearing age should be advised to avoid becoming pregnant.

Administration: Intravenous. Administered as a single course of treatment by continuous intravenous infusion for 7 consecutive days.

Preparations: Vials, 10 mg (1 mg/ml).

CLAFORAN®, see Cefotaxime sodium.

CLARITHROMYCIN—Biaxin®

Macrolide antibiotic.

Actions and Uses: Is converted, in part, to an active metabolite, 14-hydroxyclarithromycin. Inhibits protein synthesis and its spectrum of action includes many gram-positive and gram-negative bacteria, as well as organisms such as *Mycoplasma pneumoniae.* Indicated for upper respiratory tract infections, lower respiratory tract infections, and uncomplicated skin and skin structure infections caused by susceptible organisms. Is also used in combination with other agents for the treatment of disseminated infection due to *Mycobacterium avium* complex and in treatment of active duodenal ulcer associated with *H. pylori* infection in combination with omeprazole.

Warnings: Contraindicated in patients with a known hypersensitivity to any of the macrolide antibiotics. Prescribers should review drugs profile to avoid interaction with contraindicated drugs. Adverse reactions include diarrhea, nausea, abnormal taste, dyspepsia, abdominal pain or discomfort, and headache. Should not be used in pregnant women unless no alternative therapy is appropriate. Concurrent use with terfenadine should be avoided. May increase serum concentrations of theophylline, carbamazepine, and other drugs that are metabolized via liver enzyme systems; concurrent therapy should be closely monitored.

Administration: Oral.

Preparations: Tablets, 250 and 500 mg. Granules for oral suspension, 125 mg/5 ml and 250 mg/5 ml when reconstituted.

CLARITIN®, see Loratadine

CLARITIN-D®, Combination of loratidine and pseudoephedrine

CLEMASTINE FUMARATE—Tavist®

Antihistamine.

Actions and Uses: Indicated for the relief of symptoms associated with allergic rhinitis, and for the relief of mild, uncomplicated allergic skin manifestations of urticaria and angioedema.

Warnings: Contraindicated in nursing mothers and in patients being treated with a monoamine oxidase inhibitor. Should not be used to treat lower respiratory tract symptoms including asthma. Adverse reactions include drowsiness and other CNS effects; patients should be cautioned regarding activities such as drivingand operating machinery, as well as interactions with other CNS-acting drugs including alcohol. Exhibits anticholinergic activity and must be used with caution in patients with conditions such as narrow-angle glaucoma.

Administration: Oral.

Preparations: Tablets, 1.34 and 2.68 mg. Syrup, 0.67 mg/5 ml.

CLEOCIN®, see Clindamycin

CLIDINIUM BROMIDE—Quarzan®

Anticholinergic agent indicated as adjunctive therapy in peptic ulcer disease.

Preparations: Capsules, 2.5 and 5 mg.

CLIMARA®, see Estradiol

CLINDAMYCIN—Cleocin®, Cleocin T®

Antibiotic indicated for the treatment of infections caused by susceptible anaerobic bacteria including *Bacteroides fragilis,* and for the treatment of infections caused by susceptible gram-positive cocci. Topical solution, gel, and lotion formulations are indicated in the treatment of acne. Vaginal cream is indicated in the treatment of bacterial vaginosis.

Preparations: Capsules (as the hydrochloride), 75, 150, and 300 mg. For oral solution (as the palmitate), 75

mg clindamycin/5 ml. Ampules and vials (as the phosphate), 150 mg clindamycin/ml. Topical solution, gel, and lotion (as the phosphate), 1%. Vaginal cream, 2%.

CLINORIL®, see Sulindac

CLIOQUINOL—Iodochlorhydroxyquin, Vioform®

Anti-infective agent used in the topical management of inflamed conditions of the skin (e.g., eczema, athlete's foot).

Preparations: Cream and ointment, 3%.

CLOBETASOL PROPIONATE—Temovate®

Topical corticosteroid.

Actions and Uses: Indicated for the short-term treatment of inflammatory and pruritic manifestations of moderate to severe corticosteroid-responsive dermatoses.

Warnings: Is highly potent and is more likely than are less potent analogs to cause systemic effects including suppression of the hypothalamic-pituitary-adrenal (HPA) axis. Treatment period should be limited to 2 weeks, and not more than 50 g of the cream or ointment should be used per week. Occlusive dressings should not be used.

Administration: Topical.

Preparations: Cream and ointment, 0.05%.

CLOFAZIMINE—Lamprene®

Antileprosy agent.

Actions and Uses: Exerts a slow bactericidal effect on *Mycobacterium leprae.* Indicated in the treatment of lepromatous leprosy, including dapsone-resistant lepromatous leprosy and lepromatous leprosy compli-cated by erythema nodosum leprosum.

Warnings: The drug is a dye and will cause pink to brownish-black pigmentation of the skin within a few weeks of treatment. It will also cause discoloration of the cconjunctivae, lacrimal fluid,sweat, sputum, urine, and feces. Other dermatologic reactions include ichthyosis, dryness, rash, and pruritus; the application of oil to the skin may help alleviate some of these effects. Many patients experience adverse gastrointestinal effects, such as abdominal and epigastric pain, diarrhea, nausea, vomiting, and gastrointestinal intolerance; taking the medication with meals may reduce the occurrence of these effects. There have been rare reports of bowel obstruction, gastrointestinal bleeding, and splenic infarction.

Administration: Oral.

Preparations: Capsules, 50 and 100 mg.

CLOFIBRATE—Atromid-S®

Antihyperlipidemic agent indicated for primary dysbetalipoproteinemia (Type III hyperlipidemia) that does not respond adequately to diet. May be considered for the treatment of selected patients with very high serum triglyceride levels (Types IV and V).

Preparation: Capsules, 500 mg.

CLOMID®, see Clomiphene

CLOMIPHENE CITRATE—Clomid®, Milophene®, Serophene®

Ovulation stimulant indicated for the treatment of ovulatory dysfunction in patients desiring pregnancy, and whose partners are fertile and potent. Unlabeled uses include male infertility, menstrual abnormalities, gynecomastia, fibrocystic breast disease, regulation of cycles in patients using rhythm methods of contraception, endometrial hyperplasia, and persistent lactation.

Preparation: Tablets, 50 mg.

CLOMIPRAMINE HYDROCHLORIDE—Anafranil®

Antiobsessional agent.

Actions and Uses: A tricyclic antidepressant that acts primarily by inhibiting the reuptake of serotonin. Indicated for the treatment of obsessions and compulsions in patients with obsessive-compulsive disorder.

Warnings: Should not be given in combination, or within 14 days of treatment with a monoamine oxidase inhibitor. Is also contraindicated during the acute recovery period after a myocardial infarction. Adverse reactions include CNS effects and patients should be cautioned regarding activities such as driving and operating machinery, as well as interactions with other CNS-acting drugs including alcohol. Other adverse reactions include dry mouth, blurred vision, nausea, dyspepsia, increased appetite, weight gain, sweating, orthostatic hypotension, and sexual dysfunction.

Administration: Oral. During the initial titration, clomipramine should be given in divided doses with meals to reduce gastrointestinal side effects. After titration, the total daily dose may be given once daily at bedtime to minimize daytime sedation.

Preparations: Capsules, 25, 50, and 75 mg.

CLONAZEPAM—Klonopin®

Benzodiazepine anticonvulsant indicated in the treatment of the Lennox-Gastaut syndrome (petit mal variant), akinetic and myoclonic seizures and panic disorder. May also be useful in absence seizures (petit mal).

Preparations: Tablets, 0.5, 1, and 2 mg.

CLONIDINE HYDROCHLORIDE—Catapres®, Catapres-TTS®

Antihypertensive agent.

Actions and Uses: Is a centrally-acting alpha-adrenergic receptor agonist indicated in the treatment of hypertension.

Warnings: Adverse reactions include drowsiness and other CNS effects; patients should be cautioned regarding activities such as driving and operating machinery, as well as interactions with other CNS-acting drugs including alcohol. Other adverse reactions include dry mouth, headache, dizziness, and dermatological effects (primarily with the use of the transdermal formulation). Effect may be reduced by the concurrent administration of a tricyclic antidepressant. The abrupt discontinuation of therapy may be followed by a rapid rise in blood pressure; patients should be advised of the importance of complying with the instructions for using the medication and, if therapy is to be discontinued, it should be done so gradually.

Administration: Oral and transdermal.

Preparations: Tablets, 0.1, 0.2, and 0.3 mg. Transdermal system, programmed delivery of 0.1, 0.2, and 0.3 mg clonidine base per day, for 1 week.

CLONOPIN®, former name for Klonopin®—see Clonazepam

CLORAZEPATE DIPOTASSIUM—Tranxene®

Benzodiazepine antianxiety agent and anticonvulsant.

Actions and Uses: A CNS depressant indicated (1) for the management of anxiety disorders or for the short-term relief of the symptoms of anxiety, (2) for the symptomatic relief of acute alcohol withdrawal, and (3) as adjunctive therapy in the management of partial seizures.

Warnings: Contraindicated in patients with acute narrow-angle glaucoma. Adverse reactions include drowsiness and other CNS effects; patients should be cautioned regarding activities such as driving and operating machinery, as well as interactions with other CNS-acting drugs including alcohol. Can cause dependence and is included in Schedule IV.

Administration: Oral.

Preparations: Tablets, 3.75, 7.5, 11.25, 15, and 22.5 mg. Capsules, 3.75, 7.5, and 15 mg.

CLORPACTIN®, see Oxychlorosene

CLOTRIMAZOLE—Gyne-Lotrimin®, Lotrimin®, Lotrimin AF®, Mycelex®, Mycelex-G®

Imidazole antifungal agent.

Actions and Uses: Indicated for (1) dermal infections—tinea pedis, tinea cruris, tinea corporis, candidiasis, tinea versicolor, (2) vulvovaginal candidiasis, and (3) oropharyngeal candidiasis.

Warnings: Adverse reactions include pruritus, stinging, erythema, vulval irritation.

Administration: Topical and vaginal.

Preparations: Cream, lotion, and solution, 1%. Vaginal cream, 1%. Vaginal tablets, 100 and 500 mg. Troches, 10 mg.

CLOVE OIL

Local anesthetic included in some formulations used for the relief of toothache.

Preparation: Drops

CLOXACILLIN SODIUM—Tegopen®

Penicillin antibiotic indicated for the treatment of staphylococcal infections.

Preparations: Capsules, 250 and 500 mg. Powder for oral solution, 125 mg/5 ml when reconstituted.

CLOZAPINE—Clozaril®

Antipsychotic agent.

Actions and Uses: An atypical antipsychotic drug with effects on dopamine mediated behaviors that differ from those exhibited by the standard antipsychotic agents. Is much less likely than the standard antipsychotic drugs to cause extrapyramidal effects. Indicated for the management of severely ill schizophrenic patients who fail to respond adequately to standard antipsychotic drug treatment, either because of insufficient effectiveness or the inability to achieve an effective dose due to intolerable adverse effects from those drugs.

Warnings: Contraindicated in patients with myeloproliferative disorders, or a history of clozapine-induced agranulocytosis or severe granulocytopenia. Should not be used simultaneously with other agents having a well-known potential to suppress bone-marrow function. May cause agranulocytosis and, prior to initiating treatment, a white blood cell (WBC) count should be performed and subsequent WBC counts should be done at least weekly for the duration of therapy, as well as for 4 weeks past discontinuation. If the total WBC count falls below 2000/mm^3 or granulocyte count below 1000/mm^3 during clozapine therapy, the drug should be discontinued and not resumed because of an even higher risk of agranulocytosis upon rechallenge. Patients should be advised to immediately report the appearance of lethargy, fever, sore throat, flu-like symptoms, or any other signs of infection. Use has also been associated with occurrence of seizures as well as other CNS effects (e. g., drowsiness/sedation, dizziness/vertigo).Patients should be cautioned regarding activities such as driving and operating machinery, as well as interactions with other CNS-acting drugs including alcohol. Other adverse reactions include tachycardia, hypotension, constipation, nausea, hypersalivation, sweating, dry mouth, visual disturbances, and fever.

Administration: Oral.

Preparations: Tablets, 25 and 100 mg.

CLOZARIL®, see Clozapine

COAL TAR

Antipruritic and irritant used in the topical treatment of dermatologic disorders including scalp conditions.

Preparations: Solution, gel, cream, ointment, lotion, soap, and shampoo.

COCAINE

Local anesthetic applied topically to provide anesthesia for mucous membranes.

Preparations: Powder. Topical solution, 40 mg/ml and 100 mg/ml. Soluble tablets, 135 mg.

CODEINE PHOSPHATE AND SULFATE

Opioid analgesic and antitussive.

Actions and Uses: Is a centrally acting analgesic indicated for the relief of pain and the management of cough.

Warnings: Adverse reactions include sedation and other CNS effects; patients should be cautioned regarding activities such as driving and operating machinery, as well as interactions with other CNS-acting drugs including alcohol. Other adverse reactions include constipation, nausea, vomiting, rash, and, in higher doses, respiratory depression. Can cause dependence and formulations are covered under the provisions of the Controlled Substances Act.

Administration: Oral and parenteral.

Preparations: Tablets, 15, 30, and 60 mg. Vials, 30 and 60 mg/ml. Is often used in combination with other agents (e.g., acetaminophen, aspirin) in capsule, tablet, and liquid formulations.

COD LIVER OIL

Vitamins A and D used to prevent and treat deficiences of these vitamins.

Preparations: Oil, emulsion, capsules.

COGENTIN®, see Benztropine

COGNEX®, see Tacrine hydrochloride

COLACE®, see Docusate sodium

COLCHICINE

Agent for gout. Indicated for the relief of pain associated with acute attacks of gout. Has also been used in chronic gouty conditions for the prevention of acute attacks of gout.

Preparations: Tablets, 0.5 and 0.6 mg. Ampules, 1 mg.

COLESTID®, see Colestipol

COLESTIPOL HYDROCHLORIDE—Colestid®

Antihyperlipidemic agent indicated as adjunctive therapy to diet for the reduction of elevated serum cholesterol in patients with primary hypercholesterolemia.

Preparations: Tablets, 1g. Granules, packets, 5g.

COLFOSCERIL PALMITATE, CETYL ALCOHOL, AND TYLOXAPOL—Exosurf Neonatal®

Agent for respiratory distress syndrome.

Actions and Uses: A synthetic pulmonary surfactant which contains colfosceril palmitate [also known as dipalmitoylphosphatidylcholine

(DPPC)], cetyl alcohol, and tyloxapol. Replenishes surfactant and restores surface activity to the lungs. Indicated for the prophylactic treatment of infants with birth weights of less than 1350 grams who are at risk of developing (RDS); the prophylactic treatment of infants with birth weights greater than 1350 grams who have evidence of pulmonary immaturity; and the rescue treatment of infants who have developed RDS.

Warnings: Adverse reactions include pulmonary bleeding, apnea, and mucous plugging. Suctioning of infant before dosing may lessen the possibility of mucous plugs obstructing the endotracheal tube. May rapidly affect oxygenation and lung compliance.

Administration: Intratracheal. Before administration, the infant should be suctioned. Is administered in the form of a suspension by instillation into the trachea via the sideport on a special endotracheal tube adapter without interrupting mechanical ventilation. Each dose is administered in two half doses. The infant is turned from the mid-line position to the right after the first half-dose, and from the mid-line position to the left after the second half-dose.

If the suspension appears to separate, the vial should be gently shaken or swirled to resuspend the preparation.

Preparations: Vials, 108 mg colfosceril palmitate, 12 mg cetyl alcohol, 8 mg tyloxapol, and 47 mg sodium chloride.

COLISTIMETHATE SODIUM—Coly-Mycin M®, see Colistin sulfate

COLISTIN SULFATE—Coly-Mycin S®, Polymixin E®

Antibiotic indicated for the treatment of infections caused by gram-negative bacteria including *Pseudomonas aeruginosa.* Colistimethate is used in the formulation administered parenterally, and colistin is used in the formulations administered orally (for gastrointestinal infections) and as otic drops.

Preparations: Vials, 150 mg. Oral suspension, 25 mg/5 ml when reconstituted. Otic drops (in combination with other agents), 3 mg/ml.

COLLAGENASE—Santyl®

Enzmye indicated for debriding chronic dermal ulcers and severely burned areas.

Preparation: Ointment, 250 units/g.

COLLYRIUM®, see Sodium borate

COLY-MYCIN®, see Colistimethate

COLYTE®, see Polyethylene glycol 3350

COMBIVIR®—Combination agent camivudine and zidovudine

COMBIVENT®—Combination agent ipratopium bromide and albuterol

COMPAZINE®, see Prochlorperazine

CONDYLOX®, see Podofilox

CONJUGATED ESTROGENS, see Estrogens, conjugated

CORDARONE®, see Amiodarone

CORDRAN®, see Flurandrenolide

CORGARD®, see Nadolol

CORTEF®, see Hydrocortisone

CORTICOTROPIN—Adrenocorticotropic hormone, ACTH, Acthar®

Hormone indicated for parenteral use in the diagnostic testing of adrenocortical function. Is of limited value in conditions responsive to corticosteroid therapy.

Preparations: Vials, 25 and 40 units. Vials (gel for repository effect), 40 and 80 units/ml.

CORTISOL, see Hydrocortisone

CORTISONE ACETATE—Cortone acetate®

Corticosteroid indicated for oral or intramuscular use in a wide range of endocrine, rheumatic, allergic, dermatologic, respiratory, hematologic, neoplastic, and other disorders.

Preparations: Tablets, 5, 10, and 25 mg. Vials, 25 and 50 mg/ml.

CORTISPORIN OTIC®, Combination of hydrocortisone, neomycin, and polymyxin B

CORTONE®, see Cortisone acetate

CORTROSYN®, see Cosyntropin

CORVERT®, see Ibutilide Fumarate

COSMEGEN®, see Dactinomycin

COSOPT®—Combination agent dorzolamide Hcl 2% and timolol maleate 0.5%

COSYNTROPIN—Cortrosyn®

Synthetic ACTH analog indicated for parenteral use in the diagnostic testing of adrenocortical function.

Preparation: Vials, 0.25 mg.

COTRIMOXAZOLE, see Trimethoprim-sulfamethoxazole

COUMADIN®, see Warfarin

COVERA-HS®, see Verapamil

COZAAR®see Losartan potassium

CRIXIVAN®, see Indinavir

CROMOLYN SODIUM—Crolom®, Gastrocrom®, Intal®, Nasalcrom®

Antiasthmatic agent used by oral inhalation in the prophylactic management of bronchial asthma, and shortly before exposure to factors (e.g., exercise) that precipitate bronchoconstriction. Instruct patients that this agent is not for treatment of acute bronchial asthmatic attacks. Ophthalmic solution is indicated for the treatment of vernal keratoconjunctivitis, vernal conjunctivitis, and vernal keratitis. Nasal solution is indicated for the prevention and treatment of symptoms of allergic rhinitis. Capsules for oral administration are used in the treatment of mastocytosis.

Preparations: Capsules, 100 mg. Oral solution, 100 mg/5ml. Nebulizer solution (20 mg/2 ml). Metered dose inhalation unit. Nasal solution, 40 mg/ml. Ophthalmic solution, 4%.

CROTAMITON—Eurax®

Scabicide indicated for the treatment of scabies and for the symptomatic treatment of pruritic skin.

Preparations: Cream and lotion, 10%.

CRYSTICILLIN®, see Procaine Penicillin G

CUPRIMINE®, see Penicillamine

CURARE, see Tubocurarine

CUTIVATE®, see Fluticasone propionate

CYANOCOBALAMIN—Vitamin B_{12}, Nascobal®

Vitamin indicated in the treatment of pernicious anemia, dietary deficiency of Vitamin B_{12}, malabsorption of Vitamin B_{12}, and other situations in which there is inadequate utilization of Vitamin B_{12}. Also used for the Schilling test.

Preparations: Tablets, 25, 50, 100, 250, 500, and 1,000 μg. Vials, 100 and 1,000 μrg/ml. Intranasal gel, 500 μg/0.1 ml,

CYCLANDELATE—Cyclospasmol®

Vasodilator indicated for adjunctive therapy in intermittent claudication, Raynaud's phenomenon, nocturnal leg cramps, and other peripheral vascular disorders. Has also been used in selected cases in ischemic cerebral vascular disease.

Preparations: Tablets, 400 mg. Capsules, 200 and 400 mg.

CYCLIZINE—Marezine®

Antiemetic indicated in the management of nausea and vomiting of motion sickness.

Preparations: Tablets (as the hydrochloride), 50 mg. Ampules (as the lactate), 50 mg.

CYCLOBENZAPRINE HYDROCHLORIDE—Flexeril®

Skeletal muscle relaxant.

Actions and Uses: Indicated as an adjunct to rest and physical therapy for relief of muscle spasm associated with acute, painful musculoskeletal conditions.

Warnings: Contraindicated during the acute recovery phase of myocardial infarction, in patients with arrhythmias, heart block or conduction disturbances, congestive heart failure, or hyperthyroidism, and in patients being treated with a monoamine oxidase inhibitor. Adverse reactions include drowsiness and other CNS effects; patients should be cautioned regarding activities such as driving and operating machinery, as well as interactions with other CNS-acting drugs including alcohol. Has an anticholinergic effect and adverse reactions such as dry mouth are common; caution should be exercised in patients with conditions such as angle-closure glaucoma, and in those taking other anticholinergic medications.

Administration: Oral. Use for longer than 2 to 3 weeks is not recommended.

Preparation: Tablets, 10 mg.

CYCLOCORT®, see Amcinonide

CYCLOGYL®, see Cyclopentolate

CYCLOMEN®, see Danazol

CYCLOPENTOLATE HYDROCHLORIDE—Cyclogyl®

Anticholinergic agent used to produce mydriasis and cycloplegia in diagnostic procedures.

Preparations: Ophthalmic solution, 0.5% and 1%.

CYCLOPHOSPHAMIDE—Cytoxan®, Neosar®

Antineoplastic agent indicated in the oral and parenteral treatment of malignant lymphomas, leukemias, multiple myeloma, carcinoma of the breast, neuroblastoma, adenocarcinoma of the ovary, retinoblastoma, and mycosis fungoides.

Preparations: Tablets, 25 and 50 mg. Vials, 100, 200, and 500 mg, 1 and 2 g.

CYCLOSERINE—Seromycin®

Antibiotic indicated in the treatment of tuberculosis when therapy with the primary medications has not been successful. Has also been used for urinary tract infections in which conventional therapy has failed.

Preparation: Capsules, 250 mg.

CYCLOSPASMOL®, see Cyclandelate

CYCLOSPORINE—Sandimmune®, Neoral®

Immunosuppressant used orally and intravenously, in conjunction with a corticosteroid, for the prophylaxis of organ rejection in kidney, liver, and heart transplants and severe, active rheumatoid arthritis unresponsive to methotrexate alone.

Preparations: Capsules, 25 and 100 mg. Oral solution, 100 mg/ml. Ampules, 50 mg.

CYCRIN®, see Medroxyprogesterone

CYKLOKAPRON®, see Tranexamic acid

CYLERT®, see Pemoline

CYPROHEPTADINE HYDROCHLORIDE—Periactin®

Antihistamine indicated for allergic disorders. Also possesses antiserotonin and appetite-stimulating properties.

Preparations: Tablets, 4 mg. Syrup, 2 mg/5 ml.

CYSTAGON, new drug; see Cysteamine bitartrate in Part II

CYSTEAMINE BITARTRATE—Cystagon®

Cystine-depleting agent indicated in the management of nephropathic cystinosis in children and adults. Contraindicated in patients with known hypersensitivity to this agent or penicillamine. Adverse reactions include vomiting, anorexia, fever, diarrhea, lethargy, and rash. If rash develops, the drug should be withheld until the rash clears. If a severe skin rash (e.g., erythema multiforme) develops, should not be readministered. Has occasionally been associated with reversible leukopenia and abnormal liver function studies; therefore, blood counts and liver function studies should be monitored.

Administration: Oral. Usual maintenance dosage for children through the age of 12 years is 1.3 $g/m^2/day$, given in 4 divided doses. Recommended maintenance dose for patients more than 12 years old and more than 110 pounds is 2 g/day, given in 4 divided doses.

Preparations: Capsules, 50 and 150 mg.

CYTARABINE—Cytosine arabinoside, ARA-C, Cytosar-U®

Antineoplastic agent indicated for the parenteral treatment of leukemias (primarily acute myelocytic leukemia) and as part of a combination regimen in children with non-Hodgkin's lymphoma.

Preparations: Vials, 100 and 500 mg.

CYTOMEL®, see Liothyronine

CYTOSAR-U®, see Cytarabine

CYTOSINE ARABINOSIDE, see Cytarabine

CYSTOSPAZ®, see Hyoscyamine

CYTOTEC®, see Misoprostol

CYTOVENE®, see Ganciclovir

CYTOXAN®, see Cyclophosphamide

D

DACARBAZINE—DTIC®

Antineoplastic agent indicated for the parenteral treatment of metastatic malignant melanoma, refractory Hodgkin's disease, various sarcomas, and neuroblastoma.

Preparations: Vials, 100 and 200 mg.

DACTINOMYCIN—Cosmegen®

Antineoplastic agent indicated for the parenteral treatment of Wilm's tumor, testicular carcinoma, choriocarcinoma, rhabdomyosarcoma, and other neoplasms.

Preparation: Vials, 0.5 mg.

DALGAN®, see Dezocine

DALMANE®, see Flurazepam

DALTEPARIN—Fragmin®

Antithrombotic agent.

Uses and Actions: Prevention of deep vein thrombosis and pulmonary embolism following abdominal surgery in high-risk patients (age > 40, obesity, general anesthesia > 30 minutes, history of malignancy or previous thromboembolic phenomena).

Warnings: Contraindicated in active major bleeding and thrombocytopenia associated with positive *in vitro* tests for antiplatelet antibody in the presence of dalteporin, heparin, or pork allergy. Adverse effects include local hematoma, anaphylaxis, and thrombocytopenia.

Administration: 2,500 IU SC once daily starting 1–2 hours before surgery and continuing for 5–10 days postoperatively.

Preparations: 2,500 and 5,000 IU/0.2 ml single- dose, prefilled syringe.

DANAZOL—Cyclomen®, Danocrine®

Androgen indicated for the treatment of endometriosis unresponsive to more conventional treatment, fibrocystic breast disease, and hereditary angioedema.

Preparations: Capsules, 50, 100, and 200 mg.

DANOCRINE®, see Danazol

DANTRIUM®, see Dantrolene

DANTROLENE SODIUM—Dantrium®

Muscle relaxant and antispastic agent used in controlling the manifestations of spasticity resulting from upper-motor-neuron disorders (e.g., stroke, cerebral palsy, multiple sclerosis). Also used intravenously in the management of malignant hyperthermia crisis, and orally to prevent or reduce the development of signs of malignant hyperthermia in susceptible patients.

Preparations: Capsules, 25, 50, and 100 mg. Vials, 20 mg.

DAPIPRAZOLE HYDROCHLORIDE—Rejv-Eyes®

Antimydriatic agent.

Actions and Uses: An alpha-adrenergic blocking agent that reverses the mydriasis caused by agents used in ocular examinations. Indicated in the treatment of iatrogenically induced mydriasis produced by adrenergic (phenylephrine) and parasympatholytic (tropicamide) agents.

Warnings: Contraindicated in patients

in whom constriction is undesirable (e.g., acute iritis). Adverse reactions include conjunctival injection, burning on instillation, ptosis, lid erythema, lid edema, chemosis, itching, punctate keratitis, corneal edema, browache, photophobia, and headaches.

Administration: Ophthalmic.

Preparations: Ophthalmic solution, 0.5%.

DAPSONE, Avlosulfan®, DDS®

Antileprosy agent indicated for the management of all forms of leprosy. Also indicated in the treatment of dermatitis herpetiformis.

Preparations: Tablets, 25 and 100 mg.

DARANIDE®, see Dichlorphenamide

DARAPRIM®, see Pyrimethamine

DARICON®, see Oxphencyclimine

DARVOCET-N®, Combination of propoxyphene napsylate and acetaminophen

DARVON®, see Propoxyphene hydrochloride

DARVON-N®, see Propoxyphene napsylate

DAUNORUBICIN HYDROCHLORIDE—Cerubidine®

Antineoplastic agent indicated for the parenteral treatment of acute nonlymphocytic leukemia in adults and in acute lymphocytic leukemia in children.

Preparation: Vials, 20 mg (of the base).

DAYPRO®, see Oxaprozin

DDAVP®, see Desmopressin acetate

ddC, see Zalcitabine

ddI, see Didanosine

DDS®, see Dapsone

DEBRISAN®, see Dextranomer

DEBROX®, see Carbamide peroxide

DECADRON®, see Dexamethasone

DECA-DURABOLIN®, see Nandrolone decanoate

DECHOLIN®, see Dehydrocholic acid

DECLOMYCIN®, see Demeclocycline

DEFEROXAMINE MESYLATE—Desferal®

Antidote that chelates iron. Indicated for parenteral use to facilitate the removal of iron in the treatment of acute iron intoxication and in chronic iron overload due to transfusion-dependent anemias.

Preparation: Vials, 500 mg.

DEHYDROCHOLIC ACID—Decholin®

Hydrocholeretic indicated for the relief of constipation. Has also been used as an adjunct in the treatment of various biliary conditions.

Preparation: Tablets, 250 mg.

DELATESTRYL®, see Testosterone enanthate

DELAVIRDINE MESYLATE—Rescriptor®

Antiretroviral indicated in the treatment of HIV-1 infection in combination with other antiretroviral agents when therapy is warranted. When used as monotherapy viral resistance emerged rapidly.

Warnings: Discontinue if serious rash (or rash with other symptoms) occurs. Use cautiously in patients with impaired liver function or achlorhydria (take with an acidic beverage). Adverse reactions include rash, GI upset.

Administration: Always use in combination with other antiretroviral therapy to minimize the risk of resistance. Potential for cross-resistence between delavirdine and either nucleoside analogues or protease inhibitors is unlikely due to their different mechanisms of action. Take 400 mg 3 times daily. May swallow tabs or disperse them in at least 3 oz of water and drink.

Preparation: Tablets, 100 mg.

DELESTROGEN®, see Estradiol valerate

DELSYM®, see Dextromethorphan

DELTA-CORTEF®, see Prednisolone

DELTASONE®, see Prednisone

DEMADEX®, see Torsemide

DEMECARIUM BROMIDE—Humorsol®

Cholinesterase inhibitor exhibiting miotic activity. Indicated for ophthalmic use in the treatment of open-angle glaucoma, conditions obstructing aqueous outflow, accommodative esotropia, and following iridectomy.

Preparations: Ophthalmic solution, 0.125% and 0.25%.

DEMEROL®, see Meperidine

DEMECLOCYCLINE HYDROCHLORIDE —Declomycin®

Tetracycline antibiotic indicated for the treatment of infections caused by susceptible organisms.

Preparations: Tablets, 150 and 300 mg. Capsules, 150 mg.

DEMSER®, see Metyrosine

DENAVIR®, see Penciclovir

DEPAKENE®, see Valproic acid

DEPAKOTE®, see Valproic acid

DEPEN®, see Penicillamine

DEPO-ESTRADIOL®, see Estradiol cypionate

DEPO-MEDROL®, see Methylprednisolone acetate

DEPONIT®, see Nitroglycerin

DEPO-PROVERA®, see Medroxyprogesterone acetate

DEPO-TESTOSTERONE®, see Testosterone cypionate

DERIFIL®, see Chlorophyll

DERMATOP®, see Prednicarbate

DES, see Diethylstilbestrol

DESENEX®, see Undecylenic acid

DESFERAL®, see Deferoxamine mesylate

DESFLURANE—Suprane®

General Anesthetic.

Actions and Uses: Is a halogenated volatile liquid that is administered via a vaporizer as a general inhalation anesthetic. Indicated as an inhalation agent for induction or maintenance of anesthesia for inpatient and outpatient surgery in adults. Also indicated for maintenance of anesthesia in infants and children after induction of anesthesia with other agents, and for tracheal intubation.

Warnings: Contraindicated in patients with a known or suspected genetic susceptibility to malignant hyperthermia. Adverse reactions include coughing, breathholding, apnea, increased secretions, laryngospasm, pharyngitis, nausea, and vomiting. Because it may increase heart rate, it is recommended that it should not be used as the sole agent for anesthetic induction in patients with coronary artery disease or in any patients in whom increases in heart rate or blood pressure are undesirable. May trigger a skeletal muscle hypermetabolic state that results in malignant hyperthermia. Concurrent use of preanesthetic medications such as an opioid or benzodiazepine may decrease the amount of desflurane required to produce anesthesia. Use will probably reduce the dose of a neuromuscular blocking agent required during anesthesia; however, for endotracheal intubation, it is recommended that the dose of the neuromuscular blocking agent not be reduced.

Administration: Inhalation. Should be administered using a vaporizer (Tec 60) specifically designed for use with the drug.

Preparations: Bottles, 240 ml.

DESIPRAMINE HYDROCHLORIDE—Norpramin®, Pertofrane®

Tricyclic antidepressant.

Actions and Uses: Indicated for the relief of depression.

Warnings: Should not be given concomitantly with a monoamine oxidase inhibitor, or following recent myocardial infarction. Adverse reactions include drowsiness and other CNS effects; patients should be cautioned regarding activities such as driving and operating machinery, as well as interactions with other CNS-acting drugs including alcohol. Other adverse reactions include anti-cholinergic effects (e.g., dry mouth, blurred vision), GI effects (e.g., nausea), and cardiovascular effects (e.g., orthostatic hypotension). Caution should be exercised in patients with cardiovascular disorders.

Administration: Oral.

Preparations: Tablets, 10, 25, 50, 75, 100, and 150 mg. Capsules, 25 and 50 mg.

DESMOPRESSIN ACETATE—DDAVP®, Stimate®

Antidiuretic hormone indicated for the intranasal or parenteral treatment of diabetes insipidus, intranasal treatment of primary nocturnal enuresis, and parenteral treatment of patients with hemophilia A and von Willebrand's disease.

Preparations: Nasal solution (DDAVP), 0.1 mg/ml. (available as a nasal tube delivery system and as a nasal spray pump). Nasal solution (Stimate), 1.5 mg/ml. Ampules and vials, 4 µg/ml. Tablets, 0.1 mg, 0.2 mg.

DESOGEN®, see Desogestrel/ethinyl estradiol

DESOGESTREL/ETHINYL ESTRADIOL—Desogen®, Ortho-Cept®

Oral contraceptive.

Actions and Uses: Is a progestin/estrogen combination that acts primarily by the suppression of gonadotropins and inhibition of ovulation. Desogestrel exhibits a highly selective progestational action and minimal androgenicity. Indicated for the prevention of pregnancy in women who elect to use oral contraceptives as a method of contraception.

Warnings: Contraindicated in women who have thrombophlebitis or a thromboembolic disorder, a past history of such disorders, cerebral vascular or coronary artery disease, known or suspected carcinoma of the breast, carcinoma of the endometrium or other known or suspected estrogen-dependent neoplasia, undiagnosed abnormal genital bleeding, cholestatic jaundice of pregnancy or jaundice with prior oral contraceptive use, hepatic adenomas or carcinomas, or known or suspected pregnancy. Adverse reactions include bleeding irregularities (e.g., breakthrough bleeding, spotting, changes in menstrual flow), gastrointestinal effects e.g., nausea, vomiting, abdominal cramps), fluid retention, melasma, rash, reduced tolerance to carbohydrates, and vaginal candidiasis. Women should be strongly advised not to smoke because of the increased risk of cardiovascular effects.

Administration: Oral. Administered once a day at about the same time each day. Available in packages designed for a 21-day regimen (i.e., one tablet a day for 21 days, followed by 7 days in which medication is not taken) and a 28-day regimen (i.e., one tablet a day for 21 days, followed by one inactive "reminder" tablet a day for 7 days).

Preparations: Tablets, 0.15 mg of desogestrel and 30 ug of ethinyl estradiol in 21-day and 28-day regimens.

DESONIDE—Tridesilon®

Corticosteroid indicated for the topical treatment of corticosteroid-responsive dermatoses and, in combination with acetic acid in an otic solution, for the management of superficial infections of the external auditory canal.

Preparations: Cream and ointment, 0.05%. Otic solution, 0.05% with 2% acetic acid.

DESOXIMETASONE—Topicort®

Corticosteroid indicated for the topical treatment of corticosteroid-responsive dermatoses.

Preparations: Cream, 0.05% and 0.25%. Ointment, 0.25%. Gel, 0.05%.

DESOXYN®, see Methamphetamine

DESYREL®, see Trazodone

DEXAMETHASONE—Decadron®, Hexadrol®

Corticosteroid indicated in a wide range of endocrine, rheumatic, allergic, dermatologic, respiratory, hematologic, neoplastic, and other disorders.

Preparations: Tablets, 0.5, 0.75, 1, 1.5, 2, 3, and 6 mg. Liquid, 0.5 mg/5 ml. Oral concentrate, 0.5 mg/0.5 ml. Vials (as the acetate for intramuscular, intra-articular and intralesional use), 8 mg/ml. Vials and ampules (as the sodium phosphate for parenteral use), 4, 10, 20, and 24 (for IV use only) mg/ml. Topical gel, 0.1%. Topical aerosol, 10 mg/25 g. Cream (as the sodium phosphate), 0.1% Ophthalmic solution (as the sodium phosphate), 0.1%. Ophthalmic ointment (as the sodium phosphate),

0.05%. Aerosols (as the sodium phosphate) for oral inhalation and intranasal administration.

DEXATRIM®, see Phenylpropanolamine

DEXCHLORPHENIRAMINE MALEATE—Polaramine®

Antihistamine indicated in the treatment of allergic disorders.

Preparations: Tablets, 2 mg. Controlled-release tablets, 4 and 6 mg. Syrup, 2 mg/5 ml.

DEXEDRINE®, see Dextroamphetamine

DEXPANTHENOL—Ilopan®

Pantothenic acid derivative used as a GI stimulant. Indicated for parenteral treatment of intestinal atony causing abdominal distention, postoperative and postpartum retention of flatus, or postoperative delay in resumption of intestinal motility, paralytic ileus, and for prophylactic use immediately after major abdominal surgery to minimize the possibility of paralytic ileus.

Preparations: Ampules, vials, and syringes, 250 mg/ml. Has been used orally in combination with choline bitartrate.

DEXRAZOXANE—Zinecard®

Actions and Uses: Cardioprotective agent indicated for reducing the incidence and severity of cardiomyopathy associated with doxorubicin administration in women with metastatic breast cancer who have received a cumulative doxorubicin dose of 300 mg/m^2 and who would benefit from continuing doxorubicin therapy. Not recommended for use with the initiation of doxorubicin therapy.

Warnings: Contraindicated in chemotherapy regimens which do not contain an anthracycline. Additive myelosuppressive effect of this agent with antineoplastic agents requires careful blood count monitoring.

Administration: Intravenous. Recommended dosage ratio of dexrazoxane: doxorubicin is 10:1 (e.g., 500 mg/m^2 dexrazoxane: 50 mg/m^2 doxorubicin). After completing the infusion of dexrazoxane, and prior to a total elapsed time of 30 minutes (from the beginning of the dexrazoxane infusion), the intravenous injection of doxorubicin should be given. Doxorubicin should not be given prior to the administration of dexrazoxane.

Preparations: Vials, 250 and 500 mg.

DEXTRAN, LOW MOLECULAR WEIGHT—Dextran 40, Gentran 40®, Rheomacrodex®

DEXTRAN, HIGH MOLECULAR WEIGHT—Dextran 70, Dextran 75, Gentran 75®, Macrodex®

Synthetic polysaccharide administered parenterally primarily as a plasma expander as adjunctive treatment of shock or impending shock due to hemorrhage, burns, surgery, or other trauma.

Preparations: Injection, 10% low molecular weight dextran and 6% high molecular weight dextran.

DEXTRANOMER—Debrisan®, Envisan®

Applied topically for use in cleaning wet ulcers and wounds such as venous stasis ulcers, pressure ulcers, infected traumatic and surgical wounds, and infected burns.

Preparations: Beads. Paste.

DEXTROAMPHETAMINE SULFATE—Dexedrine®

Central nervous system stimulant indicated in the treatment of narcolepsy, attention-deficit disorder with hyperactivity, and in exogenous obesity as a short-term adjunct in a regimen of weight reduction based on caloric restriction.

Preparations: Tablets, 5 mg. Controlled-release capsules, 15 mg.

DEXTROMETHORPHAN—Benylin DM®, Delsym®

Antitussive indicated for the relief of cough.

Preparations: Syrup (as the hydrobromide) 5, 10, and 15 mg/5 ml. Sustained-action liquid (as the polistirex), 30 mg/5 ml.

DEXTROSE—Glucose, Glutose®, Instaglucose®

Carbohydrate administered parenterally as a source of calories. Oral forms are used to correct hypoglycemia in conscious patients.

Preparations: Solutions, 2.5%, 5%, 10%, 20%, 25%, 30%, 40%, 50%, 60%, and 70%. Oral gel, 40% in 25-g and 30-g tubes and 80-g bottle. Chewable tablets, 5g.

DEXTROTHYROXINE SODIUM—Choloxin®

Antihyperlipidemic agent used as an adjunct to diet and other measures for the reduction of elevated serum cholesterol levels. May also reduce beta lipoprotein and triglyceride levels.

Preparations: Tablets, 1, 2, and 4 mg.

DEZOCINE—Dalgan®

Analgesic.

Actions and Uses: An opioid agonist-antagonist analgesic that exhibits analgesic efficacy, as well as an onset and duration of action, that are comparable to those of morphine. Is most often used in the management of postoperative pain and pain associated with surgery and orthopedic trauma.

Warnings: Adverse reactions include sedation, dizziness/vertigo, and psychotomimetic effects. Patients should be cautioned regarding activities such as driving and operating machinery, as well as interactions with other CNS-acting drugs including alcohol. Other adverse reactions include nausea, vomiting, and injection site reactions. Should not be used in patients who are physically dependent on narcotics because its antagonist action may precipitate withdrawal symptoms.

Administration: Intramuscular and intravenous.

Preparations: Single-dose vials and syringes, 5,

10, and 15 mg. Multiple-dose vials, 10 mg/ml.

DHE 45®, see Dihydroergotamine

DHT®, see Dihydrotachysterol

DIAβETA®, see Glyburide

DIABINESE®, see Chlorpropamide

DIACETYLMORPHINE, see Heroin

DIAMOX®, see Acetazolamide

DIASTAT®, see Diazepam

DIAZEPAM—Diastat®, Valium®, Valrelease®

Benzodiazepine antianxiety agent and anticonvulsant.

Actions and Uses: A CNS depressant indicated (1) for the management of anxiety disorders or for the short-term relief of the symptoms of anxiety; (2) in acute alcohol withdrawal; (3) as an adjunct for the relief of skeletal muscle spasm due to reflex spasm to local pathology; athetosis; stiff-man syndrome; and tetanus; (4) as an adjunct in convulsive disorders; (5) as an adjunct in status epilepticus and severe recurrent convulsive seizures; (6) as an adjunct prior to endoscopic procedures; and (7) as a premedication in patients who are to undergo surgical procedures.

Warnings: Contraindicated in patients with acute narrow-angle glaucoma. Adverse reactions include drowsiness and other CNS effects; patients should be cautioned regarding activities such as driving and operating machinery, as well as interactions with other CNS-acting drugs including alcohol. Can cause dependence and is included in Schedule IV. Intramuscular injections are painful and erratically absorbed. If IM route is essential for administration, inject deeply into a large muscle mass and rotate sites.

Administration: Oral, intravenous, and intramuscular.

Preparations: Tablets, 2, 5, and 10 mg. Controlled-release capsules, 15 mg. Oral solution, 5 mg/5 ml. Concentrated oral solution, 5 mg/ml. Ampules, vials, and syringes, 5 mg/ml. Rectal gel, 2.5, 5, 10, 15, and 20 mg. Sterile emulsion for injection, 5 mg/ml (contains egg phospholipids, and soybean oil).

DIAZOXIDE—Hyperstat®, Proglycem®

Antihypertensive agent administered intravenously for short-term use in the emergency reduction of blood pressure in severe hypertension. Also used orally in the management of hypoglycemia due to hyperinsulinism associated with various conditions (e.g., inoperable islet cell carcinoma or adenoma).

Preparations: Ampules, 300 mg. Capsules, 50 mg. Oral suspension, 50 mg/ml.

DIBENT®, see Dicyclomine

DIBENZYLINE®, see Phenoxybenzamine

DIBUCAINE—Nupercainal®

Local anesthetic used for painful skin conditions

and hemorrhoids.

Preparations: Cream, 0.5%. Ointment, 1%.

DICHLORPHENAMIDE—Daranide®, Oratrol®

Carbonic anhydrase inhibitor indicated for adjunctive treatment of open-angle glaucoma, secondary glaucoma, and preoperatively in acute angle-closure glaucoma.

Preparation: Tablets, 50 mg.

DICLOFENAC POTASSIUM—Cataflam®

DICLOFENAC SODIUM—Voltaren®

Nonsteroidal anti-inflammatory drug.

Actions and Uses: Inhibits prostaglandin synthesis. Diclofenac sodium is indicated for the treatment of rheumatoid arthritis, osteoarthritis, and ankylosing spondylitis. Also indicated for ophthalmic use for the treatment of postoperative inflammation following cataract extraction and in photophobia due to incisional refractive surgery. Diclofenac potassium is indicated for the management of pain and primary dysmenorrhea.

Warnings: Should not be given to patients in whom aspirin or another NSAID causes asthma, rhinitis, urticaria, or other allergic-type reactions. May cause GI effects, and use should be avoided in patients with active GI tract disease and closely monitored in patients with a previous history of such disorders. Other adverse reactions include headache, dizziness, rash, pruritus, tinnitus, and fluid retention. Elevations in liver function tests have occurred and it is recommended that hepatic function tests be performed no later than 8 weeks after starting therapy and periodically thereafter.

Administration: Oral and ophthalmic.

Preparations: Tablets (Cataflam), 25, 50, and 75 mg. Enteric coated tablets (Voltaren)), 25, 50, and 75 mg. Entericcoated tablets (Cataflam), 75 mg and 100 mg. Ophthalmic solution, 0.1%. Suppositories, 50 and 100 mg, 100 mg extended-release tabs (Voltarum-XR).

DICLOXACILLIN SODIUM—Dycill®, Dynapen®, Pathocil®

Penicillin antibiotic indicated for the treatment of staphylococcal infections.

Preparations: Capsules, 125, 250, and 500 mg. Powder for oral solution, 62.5 mg/5 ml when reconstituted.

DICUMAROL

Coumarin anticoagulant indicated for conditions such as prophylaxis and treatment of venous thrombosis and its extension. During period of dosage adjustment, prothrombin activity should be measured daily and dose order obtained.

Preparations: Tablets, 25 and 50 mg.

DICYCLOMINE HYDROCHLORIDE—Antispas®, A-spas®, Bentyl®, Dibent®, Di-Spaz®, Spasmoject®

Anticholinergic agent.

Actions and Uses: Relieves smooth muscle spasm of the GI tract and is indicated for the treatment of functional bowel/irritable bowel syndrome (irritable colon, spastic colon, and mucous colitis).

Warnings: Contraindicated in patients with obstructive uropathy, obstructive disease of the GI tract, paralytic ileus, intestinal atony, unstable cardiovascular status in acute hemorrhage, severe ulcerative colitis, myasthenia gravis, and glaucoma. Adverse reactions include dry mouth, blurred vision, and nausea. Anticholinergic psychosis, and heat prostration (in the presence of a high environmental temperature) have been reported in sensitive patients. May cause drowsiness and other CNS effects; patients should be cautioned regarding activities such as driving and operating machinery, as well as interactions with other CNS-acting drugs including alcohol.

Administration: Oral and intramuscular.

Preparations: Tablets, 10 and 20 mg. Extended release tablets, 30 mg. Capsules, 10 and 20 mg. Syrup, 10 mg/5 ml. Solution for injection, 10 mg/ml.

DIDANOSINE—Videx®

Antiviral agent.

Actions and Uses: Also known as dideoxyinosine or ddI. It inhibits the replication of the human immunodeficiency virus (HIV). Is converted by cellular enzymes to the active antiviral metabolite that inhibits viral replication, in part, by interfering with reverse transcriptase. Indicated for adult and pediatric patients (over 6 months of age) with advanced HIV infection who are intolerant of zidovudine therapy or who have demonstrated significant clinical or immunologic deterioration during zidovudine therapy. Also indicated for adult patients with advanced HIV infection who have received prolonged prior zidovudine therapy.

Warnings: May cause pancreatitis and, if a patient develops abdominal pain and nausea, vomiting, or elevated amylase levels, use of the drug should be interrupted until the possibility of pancreatitis is excluded. Use of didanosine in patients with a history of pancreatitis or alcoholism is best avoided as is the concurrent use with other agents known to be associated with pancreatic toxicity (e.g., intravenous pentamidine). May cause peripheral neuropathy, particularly in patients with a history of neuropathy or neurotoxic drug therapy; patients should be advised to report symptoms such as tingling, burning, pain, or numbness in the hands or feet. Other adverse reactions include headache, diarrhea, insomnia, rash, pruritus, depression, pain, constipation, stomatitis, taste disturbance, myalgia, arthritis, hepatic enzyme elevations, leukopenia, granulocytopenia, and thrombocytopenia. Because 2 of the 3 formulations contain (or have added) magnesium and aluminum antacids (to reduce the degradation of the drug by gastric acid), tetracyclines, fluoroquinolones, or other drugs that interact with metals should not be administered within 2 hours of taking didanosine. Ketoconazole should be administered at least 2 hours before dosing with didanosine. Each tablet contains 15.7 mEq of magnesium, 264.5 mg of sodium, as well as a quantity of phenylalanine; caution should be exercised in patients with significant renal impairment, on a sodium-restricted diet, and/or who are phenylketonuric.

Administration: Oral. Food reduces absorption by as much as 50%; therefore, the drug should be administered on an empty stomach (i.e., having nothing to eat or drink, except water, for 1 hour before and 1 to 2 hours after taking the drug). Each dose of the tablet formulation must consist of 2 tablets to achieve adequate acid-neutralizing capacity for maximal absorption. The tablets should be thoroughly chewed, manually crushed, or dispersed in water. The buffered powder for oral solution is provided in packets, the contents of which should be poured into a container with about 4 ounces of water. The drug must not be mixed with fruit juice or other acid-containing liquid. The pediatric powder for oral solution is initially constituted with purified water, to which the pharmacist then adds an appropriate quantity of an antacid (Mylanta Double Strength Liquid or Maalox TC Suspension).

Preparations: Chewable/dispersible buffered tablets, 25, 50, 100, and 150 mg. Packets of powder for oral solution, 100, 167, 250, and 375 mg. Bottles of pediatric powder for oral solution, 2 and 4 grams.

DIDREX®, see Benzphetamine

DIDRONEL®, see Etidronate

DIENESTROL

Estrogen indicated for intravaginal use in the treatment of atrophic vaginitis and kraurosis vulvae.

Preparation: Vaginal cream, 0.01%.

DIETHYLPROPION HYDROCHLORIDE—Tenuate®, Tepanil®

Anorexiant indicated in the management of exogenous obesity as a short-term adjunct in a regimen of weight reduction based on caloric restriction.

Preparations: Tablets, 25 mg. Controlled-release tablets, 75 mg.

DIETHYLSTILBESTROL—DES

DIETHYLSTILBESTROL DIPHOSPHATE—Stilphostrol®

Estrogen indicated in the treatment of moderate to severe vasomotor symptoms associated with the menopause, atrophic vaginitis, kraurosis vulvae, female hypogonadism, female castration, primary ovarian failure, and breast cancer. Both oral and parenteral (diphosphate) dosage forms are indicated in the treatment of prostatic carcinoma.

Preparations: Tablets, 1 and 5 mg. Enteric-coated tablets, 0.1, 1, and 5 mg. Tablets (diphosphate), 50 mg. Ampules (diphosphate), 250 mg/ 5 ml.

DIFENOXIN HYYDROCHLORIDE/ ATROPINE SULFAT—Motofen®

Antidiarrheal agent.

Actions and Uses: Difenoxin is the principal active metabolite of diphenoxylate. A subtherapeutic dose of atropine is included in the formulation to discourage abuse of difenoxin. Indicated as adjunctive therapy in the management of diarrhea.

Warnings: Contraindicated in patients with diarrhea associated with pseudomembranous colitis. Is also contraindicated in children under 2 years of age because of an increased risk of adverse reactions. Adverse reactions include drowsiness and other CNS effects; patients should be cautioned regarding activities such as driving and operating machinery, as well as interactions with other CNS-acting drugs including alcohol. Should not be administered to patients being treated with a monoamine oxidase inhibitor. Is inluded in Schedule IV.

Administration: Oral.

Preparation: Tablets containing 1 mg difenoxin hydrochloride and 0.025 mg atropine sulfate.

DIFFERIN®, see Adaplalene

DIFLORASONE DIACETATE—Florone®, Maxiflor®

Corticosteroid used topically in the treatment of corticosteroid-responsive dermatoses.

Preparations: Cream and ointment, 0.05%.

DIFLUCAN®, see Fluconazole

DIFLUNISAL—Dolobid®

Nonsteroidal anti-inflammatory drug.

Actions and Uses: A salicylate analog that exhibits analgesic, antipyretic, and anti-inflammatory effects. Indicated for the treatment of mild to moderate pain, rheumatoid arthritis, and osteoarthritis.

Warnings: Contraindicated in patients in whom acute asthmatic attacks, urticaria, or rhinitis are precipitated by aspirin or other nonsteroidal anti-inflammatory drugs. May cause GI effects and use should be avoided in patients with active GI tract disease and closely supervised in patients with a previous history of such disorders. Other adverse reactions include headache and rash. Effect may be reduced by antacids.

Administration: Oral.

Preparations: Tablets, 250 and 500 mg.

DIGIBIND®, see Digoxin immune FAB

DIGITALIS

Cardiac glycosides primarily used in the treatment of congestive heart failure.

Preparation: Tablets, 100 mg.

DIGITOXIN

Cardiac glycoside indicated in the treatment of heart failure, atrial flutter, atrial fibrillation, and supraventricular tachycardia.

Preparations: Tablets, 0.1 and 0.2 mg.

DIGOXIN—Lanoxicaps®, Lanoxin®

Cardiac (digitalis) glycoside.

Actions and Uses: Exhibits a positive inotropic action and also causes a slowing of heart rate and decreased conduction velocity through the AV node. Indicated in the management of heart failure, atrial fibrillation, atrial flutter, and paroxysmal atrial tachycardia.

Warnings: Contraindicated in patients in ventricular fibrillation. May cause serious cardiac toxicity (e.g., arrhythmias) and therapy must be closely supervised. Other adverse reactions include anorexia, nausea, and vomiting, visual disturbances, headache, weakness, apathy, psychosis, and gynecomastia. Certain diuretics and corticosteroids may cause potassium depletion and increase the risk of digoxin toxicity. Simultaneous administration of antacids, cholestyramine, or colestipol may reduce absorption, and as long an interval as possible should separate the administration of digoxin and one of these agents.

Administration: Oral, intravenous, and intramuscular.

Preparations: Tablets, 0.125, 0.25, and 0.5 mg. Liquid in caps, 0.05, 0.1, and 0.2 mg. Elixir (pediatric), 0.05 mg/ml. Ampules, 0.1 mg/ml (pediatric) and 0.25 mg/ml.

DIGOXIN IMMUNE FAB (OVINE)—Digibind®

Antidote for digoxin toxicity.

Actions and Uses: Indicated for the treatment of potentially life-threatening digoxin or digitoxin intoxication.

Warnings: A potential for hypersensitivity reactions exists. Low-cardiac-output states and congestive heart failure may be exacerbated by the withdrawal of the inotropic effects of digoxin. Hypokalemia may result from the rapid reversal of the hyperkalemia associated with digoxin intoxication, and potassium concentrations should be monitored closely.

Administration: Intravenous.

Preparation: Vials, 40 mg.

DIHYDROCODEINE BITARTRATE

Opioid analgesic indicated for the relief of moderate to moderately severe pain. Used in combination with other analgesics.

DIHYDROERGOTAMINE MESYLATE—DHE 45®

Vasoconstrictor administered parenterally to abort or prevent vascular headaches (e.g., migraine). In conjunction with low-dose heparin to prevent post-operative deep vein thrombosis and pulmonary embolism.

Preparation: Ampules, 1 mg.

DIHYDROTACHYSTEROL—DHT®, Hytakerol®

Vitamin D analog indicated for the treatment of hypoparathyroidism, postoperative tetany, and idiopathic tetany.

Preparations: Capsules, 0.125 mg. Tablets, 0.125, 0.2, and 0.4 mg. Solution, 0.2 mg/5 ml. Concentrated solution, 0.2 mg/ml. Solution in oil, 0.25 mg/ml.

DILACOR XR®, see Diltiazem.

DILANTIN®, see Phenytoin.

DILAUDID®, see Hydromorphone

DILOR®, see Dyphylline

DILTIAZEM HYDROCHLORIDE—Cardizem®, Cardizem SR®, Cardizem CD®, Dilacor XR®, Tiazac®

Antianginal, antiarrhythmic, and antihypertensive agent.

Actions and Uses: Is a calcium-channel-blocking agent that is indicated in the treatment of (1) angina pectoris due to coronary artery spasm; (2)

chronic stable angina in patients who cannot tolerate therapy with beta blockers and/or nitrates or who remain symptomatic despite adequate doses of these agents; (3) hypertension Cardizem SR, Cardizem CD, Dilacor XR); (4) atrial fibrillation or flutter (intravenously); and (5) paroxysmal supraventricular tachycardia (intravenously).

Warnings: Contraindicated in patients with sick sinus syndrome (except in the presence of a functioning ventricular pacemaker), second- or third-degree AV block, and hypotension. Adverse reactions include edema, headache, nausea, dizziness, and rash. Although usually well tolerated, concomitant therapy with a beta-adrenergic blocking agent or digitalis glycoside should be monitored closely because there may be additive effects in prolonging AV conduction.

Administration: Oral and intravenous.

Preparations: Tablets, 30, 60, 90, and 120 mg. Sustained-release capsules, 60, 90, and 120 mg (Cardizem SR); 180, 240, and 300 mg (Cardizem CD); 180 and 240 mg (Dilacor XR); 120, 180, 240, 300, and 360 (Tiazac). Vials, 25 and 50 mg.

DIMENHYDRINATE—Dramamine®

Antinauseant/antiemetic indicated for the prevention and treatment of the nausea, vomiting, or vertigo of motion sickness. When used for prophylaxis of motion sickness, administer at least 30 minutes and preferably 1–2 hr before exposure to conditions that may precipitate motion sickness.

Preparations: Tablets and capsules, 50 mg. Extended-release capsules, 25 mg. Chewable tablets, 50 mg. Liquid, 12.5 mg/4 ml. Elixir, 12.5 mg/5 ml and 15 mg/5 ml. Ampules and vials, 50 mg/ml. Suppositories, 50 mg.

DIMERCAPROL—BAL

Antidote indicated in the parenteral treatment of arsenic, gold, and mercury poisoning. As an adjunct with edetate calcium disodium in the treatment of severe lead poisoning accompanied by encephalopathy.

Preparation: Ampules, 100 mg/ml.

DIMETANE®, see Brompheniramine

DIMETHYL SULFOXIDE—Rimso-50®, DMSO

Agent for symptomatic relief of interstitial cystitis and is instilled directly into the bladder. Is being evaluated for the topical treatment of conditions such as scleroderma and a wide range of musculoskeletal disorders. Also used to protect living cells and tissues during cold storage (cryoprotection).

Preparation: Aqueous solution, 50%.

DINOPROST TROMETHAMINE—Prostaglandin F_2 alpha, Prostin F2 alpha®

Abortifacient injected into the amniotic sac for the termination of pregnancy during the period from 16 to 20 gestational weeks.

Preparation: Ampules, 5 mg/ml.

DINOPROSTONE—Prostaglandin E_2, Cervidil®, Prepidil®,Prostin E2®

Abortifacient (Prostin E2) indicated for intravaginal use for the termination of pregnancy during the period from 12 to 20 gestational weeks. Used for the evacuation of the uterine content in the management of missed abortion or intrauterine fetal death up to 28 weeks gestational age. Indicated in the management of nonmetastatic gestational trophoblastic disease (benign hydatiform mole).

Agent for cervical ripening (Cervidil®, Prepidil®) used to ripen an unfavorable cervix in pregnant women at or near term with a medical or obstetrical need for labor induction.

Preparation: Vaginal suppositories (Prostin E2), 20 mg. Gel (Prepidil), 0.5 mg. Vaginal insert (Cervidil®), 10 mg.

DIOVAN®, see Valsartan

DIOVAN HCT®—Combination agent valsartan and hydrochlorothiaride (angiotensin II recrptor antagonist and diuretic)

DIPENTUM®, see Olsalazine sodium

DIPHENHYDRAMINE HYDROCHLORIDE—Benadryl®, Benylin cough®, Nytol®, Sominex®

Antihistamine, hypnotic, and antitussive used in the treatment of various allergic disorders, management of cough, treatment of insomnia, prevention of motion sickness, and drug-induced Parkinson's Disease or dystonic reactions.

Preparations: Capsules and tablets, 25 and 50 mg. Chewable tablets, 25 mg. Liquid, 12.5 mg/5 ml. Ampules and vials, 10 and 50 mg/ml. Cream and gel, 1%, 2%. Spray, 1%.

DIPHENATOL, see Diphenoxylate hydrochloride with atropine sulfate

DIPHENIDOL—Vontrol®

Antiemetic indicated in the treatment of peripheral vertigo and associated nausea and vomiting, and in the control of nausea and vomiting as seen in conditions such as postoperative states, malignant neoplasms, and labyrinthe disturbances.

Preparation: Tablets, 25 mg.

DIPHENOXYLATE HYDROCHLORIDE WITH ATROPINE SULFATE—Lomotil®, Diphenatol®, Lofene®, Lomanate®, Lonox®, Lo-Trol®, Low Qual®, Nor-Mil®

Antidiarrheal.

Actions and Uses: Diphenoxylate is structurally related to meperidine. Indicated as adjunctive therapy in the management of diarrhea.

Warnings: Contraindicated in patients with obstructive jaundice, and in diarrhea associated with pseudomembranous enterocolitis. Adverse reactions include drowsiness and other CNS effects; patients should be cautioned regarding activities such as driving and operating machinery, as well as interactions with other CNS-acting drugs including alcohol. Effects attributed to the atropine include dry mouth. Use is not recommended for children under 2 years of age because of an increased risk of adverse reactions. Should not be administered to patients being treated with a monoamine oxidase inhibitor. Is included in Schedule V.

Administration: Oral.

Preparations: Tablets and liquid. Each tablet and 5 ml of liquid contains 2.5 mg and 0.025 mg atropine sulfate.

DIPHENYLHYDANTOIN—former name for Phenytoin

DIPIVEFRIN HYDROCHLORIDE—Propine®

Sympathomimetic agent. A prodrug that is converted to epinephrine following administration. Indicated for ophthalmic use in the treatment of chronic open angle glaucoma.

Preparation: Ophthalmic solution, 0.1%.

DIPRIVAN®, see Propofol

DIPROLENE®, see Betamethasone dipropionate augmented

DIPROLENE AF®, see Betamethasone dipropionate augmented

DIPROSONE®, see Betamethasone dipropionate

DIPYRIDAMOLE—Persantine®, Persantine IV®

Agent to prevent postoperative thromboembolic complications.

Actions and Uses: Indicated as an adjunct to coumarin anticoagulants in the prevention of postoperative thromboembolic complications of cardiac valve replacement. Also indicated for intravenous use as an alternative to exercise in thallium myocardial perfusion imaging for the evaluation of coronary artery disease in patients who cannot exercise regularly.

Warnings: Adverse reactions include dizziness, abdominal distress, headache, and rash.

Administration: Oral and intravenous.

Preparations: Tablets, 25, 50, and 75 mg.Ampules, 10 mg/2 ml.

DIRITHROMYCIN—Dynabac®

Antiinfective agent. Macrolide antibiotic indicated in the treatment of mild to moderate susceptible infections including acute and chronic bronchitis, secondary bacterial infection of acute bronchitis, community acquired pneumonia, pharyngitis/tonsillitis, uncomplicated skin and skin structure infections. Should not be used in patients with bacteremia.

Warnings: Adverse reactions include abdominal pain, headache, GI upset, dizziness, pain, asthenia, cough, rash, dyspnea, pruritus, insomnia, blood dyscrasias, electrolyte imbalance and pseudomembranous colitis.

Administration: Oral. Take with food. Do not crush, chew, or cut.

Preparations: Enteric-coated tablets, 250 mg.

DISALCID®, see Salsalate

DISODIUM EDTA®, see Edetate

DISOPYRAMIDE PHOSPHATE—Norpace®, Norpace CR®

Antiarrhythmic agent indicated for the prevention

and suppression of premature ventricular contractions, and episodes of ventricular tachycardia.

Preparations: Capsules and controlled-release capsules, 100 and 150 mg.

DISOTATE, see Edetate

DI-SPAZ®, see Dicyclomine

DISULFIRAM—Antabuse®

Agent for alcoholism indicated as an aid in the management of selected chronic alcoholic patients who want to remain in a state of enforced sobriety.

Preparations: Tablets, 250 and 500 mg.

DITHRANOL, see Anthralin

DITROPAN®, see Oxybutynin

DIUCARDIN®, see Hydroflumethiazide

DIURIL®, see Chlorothiazide

DIVALPROEX SODIUM, see Valproic acid

DMSO®, see Dimethyl sulfoxide

DOAN'S PILLS®, see Magnesium salicylate

DOBUTAMINE HYDROCHLORIDE—Dobutrex®

Inotropic catecholamine indicated in the short-term intravenous treatment of adults with cardiac decompensation due to depressed contractility resulting either from organic heart disease or from cardiac surgical procedures.

Preparation: Vials, 250 mg.

DOBUTREX®, see Dobutamine hydrochloride

DOCETAXEL—Taxotere®

Antineoplastic Agent.

Actions and Uses: Antineoplastic agent used in the treatment of patients with locally advanced or metastatic breast cancer who have progressed during anthracyline-based adjuvant therapy.

Warnings: Contraindicated in patients with history of severe hypersensitivity reactions to docetaxel or to other drugs formulated with polysorbate 80 or neutrophil counts < 1,500 cells/mm^3. Toxic deaths have occurred when docetaxel was administered at doses of 100 mg/m^2 in patients with and without impaired liver function. Sepsis accounted for the majority of these deaths. Fatal G.I. bleeds in patients with severe liver impairment has been associated with drug-induced thrombocytopenia. Fluid retention, neutropenia, and cutaneous reactions have also been reported with docetaxel. Careful monitoring of blood counts, liver, and renal functions is recommended.

Administration: 60–100 mg/m^2 I.V. over 1 hour every 3 weeks. Premedicate patients with oral corticosteroids.

Preparations: Injection, 20 and 80 mg in single dose vials with diluent.

DOCUSATE CALCIUM—Dioctyl calcium sulfosuccinate, Surfak®

DOCUSATE POTASSIUM—Dioctyl potassium sulfosuccinate

DOCUSATE SODIUM—DSS, Dioctyl sodium sulfosuccinate, Colace®

Stool softener used in the treatment of constipation due to hard stools.

Preparations: Docusate calcium—Capsules, 50 and 240 mg. Docusate potassium—Capsules, 100 and 240 mg. Docusate sodium—Capsules, 50, 100, and 240 mg. Liquid, 50, 60, and 150 mg/ml and other potencies.

DOLOBID®, see Diflunisal

DOLOPHINE®, see Methadone

DONEPEZIL HYDROCHLORIDE—Aricept®

Reversible acetylcholinesterase inhibitor. Indicated in mild to moderate dementia of the Alzheimer's type.

Warnings: Adverse reactions include nausea, diarrhea, insomnia, vomiting, muscle cramps, fatigue and anorexia. Use cautiously in patients with sick sinus syndrome or other supraventricular cardiac conduction conditions. Monitor for G.I. bleeding, seizures, and asthma.

Administration: Initially 5 mg daily at bedtime; may increase to 10 mg daily at bedtime after 4–6 weeks.

Preparation: Tablets, 5 and 10 mg.

DONNATAL®, Combination of belladonna alkaloids and phenobarbital

DOPAMINE HYDROCHLORIDE—Intropin®

Inotropic catecholamine indicated for intravenous use in the correction of hemodynamic imbalances present in the shock syndrome due to myocardial infarctions, trauma, endotoxic septicemia, open heart surgery, renal failure, and chronic cardiac decompensation as in congestive failure.

Preparations: Ampules, vials, and syringes, 40, 80, and 160 mg/ml. Bottles (in 5% dextrose), 80, 160, and 320 mg/100 ml.

DOPAR®, see Levodopa

DORIGLUTE®, see Glutethimide

DOPRAM®, see Doxapram

DORAL®, see Quazepam

DORNASE ALFA—Pulmozyme®

Agent for cystic fibrosis, mucolytic.

Actions and Uses: Is a recombinant form of natural human deoxyribonuclease I (also known as DNase), and contains 260 amino acids in a sequence that is identical to that of the native human enzyme. Is administered by inhalation of an aerosol mist and selectively breaks down extracellular DNA, making the accumulated respiratory secretions less viscous and easier to clear. Indicated for daily use in conjunction with standard therapies, in the management of cystic fibrosis patients to reduce the frequency of respiratoryinfections requiring parenteral antibiotics, and to improve pulmonary function.

Warnings: Adverse reactions include sore throat, horseness, laryngitis, chest pain, rash, and conjunctivitis.

Administration: Inhalation, using a recommended nebulizer. The drug should not be diluted or mixed with other drugs in the nebulizer.

Preparation: Ampules, 2.5 mg in 2.5 ml of a sterile aqueous solution.

DORYX®, see Doxycycline

DORZOLAMIDE HYDROCHLORIDE—Trusopt®

Antiglaucoma agent.

Actions and Uses: Corbonic hydrase inhibitor indicated in the treatment of elevated intraocular pressure in patients with ocular hypertension or open-angle glaucoma.

Warnings: Adverse reactions include ocular burning, stinging, or discomfort and bitter taste following administration. Superficial punctate keratitis, and signs and symptoms of ocular allergic reaction may also occur. Use is not recommended in patients with a creatinine clearance of less than 30 ml/min or concurrently with orally administered carbonic anhydrase inhibitor. Do not administer while wearing soft contact lenses, as the formulation contains benzalkonium chloride as a preservative, which may damage soft contact lenses.

Administration: Ophthalmic. One drop in the affected eye(s) three times daily. Administer at least 10 minutes apart from other ophthalmic drugs.

Preparations: Ophthalmic solution, 2%.

DOSTINEX®, see Cabergoline

DOVONEX®, see Calcipotriene

DOXACURIUM CHLORIDE—Nuromax®

Nondepolarizing neuromuscular blocking agent.

Actions and Uses: Acts by competing for cholinergic receptors at the motor end-plate, resulting in a block of neuromuscular transmission. Has a long duration of action. Indicated as an adjunct to general anesthesia to provide skeletal muscle relaxation during surgery. Also used to provide skeletal muscle relaxation for endotracheal intubation.

Warnings: May cause excessive skeletal muscle weakness resulting in respiratory insufficiency and apnea. Action may be antagonized by neostigmine. Must be used with caution in patients with myasthenia gravis or myasthenic syndrome, and in patients receiving other medications that may increase neuromuscular blockade (e.g., inhalation anesthetics, aminoglycosides, quinidine, magnesium salts).

Administration: Intravenous.

Preparations: Vials, 1 mg/ml.

DOXAPRAM HYDROCHLORIDE—Dopram®

Respiratory stimulant indicated for intravenous use in the treatment of drug-induced central nervous system depression, chronic pulmonary disease associated with acute hypercapnia, and postanesthesia respiratory depression or apnea other than that due to muscle relaxant drugs.

Preparation: Vials, 20 mg/ml.

DOXAZOSIN MESYLATE—Cardura®

Antihypertensive agent.

Actions and Uses: An alpha$_1$-adrenergic blocking agent that acts on the peripheral vasculature to decrease systemic vascular resistance and lower blood pressure. Indicated for the treatment of hypertension and may be used alone or in combination with a diuretic or beta-adrenergic blocking agent. Also indicated for the treatment of benign prostatic hyperplasia.

Warnings: May cause orthostatic hypotension, resulting in symptoms such as dizziness, lightheadedness, vertigo, and syncope. Orthostatic effects are more common with the first dose (i.e., the "first-dose" effect). Treatment should be initiated at a dosage level of 1 mg daily. Patients should be advised of the need to sit or lie down when symptoms of lowered blood pressure occur, and to be careful when rising from a sitting or lying position. Other adverse reactions include edema, fatigue, and somnolence.

Administration: Oral.

Preparations: Tablets, 1, 2, 4, and 8 mg.

DOXEPIN HYDROCHLORIDE—Sinequan®, Zonalon®

Tricyclic antidepressant and antianxiety agent, and topical antipruritic.

Actions and Uses: Indicated in patients with (1) depression and/or anxiety, (2) depression and/or anxiety associated with alcoholism, (3) depression and/or anxiety associated with organic disease, and (4) psychotic depressive disorders with associated anxiety including involutional depression and manic-depressive disorders. Also indicated for the short-term topical management of moderate pruritus in adults with atopic dermatitis and lichen simplex chronicus.

Warnings: Contraindicated in patients with glaucoma or with a tendency to urinary retention. Should not be used in patients being treated with a monoamine oxidase inhibitor. Adverse reactions include CNS effects, and patients should be cautioned regarding activities such as driving and operating machinery, as well as interactions with other CNS-acting drugs including alcohol. Reportedly the most sedating of the tricyclic antidepressants. Other adverse reactions include anticholinergic effects (e.g., dry mouth, blurred vision), GI effects (e.g., nausea, vomiting), and cardiovascular effects (e.g., hypotension).

Administration: Oral and topical.

Preparations: Capsules, 10, 25, 50, 75, 100, and 150 mg. Oral concentrate, 10 mg/ml. Cream, 5%.

DOXORUBICIN HYDROCHLORIDE—Adriamycin PFS®, Adriamycin RDF®, Rubex®

Antineoplastic agent indicated for intravenous use in the treatment of a number of neoplastic disorders such as acute lymphoblastic leukemia, acute myeloblastic leukemia, Wilm's tumor, neuroblastoma, soft tissue and bone sarcomas, breast carcinoma, ovarian carcinoma, transitional cell bladder carcinoma, thyroid carcinoma, lymphomas of both Hodgkin and non-Hodgkin types, and bronchogenic carcinoma. Serious, irreversible myocar- dial toxicity with delayed CHF, ventricular arrhythmias and acute left ventricular failure may occur with use of this agent. Follow vesicant precautions for IV administration.

Preparations: Vials, 10, 20, and 50 mg.

DOXYCYCLINE CALCIUM—Vibramycin®

Preparation: Syrup, 50 mg/5 ml.

DOXYCYCLINE HYCLATE—Doryx®, Vibramycin®, Vibra-Tabs®

Tetracycline antibiotic.

Actions and Uses: Active against many gram-positive and gram-negative bacteria, mycoplasmal, chlamydial, and rickettsial organisms, and certain spirochetes. Indicated in the treatment of respiratory tract infections, urinary tract infections, sexually transmitted infections, and a number of other types of infections. Effective in the treatment of infections caused by *Chlamydia trachomatis* and *Ureaplasma urealyticum*. Also indicated for prophylaxis of malaria due to *Plasmodium falciparum* in short-term travelers (less than 4 months) to areas with chloroquine or pyrimethamine-sulfadoxine resistant strains.

Warnings: Use is best avoided during the last half of pregnancy and in childhood to the age of 8 years because of the risk of discoloration of the teeth. Other adverse reactions include nausea, vomiting, diarrhea, rash, and fungal superinfections. May cause photosensitivity reactions and patients should be cautioned to limit their exposure to sunlight and ultraviolet light. Absorption may be reduced by the simultaneous administration of antacids.

Administration: Oral and intravenous. May be administered orally without regard to meals.

Preparations: Capsules and tablets, 50 and 100 mg. Delayed-release capsules, 100 mg. Oral suspension, 25 mg/5 ml., and 50 mg/5 ml. Vials, 100 and 200 mg.

DOXYCYCLINE MONOHYDRATE—Monodox®, Vibramycin®

Preparations: Capsules, 100 mg. Powder for oral suspension, 25 mg/5 ml when reconstituted.

DOXYLAMINE SUCCINATE—Unisom®

Antihistamine and hypnotic. Primarily used for the treatment of insomnia.

Preparation: Tablets, 25 mg.

DRAMAMINE®, see Dimenhydrinate

DRISDOL®, see Ergocalciferol

DRONABINOL—Marinol®

Antiemetic and appetite stimulant.

Actions and Uses: Is the principal psychoactive substance in marijuana. Indicated for the treatment of nausea and vomiting associated with cancer chemotherapy in patients who have failed to respond adequately to conventional antiemetic treatments. Also indicated for the treatment of anorexia associated with weight loss in patients with AIDS.

Warnings: Can produce physical and psychological dependence and is included in Schedule II of the ControlledSubstances Act. CNS adverse reactions include drowsiness, dizziness, impairment of coordination, easy laughing, elation, hallucinations, and brief psychotic reactions.

Administration: Oral.

Preparations: Capsules, 2.5, 5, and 10 mg.

DROPERIDOL—Inapsine®

Neuroleptic agent indicated for parenteral use for (1) premedication, induction, and as an adjunct in the maintenance of general and regional anesthesia; (2) neuroleptanalgesia in conjunction with an opioid analgesic; and (3) to produce tranquilization and to induce the incidence of nausea and vomiting in surgical and diagnostic procedures.

Preparations: Ampules and vials, 2.5 mg/ml.

DTIC®, see Dacarbazine

DULCOLAX® see Bisacodyl

DURABOLIN®, see Nandrolone

DURAGESIC®, see Fentanyl

DURALUTIN®, see Hydroxyprogesterone

DURAMORPH®, see Morphine

DURANEST®, see Etidocaine

DURICEF®, see Cefadroxil

DYAZIDE®, Combination of triamterene and hydrochlorothiazide

DYCILL®, see Dicloxacillin

DYCLONE®, see Dyclonine

DYCLONINE HYDROCHLORIDE—Dyclone®

Local anesthetic used primarily for anesthetizing mucous membranes (e.g., mouth, pharynx) prior to endoscopic procedures. Also used to suppress gag reflex, to relieve pain of minor burns or trauma, and to alleviate itching of pruritis ani or vulvae.

Preparations: Topical solution, 0.5% and 1%.

DYFLEX®, see Dyphylline

DYLLINE®, see Dyphylline

DYMELOR®, see Acetohexamide

DYNABAC®, see Dirithromycin

DynaCirc®, see Isradipine

DYNAPEN®, see Dicloxacillin

DYPHYLLINE—Dilor®, Dyflex®, Dylline®, Lufyllin®, Neothylline, Thylline

Bronchodilator related to theophylline. Indicated for relief of acute bronchial asthma and for reversible bronchospasm associated with chronic bronchitis and emphysema.

Preparations: Tablets, 200 and 400 mg. Elixir, 33.3 mg/5 ml., 53.3 mg/5 ml, and 100 mg/15 ml. Injection, 250 mg/ml.

DYRENIUM®, see Triamterene

E

EASPRIN®, see Aspirin

ECHOTHIOPHATE IODIDE—Phospholine iodide®

Antiglaucoma agent, Cholinesterase inhibitor indicated for ophthalmic use in the treatment of glaucoma and accommodative esotropia. Use is usually reserved for patients not satisfactorily controlled by less potent miotics.

Preparations: For ophthalmic solution, 1.5 mg (0.03%), 3 mg (0.06%), 6.25 mg (0.125%), and 12.5 mg (0.25%) when reconstituted.

EC-NAPROSYN®, see Naproxen

ECONAZOLE NITRATE—Spectazole®

Imidazole antifungal agent indicated for topical use in the treatment of tinea pedis, tinea cruris, tinea corporis, cutaneous candidiasis, and tinea versicolor.

Preparation: Cream, 1%.

ECOTRIN®, see Aspirin

EDECRIN®, see Ethacrynic acid

EDETATE CALCIUM DISODIUM—EDTA, Calcium EDTA, Calcium disodium Versenate®

Antidote indicated in the parenteral management of acute and chronic lead poisoning and lead encephalopathy.

Preparation: Ampules, 200 mg/ml.

EDETATE DISODIUM—Disotate®, Disodium EDTA®, Endrate®

Indicated in selected patients for the emergency treatment of hypercalcemia and for the control of ventricular arrhythmias associated with digitalis toxicity.

Preparations: Ampules and vials, 150 mg/ml.

EDEX®, see alprostadil

EDROPHONIUM CHLORIDE—Enlon®, Tensilon®, Reversol®

Cholinesterase inhibitor administered parenterally for the differential diagnosis of myasthenia gravis and as an adjunct in the evaluation of treatment requirements in this disease. Also useful when a curare antagonist is needed to reverse the neuromuscular block produced by tubocurarine and related agents.

Preparations: Ampules and vials, 10 mg/ml.

EDTA, see Edetate calcium disodium

EES®, see Erythromycin ethylsuccinate

EFEDRON®, see Ephedrine

EFFEXOR®, see Venlafaxine hydrochloride

EFIDAC/24®, see Pseudoephedrine hydrochloride

EFUDEX®, see Fluorouracil

ELAVIL®, see Amitriptyline

ELASE®, see Fibrinolysin

ELDEPRYL®, see Selegiline

ELDOQUIN®, see Hydroquinone

ELMIRON®, see Pentosan Polysulfate Sodium

ELIMITE®, see Permethrin

ELIXOPHYLLIN®, see Theophylline

ELOCON®, see Mometasone furoate

ELSPAR®, see Asparaginase

ELTROXINE®, see Levothyroxine

EMCYT®, see Estramustine

EMINASE®, see Anistreplase

EMKO®, see Nonoxynol 9

EMLA®

Eutectic mixture of local anesthetics (lidocaine and prilocaine) that is applied topically. Apply thick layer of cream over selected site one hour prior to routine procedures and two hours prior to painful procedures. Cover with an occlusive dressing. Prior to procedure remove cream and cleanse area with antiseptic.

E-MYCIN®, see Erythromycin base

E-MYCIN 333®, see Erythromycin base

ENALAPRIL MALEATE—Vasotec®

Antihypertensive agent and agent for treatment of heart failure.

Actions and Uses: Is a prodrug that, after oral administration, is hydrolyzed to enalaprilat, a potent angiotensin-converting enzyme (ACE) inhibitor. Indicated for the treatment of hypertension and as adjunctive therapy in the management of heart failure, in patients who are not responding adequately to diuretics and digitalis. Also indicated for clinically stable asymptomatic patients with left ventricular dysfunction.

Warnings: Angioedema has occurred infrequently, sometimes after the first dose. Adverse reactions include headache, dizziness, fatigue, cough, proteinuria, and hyperkalemia. Excessive hypotension may occur, particularly in patients with severe salt/volume depletion (e.g., those being treated vigorously with diuretics). Use during pregnancy should be avoided.

Administration: Oral.

Preparations: Tablets, 2.5, 5, 10, and 20 mg.

ENALAPRILAT—Vasotec IV®, see discussion of enalapril.

Administration: Intravenous.

Preparation: Vials, 1.25 mg/ml.

ENDRATE®, see Edetate disodium

ENDURON®, see Methyclothiazide

ENFLURANE—Ethrane®

General anesthetic administered by inhalation in the induction and maintenance of general anesthesia.

Preparations: Bottles, 125 and 250 ml.

ENLON®, see Edrophonium

ENOXACIN—Penetrex®

Fluoroquinolone anti-infective agent.

Actions and Uses: Inhibits DNA gyrase, an essential bacterial enzyme, and exhibits a bactericidal action against many gram-positive and gram-negative bacteria. Indicated for urinary tract infections caused by susceptible organisms. Also indicated for uncomplicated urethral or cervical gonorrhea.

Warnings: Contraindicated in patients with a known hypersensitivity to any of the fluoroquinolones or the related quinolone antibacterial agents (i.e., nalidixic acid, cinoxacin). Fluoroquinolones have caused erosion of cartilage in weight-bearing joints and other signs of arthropathy in juvenile animals, and use in children under 18, pregnant women, and women who are nursing is best avoided. Adverse reactions include nausea and/or vomiting, abdominal pain, diarrhea, dyspepsia, dizziness, and headache. Because of the possibility of photosensitivity reactions, patients should be advised to avoid excessive sunlight and artificial ultraviolet light during the period of treatment. May cause dizziness, lightheadedness, and other central nervous system effects, and patients should know how they tolerate the drug before they engage in activities that require mental alertness and coordination.

Administration: Oral. Should be administered at least one hour before or two hours after a meal.

Preparations: Tablets, 200 and 400 mg.

ENOXAPARIN—Lovenox®

Antithrombotic agent.

Actions and Uses: Is a low molecular weight heparin fraction that is prepared by the degradation of heparin benzyl ester derived from porcine intestinal mucosa. Does not significantly influence platelet aggregation or the plasma fibrinogen concentration, and does not affect global blood clotting tests [i.e., prothrombin time (PT) or activated partial thromboplastin time (APTT)]. Indicated for the prevention of deep vein thrombosis (DVT) following hip replacement surgery and knee replacement surgery.

Warnings: Contraindicated in patients who are hypersensitive to the drug, heparin, or pork products. Also contraindicated in patients with active major bleeding and in patients with thrombocytopenia associated with a positive in vitro test for anti-platelet antibody in the presence of enoxaparin. May cause bleeding episodes although the incidence of such reactions was similar to that with placebo in the clinical studies. Should be used with extreme caution in patients with conditions that are associated with an increased risk of hemorrhage (e.g., congenital or acquired bleeding disorders, active ulceration or a history of recent gastrointestinal ulceration and hemorrhage, uncontrolled arterial hypertension, and hemorrhagic stroke). May cause thrombocytopenia. Periodic complete blood counts, including platelet count, and stool occult blood tests should be conducted during the course of treatment with enoxaparin.

Administration: Subcutaneous. The initial dose should be given as soon as possible after surgery, but not more than 24 hours post-operatively. The average duration of administration is 7 to 10 days. Must not be administered by intramuscular injection.

Preparations: Prefilled syringes, 30 mg.

ENTEX LA®, Combination of phenylpropanolamine and guaifenesin

ENVISAN®, see Dextranomer

EPHEDRINE HYDROCHLORIDE—Efedron®

Nasal decongestant often used in combination with other agents. See also pseudoephedrine. Has also been used as a central nervous system stimulant to counteract the depressant effect of certain other agents with which it may be used in combination.

Preparations: Capsules, 25 and 50 mg.

EPHEDRINE SULFATE

Pressor agent administered parenterally in the management of hypotensive states.

Preparations: Ampules, 25 and 50 mg/ml.

EPI E-Z PEN®, see Epinephrine

EPINEPHRINE—Adrenalin®, Bronkaid mist®, Epinephrine Pediatric®, Epi E-Z Pen®, Epipen AutoInjector®, Primatene Mist Suspension®

Sympathomimetic agent used to relieve respiratory distress due to bronchospasm, to provide rapid relief of hypersensitivity reactions to drugs and other allergens, to restore cardiac rhythm in cardiac arrest due to various causes, and to prolong the action of infiltration anesthetics. Also used in the treatment of mucosal congestion of hay fever and rhinitis, to relieve bronchial asthmatic paroxysms, for symptomatic relief of serum sickness, urticaria, and angioneurotic edema, for the management of glaucoma and other ocular conditions, and selected other disorders.

Preparations: Ampules and vials (as the hydrochloride), 1:1000, 1:10,000, and 1:100,000. Solution for nebulization (as the hydrochloride), 1.25% and 2.25%. Aerosol, 0.2 and 0.27 mg per spray. Aerosol (as the bitartrate), 0.16 mg per spray. Solution for nasal administration (as the hydrochloride), 0.1%. Ophthalmic solution (as the bitartrate, borate, and hydrochloride), 0.1%, 0.25%, 0.5%, 1%, and 2%. Autoinjector syringes, 0.3 mg and 0.15 mg.

EPIPEN AUTOINJECTOR®—see Epinephrine

EPIVIR®—see Lamivudine

EPO, see Epoetin alfa

EPOETIN ALFA—EPO, Epogen®, Procrit®

Agent for anemia.

Actions and Uses: Also known as recombinant human erythropoietin or EPO. Stimulates red blood cell production in anemic patients decreasing the need for transfusions in these patients. Indicated in the treatment for anemia associated with chronic renal failure, management of anemia secondary to zidovudine (AZT) therapy in HIV-infected patients, and the management of anemia from chemotherapy in patients with nonmyeloid malignancies.

Warnings: Contraindicated in patients with uncontrolled hypertension. Adverse reactions include hypertension, headache, arthralgias, nausea, vomiting, diarrhea, and seizures. For patients who respond to epoetin alfa with a rapid increase in hematocrit (e.g., more than 4 points in any 2-week period), the dose should be decreased to reduce the risk of hypertension. Because of the risk of seizures, patients should be cautioned to avoid potentially hazardous activities such as driving or operating machinery. During hemodialysis, patients treated with epoetin alfa may require increased anticoagulation with heparin to prevent clotting of the artificial kidney.

Administration: Intravenous or subcutaneous. In patients on dialysis, epoetin alfa is usually administered as an intravenous bolus and, in patients with chronic renal failure not on dialysis, the drug is given by intravenous or subcutaneous injection. The vials should not be shaken as shaking may denature the glycoprotein, rendering it biologically inactive.

Preparations: Vials, 2,000, 3,000, 4,000, and 10,000 units.

EPOGEN®, see Epoetin alfa

EPOPROSTENOL—Flolan®, Prostacyclin®, Prostaglandin 12 (PG 12)®, Prostaglandin X (PGX)®

Prostaglandin, vasodilator.

Actions andUses: Directly dilates pulmonary and systemic arterial vasculature. Also inhibits platelet aggregation. Indicated in the management of primary pulmonary hypertension in selected patients.

Warnings: Side effects include headache, anxiety, dizziness, tachycardia, nausea, vomiting, flushing, myalgia, hypesthesia, hyperesthesia/ paresthesia, and flulike symptoms. Dosage adjustments may be necessary in geriatric patients. Unless contraindicated concurrent anticoagulant therapy is usually administered to decrease the risk of pulmonary or systemic embolism.

Administration: Intravenously via continuous infusion.

Preparation: Powder for injection, 0.5-mg and 1.5-mg vials.

EQUALACTIN®, see Polycarbophil

EQUANIL®, see Meprobamate

ERGAMISOL®, see Levamisole

ERGOCALCIFEROL—Vitamin D_2, Drisdol®

A form of Vitamin D indicated in the treatment of rickets, familial hypophosphatemia, hypoparathyroidism, osteomalacia, anticonvulsant induced rickets, osteoporosis, and renal osteodystrophy.

Preparations: Capsules, 25,000 and 50,000 IU. Liquid, 8,000 IU/ml. Ampules, 500,000 IU/ml and 500,000 IU/5 ml.

ERGOLOID MESYLATES—Hydergine®

Ergot derivatives indicated in patients over 60 years of age who manifest signs and symptoms of an idiopathic decline in mental capacity (i.e., cognitive and interpersonal skills, mood).

Preparations: Sublingual tablets, 0.5 and 1 mg. Capsules (liquid) and tablets, 1 mg. Liquid, 1 mg/ml.

ERGOMETRINE, see Ergonovine

ERGONOVINE MALEATE—Ergometrine®, Ergotrate®

Ergot derivative indicated for the prevention and treatment of postpartum and postabortal hemorrhage due to uterine atony.

Preparations: Tablets, 0.2 mg. Ampules, 0.2 mg/ml.

ERGOSTAT®, see Ergotamine

ERGOTAMINE TARTRATE—Ergostat®

Ergot derivative indicated to abort or prevent vascular headache such as migraine and cluster.

Preparations: Sublingual tablets, 2 mg, tablets, 1 mg.

ERGOTRATE®, see Ergonovine

ERYC®, see Erythromycin base

ERYCETTE®, see Erythromycin base (topical)

EryDerm®, see Erythromycin base (topical)

ERYGEL®, see Erythromycin base (topical)

ERYMAX®, see Erythromycin base (topical)

ERYPED®, see Erythromycin ethylsuccinate

ERY-TAB®, see Erythromycin base

ERYTHRITYL TETRANITRATE—Cardilate®

Antianginal agent indicated for the prophylaxis and treatment of patients with frequent or recurrent anginal pain.

Preparations: Oral/sublingual tablets, 10 mg.

ERYTHROMYCIN BASE—E-Mycin®, E-Mycin 333®, Ery-Tab®, Ilotycin®, Robimycin®, ERYC®, PCE®

Macrolide antibiotic.

Actions and Uses: Active against most gram-positive and a number of gram-negative bacteria, mycoplasmal and chlamydial organisms, and certain spirochetes. Indicated in the treatment of respiratory tract and a number of other types of infections. Effective in the treatment of primary atypical pneumonia, Legionnaires' disease, infections caused by *Chlamydia trachomatis* and *Ureaplasma urealyticum,* and GI infections caused by *Campylobacter jejuni.* Used with neomycin for prophylaxis in colorectal surgery.

Warnings: Adverse reactions include nausea, vomiting, abdominal cramps, and hepatic dysfunction (primarily associated with the use of the estolate). Should not be used concurrently with terfenadine or astemizole.

Administrationn: Oral. Some formulationsmay be administered without regard to meals whereas others should be administered apart from meals. Labeling for individual product should be consulted.

Preparations: Enteric-coated tablets, 250, 333, and 500 mg. Capsules with enteric-coated pellets (ERYC), 125 and 250 mg. Tablets with polymer-coated particles (PCE), 333 and 500 mg. Film-coated tablets, 250 and 500 mg.

ERYTHROMYCIN BASE (for topical use)—Akne-mycin®, Erycette®, EryDerm®, Erygel®, Erymax®, Staticin®

Antibiotic for the topical treatment of acne.

Administration: Topical.

Preparations: Solution, 1.5% and 2%. Gel, 2%.

ERYTHROMYCIN ESTOLATE—Ilosone®

See discussion of erythromycin base.

Administration: Oral. May be administered without regard to meals.

Preparations: Capsules, 250 mg. Tablets, 500 mg. Suspension, 125 and 250 mg/5 ml.

ERYTHROMYCIN ETHYLSUCCINATE—EES®,EryPed®

See discussion of erythromycin base.

Administration: Oral. May be administered without regard to meals.

Preparations: Suspension, 200 and 400 mg/5 ml. Powder for oral suspension, 200 and 400 mg/5 ml when reconstituted. Tablets, 400 mg. Chewable tablets, 200 mg.

ERYTHROMYCIN GLUCEPTATE—Ilotycin gluceptate®

See discussion of erythromycin base.

Administration: Intravenous. Pain, discomfort, and phlebitis may be associated with IV administration.

Preparations: Vials, 250 and 500 mg, 1g.

ERYTHROMYCIN LACTOBIONATE

See discussion of erythromycin base.

Administration: Intravenous. Pain, discomfort, and phlebitis may be associated with IV administration.

Preparations: Vials, 500 mg, 1 g.

ERYTHROMYCIN STEARATE

See discussion of erythromycin base.

Administration: Oral. Should be administered apart from meals.

Preparations: Tablets, 250 and 500 mg.

ERYTHROPOIETIN, see Epoetin alfa

ESERINE, see Physostigmine

ESGIC-PLUS—Combination barbituate and analgesic. Butalbital, Acetaminophen, and Caffeine.

ESIDRIX®, see Hydrochlorothiazide

ESKALITH®, see Lithium carbonate

ESMOLOL HYDROCHLORIDE—Brevibloc®

Antiarrhythmic agent.

Actions and Uses: A beta-adrenergic blocking agent indicated for the rapid control of ventricular rate in patients with atrial fibrillation or atrial flutter in perioperative, postoperative, or other emergent circumstances where short-term control of ventricular rate with a short-acting agent is desirable. Also indicated in noncompensatory sinus tachycardia, where the rapid heart rate requires specific intervention.

Warnings: Contraindicated in patients with sinus bradycardia, heart block greater than first degree, cardiogenic shock, or overt heart failure. Hypotension is the most important adverse reaction, and some patients experience manifestations such as dizziness and diaphoresis. Other adverse reactions include peripheral ischemia, sedation, agitation, nausea, and local reactions at the infusion site; to reduce the incidence of venous irritation and thrombophlebitis, infusion concentrations greater than 10 mg/ml should be avoided. Therapy must be closely monitored in patients with bronchospastic diseases. It must also be used with caution in diabetic patients.

Administration: Intravenous infusion.

Preparation: Ampules, 10 mg/ml, 250 mg/ml.

ESTAZOLAM—ProSom®

Benzodiazepine hypnotic.

Actions and Uses: Usually initiates sleep within 15 to 30 minutes following administration and action continued for an average of 6 to 8 hours. Classified as an intermediate-acting benzodiazepine hypnotic. Indicated for the short-term management of insomnia characterized by difficulty in falling asleep, frequent nocturnal awakenings, and/or early morning awakenings.

Warnings: Contraindicated in pregnancy. Adverse reactions include daytime sedation, hypokinesia, dizziness, and abnormal coordination. Patients should be cautioned regarding activities such as driving and operating machinery, as well as interactions with other CNS-acting drugs including alcohol. Can cause dependence and is included in Schedule IV.

Administration: Oral.

Preparations: Tablets, 1 and 2 mg.

ESTINYL®, see Ethinyl Estradiol

ESTRACE®, see Estradiol

ESTRADERM®, see Estradiol

ESTRADIOL—Alora®, Climara®, Estrace®, Estraderm®, Estring®, Vivelle®

Estrogen indicated in the treatment of moderate to severe vasomotor symptoms associated with the menopause, atrophic vaginitis, kraurosis vulvae, female hypogonadism, female castration, primary ovarian failure, breast cancer, and prostatic cancer. Transdermal system is also indicated for postmenopausal osteoporosis. Remove vaginal ring when treating vaginal infections and during treatment with other vaginally-administered preparations.

Preparations: Tablets, 1 and 2 mg. Transdermal systems, 0.0375 mg, 0.05 mg, 0.075 mg, 0.1 mg, 4 and 8 mg. Vaginal cream, 0.1 mg/g. Vaginal ring (Estring®) 2 mg Estradiol/90 days.

ESTRADIOL CYPIONATE—Depo-Estradiol cypionate®

See discussion of estradiol.

Preparations: Vials (for intramuscular administration), 1 mg/ml and 5 mg/ml.

ESTRADIOL VALERATE—Delestrogen®

See discussion of estradiol.

Preparations: Vials (for intramuscular administration), 10 mg/ml, 20 mg/ml, and 40 mg/ml.

ESTRAMUSTINE PHOSPHATE SODIUM—Emcyt®

Antineoplastic agent indicated in the treatment of metastatic and/or progressive carcinoma of the prostate.

Preparation: Capsules, 140 mg.

ESTROGENS, CONJUGATED—Premarin®

Estrogen.

Actions and Uses: Indicated in the treatment of (1) moderate-to-severe vasomotor symptoms associated with the menopause, and (2) osteoporosis in postmenopausal women. Intravenous dosage form is indicated in the treatment of abnormal uterine bleeding due to hormonal imbalance in the absence of organic pathology. Vaginal cream is indicated in the treatment of atrophic vaginitis and kraurosis vulvae.

Warnings: Contraindicated (1) during pregnancy; (2) in patients with known or suspected cancer of the breast, except in appropriately selected patients being treated for metastatic disease; (3) in patients with known or suspected estrogen-dependent neoplasia; (4) in patients with undiagnosed abnormal genital bleeding; (5) in patients with thrombophlebitis or thromboembolic disorders; and (6) in patients with a past history of thrombophlebitis, thrombosis, or thromboembolic disorders associated with previous estrogen use (except when used in treatment of breast or prostatic malignancy). Estrogens have been reported to increase the risk of endometrial carcinoma. Adverse reactions include thromboembolic effects, increased incidence of gallbladder disease, edema, headache, nausea, vomiting, abdominal cramps, tenderness and enlargement of the breasts, and genitourinary effects.

Administration: Oral, intravenous, and vaginal.

Preparations: Tablets, 0.3, 0.625, 0.9, 1.25, and 2.5 mg. Vials, 25 mg. Vaginal cream, 0.625 mg/g.

ESTROGENS, ESTERIFIED—Menest®

Estrogen indicated for moderate to severe vasomotor symptoms of menopause, atrophic vaginitis, kraurosis vulvae, female hypogonadism, female castration, primary ovarian failure, prostatic carcinoma, and breast cancer.

Preparations: Tablets, 0.3, 0.625, 1.25, and 2.5 mg.

ESTRONE—Theelin®

Estrogen indicated for intramuscular use for moderate to severe vasomotor symptoms associated with the menopause, atrophic vaginitis, kraurosis vulvae, female hypogonadism, female castration, primary ovarian failure, and prostatic carcinoma.

Preparations: Vials, 2 mg/ml and 5 mg/ml.

ESTROPIPATE—Piperazine estrone sulfate, Ogen®

Estrogen indicated for moderate to severe vasomotor symptoms of menopause, atrophic vaginitis, kraurosis vulvae, female hypogonadism, female castration, primary ovarian failure, and postmenopausal osteoporosis.

Preparations: Tablets, 0.625, 1.25, 2.5, and 5 mg (equivalent, respectively to 0.75, 1..5, 3, and 6 mg estropipate). Vaginal cream, 1.5 mg/g.

ESTROSTEP 21®—Oral contraceptive with progestin & estrogen. Also, Estrostep®.

ESTROVIS®, see Quinestrol

ETHACRYNIC ACID—Edecrin®

Diuretic indicated for the treatment of edema associated with various conditions including the nephrotic syndrome, the short-term management of ascites, the short-term management of hospitalized pediatric patients with congenital heart disease or the nephrotic syndrome, and, intravenously, when a rapid onset of diuresis is desired.

Preparations: Tablets, 25 and 50 mg. Vials (using ethacrynate sodium), 50 mg.

ETHAMBUTOL HYDROCHLORIDE—Myambutol®

Antitubercular agent indicated in the treatment of tuberculosis or other mycobacterial diseases in conjunction with at least one other antitubercular drug.

Preparations: Tablets, 100 and 400 mg.

ETHAMOLIN®, see Ethanolamine oleate

ETHANOLAMINE OLEATE—Ethamolin®

Sclerosing agent.

Actions and Uses: Acts primarily by irritation of the intimal endothelium of the vein and produces a sterile inflammatory response which results in fibrosis and occlusion of the vein. Indicated for the treatment of patients with esophageal varices that have recently bled, to prevent rebleeding.

Warnings: Adverse reactions include pleural effusion/infiltration, esophageal ulcer, pyrexia, retrosternal pain, esophageal stricture, and pneumonia. Anaphylactic reactions have occurred infrequently.

Administration: Intravenous (directly into the varix). The maximum total dose per treatment session should not exceed 20 ml or 0.4 ml/kg for a 50 kg patient. To obliterate the varix, injections may be made at the time of the acute bleeding episode and then after 1 week, 6 weeks, 3 months, and 6 months as indicated.

Preparation: Ampules, 5%.

ETHAQUIN®, see Ethautrine

ETHATAB®, see Ethaverine

ETHAVERINE HYDROCHLORIDE—Ethaquin®, Ethatab®, Ethavex-100®, Isovex®

Peripheral vasodilator indicated in the management of peripheral and cerebral vascular insufficiency associated with arterial spasm. Also used as a smooth muscle spasmolytic in spastic conditions of the gastrointestinal and genitourinary tracts.

Preparation: Tablets, 100 mg.

ETHAVEX-100®, see Ethaverine

ETHCHLORVYNOL—Placidyl®

Hypnotic indicated for short-term use in the management of insomnia for periods of up to one week.

Preparations: Capsules, 200, 500, and 750 mg.

ETHER

General anesthetic administered by inhalation to produce anesthesia.

Preparation: Liquid.

ETHINYL ESTRADIOL—Estinyl®

Estrogen indicated in the treatment of moderate to severe vasomotor symptoms associated with the menopause, female hypogonadism, prostatic carcinoma, and breast cancer in appropriately selected women. Also used as the estrogen component of many oral contraceptive formulations.

Preparation: Tablets, 0.02, 0.05, and 0.5 mg.

ETHIONAMIDE—Trecator-SC®

Antitubercular agent indicated in the treatment of tuberculosis in conjunction with other drugs after failure of treatment with the primary antitubercular agents.

Preparation: Tablets, 250 mg.

ETHMOZINE®, see Moricizine

ETHOPROPAZINE HYDROCHLORIDE—Parsidol®

Antiparkinson agent indicated in the treatment of parkinsonism and to control extrapyramidal reactions due todrugs such as the pheno-thiazines.

Preparations: Tablets, 10 and 50 mg.

ETHOSUXIMIDE—Zarontin®

Anticonvulsant indicated in the treatment of absence (petit mal) epilepsy, myocolonic seizures, and akinetic epilepsy.

Preparations: Capsules, 250 mg. Syrup, 250 mg/5 ml.

ETHOTOIN—Peganone®

Anticonvulsant indicated for the control of tonic-clonic (grand mal) and complex partial (psychomotor) seizures.

Preparations: Tablets, 250 and 500 mg.

ETHRANE®, see Enflurane

ETHYL ALCOHOL, see Alcohol

ETHYL AMINOBENZOATE, see Benzocaine

ETHYL CHLORIDE

Local anesthetic used to provide local anesthesia and analgesia when sprayed on the skin.

Preparation: Topical spray.

ETHYLENE

General anesthetic administered by inhalation to produce anesthesia.

Preparation: Gas.

ETHYLNOREPINEPHRINE HYDROCHLORIDE—Bronkephrine®

Bronchodilator indicated for parenteral use in the treatment of bronchial asthma and for reversible bronchospasm that may occur in association with bronchitis and emphysema.

Preparation: Ampules, 2 mg/ml.

ETHYNODIOL DIACETATE

Progestin included in certain oral contraceptive formulations.

ETHYOL®, see Amifostine

ETIDOCAINE HYDROCHLORIDE—Duranest®

Local anesthetic indicated for infiltration anesthesia, peripheral nerve blocks, and central neural blocks (i.e., lumbar or caudal epidural blocks).

Preparations: Vials, 1% solution. Vials, 1% and

1.5% solutions, both with epinephrine bitartrate, 1:200,000.

ETIDRONATE DISODIUM—Didronel®

Acts primarily on bone and is indicated for the treatment of symptomatic Paget's disease of bone, and for the prevention and treatment of heterotopic ossification following total hip replacement or due to spinal cord injury. Also used parenterally for the management of hypercalcemia of malignancy inadequately managed by dietary modification or oral hydration, and in the hypercalcemia of malignancy that persists after adequate hydration has been restored.

Preparations: Tablets, 200 and 400 mg. Ampules, 300 mg.

ETODOLAC—Lodine®

Nonsteroidal anti-inflammatory drug.

Actions and Uses: Inhibits prostaglandin synthesis and is indicated for the management of osteoarthritis and rheumotoid arthritis. Is also indicated for the management of pain.

Warnings: Should not be given to patients in whom aspirin or another NSAID causes asthma, rhinitis, urticaria, or other allergic-type reactions. May cause GI effects and use should be avoided in patients with active GI tract disease and closely monitored in patients with a previous history of such disorders.

Administration: Oral.

Preparations: Capsules, 200 and 300 mg. Tablets, 400 and 500 mg. Extended release Tabs, 400, 500, and 600 mg.

ETOPOSIDE—VePesid®, VP-16®

Antineoplastic agent used in treatment of refractory testicular neoplasms in patients who have already received appropriate surgical, chemotherapeutic and radiation therapy. Indicated for the treatment of choriosarcoma in women and small cell carcinoma.

Administration: Oral, intravenous.

Preparations: Capsules, 50 mg. Injection, 50 mg/ml.

ETOMIDATE—Amidate®

General anesthetic indicated for induction of general anesthesia and for supplementation of subpotent anesthetic agents (e.g., nitrous oxide in oxygen) during maintenance of anesthesia for short surgical procedures.

Preparation: Ampules, 2 mg/ml.

EUGENOL

Local anesthetic used in some formulations used for the relief of toothache.

Preparation: Drops.

EULEXIN®, see Flutamide

EURAX®, see Crotamiton

EXCEDRIA MIGRAINE®—Combination agent acetominophen, aspirin, and caffeine (analgesic and salicylate)

EXELDERM®, see Sulconazole nitrate

EX-LAX®, see Phenolphthalein

EXNA®, see Benzthiazide

EXOSURF NEONATAL®, see Colfosceril palmitate

F

FACTREL®, see Gonadorelin

FAMCICLOVIR—Famvir®

Antiviral agent.

Actions and Uses: Is a prodrug that is rapidly converted following administration to the antiviral compound penciclovir. Indicated for the management of acute herpes zoster (shingles), and recurrent episodes of genital herpes.

Warnings: Adverse reactions include headache, nausea, and fatigue.

Administration: Oral.

Preparations: Tablets, 125, 250, and 500 mg.

FAMOTIDINE—Mylanta AR®, Pepcid®, Pepcid AC®

Antiulcer agent.

Actions and Uses: Indicated in (1) short-term treatment of active duodenal ulcer, (2) maintenance therapy for duodenal ulcer patients at reduced dosage after healing of an active ulcer, (3) short-term treatment of active, benign gastric ulcer, (4) treatment of gastroesophageal reflux disease including erosive esophagitis, and (5) treatment of pathological hypersecretory conditions (e.g., Zollinger-Ellison syndrome, multiple endocrine adenomas). Available without a prescription (Pepcid AC®) to relieve and prevent acid indigestion.

Warnings: Adverse reactions include headache, dizziness, constipation, diarrhea, and transient irritation at the injection site when administered intravenously.

Administration: Oral and intravenous.

Preparations: Tablets, 10 (Pepcid AC®), 20 and 40 mg. Oral suspension containing 40 mg/5ml when reconstituted. Vials, 10 mg/ml.

FAMVIR®, see Famciclovir

FANSIDAR®, Combination of sulfadoxine and pyrimethamine

FASTIN®, see Phentermine

FELBAMATE—Felbatol®

Antiepileptic agent.

Actions and Uses: Because of the risks ofaplastic anemia and acute liver failure, should only be used in patients whose epilepsy is so severe that the risk is deemed acceptable in light of the benefits conferred by its use. Indicated as monotherapy and adjunctive therapy in the treatment of partial seizures with and without generalization in adults with epilepsy, and as adjunctive therapy in the treatment of partial and generalized seizures associated with Lennox-Gastaut syndrome in children.

Warnings: Adverse reactions include aplastic anemia, acute liver failure, anorexia, nausea, vomiting, insomnia, somnolence, dizziness, and headache. Do full baseline hematologic evaluation and hepatic function tests before, during and after therapy. Discontinue if hepatic tests are abnormal or bone marrow depression occurs. Consult hematologist if hematologic abnormalities occur.

Administration: Oral. When felbamate is added to or substituted for existing antiepileptic drugs, it is necessary to reduce the dosage of those drugs in the range of 20–33% to minimize side effects. Avoid abrupt cessation.

Preparations: Tablets, 400 and 600 mg. Oral suspension, 600 mg/5 ml.

FELBATOL®, see Felbamate

FELDENE®, see Piroxicam

FELODIPINE—Plendil®

Antihypertensive agent.

Actions and Uses: A calcium channel blocking agent that is indicated in the management of hypertension. May be used alone or concurrently with other antihypertensive agents.

Warnings: Adverse reactions include peripheral edema, headache, flushing, dizziness, asthenia, cough, paresthesia, dyspepsia, chest pain, nausea, muscle cramps, and palpitation. Mild gingival hyperplasia has been reported and may be reduced by good dental hygiene. Caution should be exercised in patients with congestive heart failure, particularly if a beta-blocker is used concurrently. Action may be increased by the concurrent use of cimetidine. Bioavailability of the drug has been reported to be significantly increased when taken with doubly concentrated grapefruit juice.

Administration: Oral.

Preparations: Extended-release tablets, 2.5, 5, and 10 mg.

FEMSTAT®, see Butoconazole

FENOPROFEN CALCIUM—Nalfon®

Nonsteroidal anti-inflammatory drug.

Actions and Uses: Inhibits prostaglandin synthesis and is indicated for the relief of mild to moderate pain, rheumatoid arthritis, and osteoarthritis.

Warnings: Should not be used in patients with a history of significantly impaired renal function. Should not be given to patients in whom aspirin or another NSAID causes asthma, rhinitis, urticaria, or other allergic-type reactions. May cause GI effects and use should be avoided in patients with active GI tract disease and closely monitored in patients with a previous history of such disorders. Other adverse reactions include dizziness, pruritus, palpitations, and nervousness.

Administration: Oral.

Preparations: Capsules, 200 and 300 mg. Tablets, 600 mg.

FENTANYL—Duragesic® -25, -50, -75, -100

Opioid analgesic indicated for the management of chronic pain. Transdermal system provides analgesic activity for up to 72 hours.

Preparations: Transdermal system, 25 ug/hour (2.5 mg), 50 ug/hour (5 mg), 75 ug/hour (7.5 mg), and 100 ug/hour (10 mg).

FENTANYL CITRATE—Sublimaze®, Oralet®

Opioid analgesic/anesthetic indicated for parenteral use for (1) analgesic action before, during, and following surgery; (2) use as an analgesic supplement in general or regional anesthesia; (3) administration with a neuroleptic in conjunction with anesthesia; and (4) as an anesthetic agent with oxygen in selected high risk patients. Also indicated for oral transmucosal use (as a lozenge) for anesthetic premedication in children and adults, and for use in anesthesia or monitored anesthesia care.

Preparations: Ampules, 50 µg/ml. Lozenges, 200, 300, and 400 µg

FEOSOL®, see Ferrous sulfate exsiccated

FEOSTAT®, see Ferrous fumarate

FERGON®, see Ferrous gluconate

FER-IN-SOL.®, see Ferrous sulfate

FERO-GRADUMET®, see Ferrous sulfate

FERROUS FUMARATE—Feostat®

Hematinic indicated for the prevention and treatment of iron deficiency anemias.

Preparations: Tablets, 100, 200, and 325 mg. Suspension, 100 mg/5 ml. Drops, 45 mg/0.6 ml.

FERROUS GLUCONATE—Fergon®

Hematinic indicated for the prevention and treatment of iron deficiency anemias.

Preparations: Tablets, 325 mg. Capsules, 325 and 435 mg. Elixir, 300 mg/5 ml.

FERROUS SULFATE—Fero-Gradumet®, Fer-In-Sol®

Hematinic indicated for the prevention and treatment of iron deficiency anemias.

Preparations: Controlled-release tablets, 525 mg. Syrup, 90 mg/5 ml. Drops, 75 mg/0.6 ml.

FERROUS SULFATE, EXSICCATED—Feosol®, Slow FE®

Hematinic indicated for the prevention and treatment of iron deficiency anemias.

Preparations: Tablets, 200 mg. Controlled-release capsules and tablets, 160 mg.

FEXOFENADINE HYDROCHLORIDE—Allegra®

A nonsedating antihistamine with selective peripheral H_1-receptor antagonist activity indicated in the treatment of seasonal allergic rhinitis.

Warnings: Adverse reactions include viral infection, nausea, dysmenorrhea, drowsiness, dyspepsia, and fatigue. Use cautiously in patients with renal impairment.

Administration: 60 mg twice daily.

Preparation: Capsules, 60 mg.

FIBERCON®see Polycarbophil

FIBRINOLYSIN—in Elase®

Fibrinolytic agent used in combination with desoxyribonuclease for topical use as debriding agents in a variety of inflammatory and infected lesions.

Preparations: Ointment and powder for solution.

FILGRASTIM—Neupogen®

Colony stimulating factor.

Actions and Uses: A human granulocyte colony stimulating factor (G-CSF) produced by recombinant DNA technology. Regulates the production of neutrophils within the bone marrow and is indicated to decrease the incidence of infection, as manifested by febrile neutropenia, in patients with non-myeloid malignancies receiving myelosuppressive anti-cancer drugs associated with a significant incidence of severe neutropenia with fever. may be used to reduce the time of neutrophl recovery and fever duration after induction and consolidation chemotherapy treatment of adults with AML. Also indicated in patients with non-myeloid malignancies undergoing chemotherapy followed by marrow transplantation. Also indicated to reduce the incidence and duration of sequelae of severe chronic neutropenia.

Warnings: May cause bone pain and leukocytosis. Caution must be exercised in patients with any malignancy with myeloid characteristics because of the possibility that the drug may act as a growth factor for the tumor.

Administration: Intravenous and subcutaneous. Should be administered no earlier than 24 hours after the administration of cytotoxic chemotherapy, and should not be administered in the period 24 hours before the administration of chemotherapy. Vials should not be shaken.

Preparations: Vials, 300 and 480 ug.

FINASTERIDE—Proscar®

Agent for benign prostatic hyperplasia (BPH).

Actions and Uses: Inhibits steroid 5α-reductase that converts testosterone into 5α-dihydrotestosterone (DHT), a potent androgen. Indicated for the treatment of symptomatic benign prostatic hyperplasia to improve symptoms and reduce risks of acute urinary retention and the need for prostate surgery.

Warnings: Contraindicated during pregnancy and in nursing mothers. Adverse reactions include impotence, decreased libido, and decreased volume of ejaculate. May cause harm to a male fetus and women who are pregnant should avoid exposure to the drug—crushed tablets should not be handled by a woman who is pregnant and, when the patient's sexual partner is or may become pregnant, the patient should avoid exposure of his partner to semen or discontinue the medication. May cause a decrease in serum prostate-specific antigen (PSA).

Administration: Oral. A minimum of 6 months of treatment may be necessary to determine whether an individual will respond to the drug.

Preparations: Tablets, 5 mg.

FIORICET®, Combination of butalbital, acetaminophen, and caffeine

FIORINAL®, Combination of butalbital, aspirin, and caffeine

5 FU®, see Fluorouracil

FLAGYL®, see Metronidazole

FLAVOXATE HYDROCHLORIDE —Urispas®

Spasmolytic agent indicated for the symptomatic relief of urinary tract problems such as dysuria, urgency, nocturia, suprapubic pain, frequency, and incontinence.

Preparation: Tablets, 100 mg.

FLAXEDIL®, see Gallamine

FLECAINIDE ACETATE—Tambocor®

Antiarrhythmic agent.

Actions and Uses: A class IC antiarrhythmic agent. Indicated for the treatment of life-threatening ventricular arrhythmias such as sustained ventricular tachycardia. Also indicated for paroxysmal atrial fibrillation/flutter associated with disabling symptoms and paroxysmal supraventricular tachycardias associated with disabling symptoms in patients without structural heart disease.

Warnings: Contraindicated in patients with second- or third-degree AV block, with right bundle branch block when associated with a left hemiblock (unless a pacemaker is present), or in the presence of cardiogenic shock. Adverse reactions include proarrhythmic events, worsening of congestive heart failure, dizziness, visual disturbances, dyspnea, headache, nausea, fatigue, and palpitation.

Administration: Oral.

Preparation: Tablets, 50, 100, and 150 mg.

FLEXERIL®, see Cyclobenzaprine

FLOLAN®, see Epoprostenol

FLORINEF®, see Fludrocortisone

FLORONE®, see Diflorasone

FLOROPRYL®, see Isoflurophate

FLOXIN®, see Ofloxacin

FLOXIN IV®, see Ofloxacin

FLOXURIDINE—FUDR®

Antineoplastic agent administered by intra-arterial infusion in the management of gastrointestinal adenocarcinoma metastatic to the liver.

Preparation: Vials, 5 mg.

FLUCONAZOLE—Diflucan®

Antifungal agent.

Actions and Uses: Indicated for the treatment of cryptococcal meningitis, serious systemic candidal infections including urinary tract infection, peritonitis, and pneumonia, as well as oropharyngeal and esophageal candidiasis. Also indicated as a single-dose treatment for vaginal candidiasis.

Warnings: Adverse reactions include nausea, vomiting, abdominal pain, diarrhea, headache, rash, and hepatic reactions. May increase the plasma concentrations and/or activity of warfarin, phenytoin, cyclosporine, and oral hypoglycemic agents. Rifampin may increase the rate of metabolism and it may be necessary to increase the dosage of the antifungal agent during the period of concurrent therapy.

Administration: When administered intravenously, it should be given as a continuous infusion at a maximum rate of 200 mg/hour.

Preparations: Tablets, 50, 100 and 200 mg. Oral suspension, 10 mg/ml. Glass bottles and plastic containers, 200 mg/100 ml and 400 mg/200 ml.

FLUCYTOSINE—Ancobon®

Antifungal agent indicated for systemic infections caused by *Candida* and *Cryptococcus.*

Preparations: Capsules, 250 and 500 mg.

FLUDARA®, see Fludarabine

FLUDARABINE PHOSPHATE—Fludara®

Antineoplastic agent.

Actions and Uses: Is an analog of the antiviral agent vidarabine. Indicated for the treatment of patients with B-cell chronic lymphocytic leukemia who have not responded to or have progressed during treatment with at least one standard regimen containing an alkylating agent.

Warnings: May cause fetal harm and should not be used during pregnancy unless safer alternatives are not available.

Administration: Intravenous.

Preparations: Vials, 50 mg.

FLUDROCORTISONE ACETATE—Florinef®

Mineralocorticoid indicated for the treatment of Addison's disease and salt-losing adrenogenital syndrome.

Preparation: Tablets, 0.1 mg.

FLUMADINE®, see Rimantadine hydrochloride

FLUMAZENIL—Romazicon®

Benzodiazepine antagonist.

Actions and Uses: Reverses the sedating and psychomotor effects of benzodiazepines (e.g., diazepam, midazolam); however, amnesia is less completely and less consistently reversed. Indicated for the complete or partial reversal of the sedative effects of benzodiazepines in cases where general anesthesia has been induced and/or maintained with benzodiazepines, where sedation has been produced with benzodiazepines for diagnostic and therapeutic procedures, and for the management of benzodiaze-pine overdose.

Warnings: Contraindicated in patients who may be relying on the effects of a benzodiazepine to control potentially life-threatening conditions (e.g., status epilepticus, increased intracranial pressure). Is also contraindicated in cases of serious cyclic antidepressant (e.g., amitriptyline) overdose. May cause seizures including withdrawal seizures in patients who are physically dependent on benzodiazepines. Other adverse reactions include nausea, vomiting, dizziness, agitation, and injection-site pain. In situations in which a patient has received a neuromuscular blocking agent, flumazenil should not be used until the effects of neuromuscular blockade have been fully reversed. Duration of action is shorter than that of the benzodiazepines and a return of sedation (resedation) may occur following initial reversal; patients should be monitored for resedation, as well as respiratory depression and other residual benzodiazepine effects. Patients should be advised not to engage in any activities requiring complete alertness until at least 18 to 24 hours after discharge and not to take any alcohol or nonprescription drugs for 18 to 24 hours after flumazenil administration or if the effects of the benzodiazepine persist. Because flumazenil does not consistently reverse amnesia, patients cannot be expected to remember information told to them in the post-procedure period, and instructions given to patients should be reinforced in writing or given to a responsible family member.

Administration: Intravenous. Should be administered through a freely running intravenous infusion into a large vein to minimize the likelihood of pain or inflammation at the injection site.

Preparations: Vials, 0.1 mg/ml.

FLUMETHIAZIDE

Thiazide diuretic used in combination with other agents in the treatment of hypertension.

FLUNISOLIDE—Aerobid®, Aerobid-M® (menthol flavor), Nasalide®, Nasarel®

Corticosteroid.

Actions and Uses: Nasalide: Indicated for the topical treatment of the symptoms of seasonal or perennial rhinitis when effectiveness of or tolerance of conventional treatment is unsatisfactory. Nasarel: Treatment of seasonal or perennial rhinitis. Aerobid®: Maintenance treatment of asthma as prophylactic therapy or to reduce the need for systemic corticosteroids in individuals requiring systemic steroid therapy.

Warnings: Adverse reactions include transient nasal burning and stinging, and nasal congestion. Caution must be exercised when transferring a patient from systemic corticosteroid therapy to flunisolide therapy. Contraindicated as primary treatment of an acute attack, in varicella and vaccinia.

Administration: Nasal spray.

Preparation: Nasal solution spray bottle, 6.25 mg, metered dose inhaler 250 μg/inh.

FLUOCINOLONE ACETONIDE—Synalar®

Corticosteroid applied topically for relief of inflammatory and pruritic manifestations of corticosteroid-responsive dermatoses.

Preparations: Cream, 0.01%, 0.025%, and 0.2%. Ointment, 0.025%. Topical solution, 0.01%.

FLUOCINONIDE—Lidex®, Lidex-E®

Topical corticosteroid.

Actions and Uses: Indicated for the relief of the inflammatory and pruritic manifestations of corticosteroid-responsive dermatoses.

Warnings: Adverse reactions include burning, itching, dryness, irritation, and a potential for systemic effects.

Administration: Topical.

Preparations: Cream, gel, ointment, and solution, 0.05%. Lidex-E cream utilizes water-washable aqueous base.

FLUORESCEIN SODIUM

Diagnostic aid used in various ocular conditions.

Preparations: Solution, 2%. Strips, 0.6 and 1 mg. Ampules, 10% and 25%.

FLUOROMETHOLONE—FML®

Corticosteroid indicated for ophthalmic use in the treatment of inflammatory conditions of the eye.

Preparations: Ophthalmic suspension and ointment, 0.1%.

FLUOROPLEX®, see Fluorouracil

FLUOROURACIL—Adrucil®, Efudex®, 5 FU®, Fluoroplex®

Antineoplastic agent indicated for intravenous use in the management of carcinoma of the colon, rectum, breast, stomach, and pancreas, and for the topical treatment of active or solar keratoses, and superficial basal cell carcinomas.

Preparations: Ampules, 500 mg. Cream, 1% and 5%. Topical solution, 1%, 2%, and 5%.

FLUOTHANE®, see Halothane

FLUOXETINE HYDROCHLORIDE—Prozac®

Antidepressant.

Actions and Uses: Indicated for the treatment of depression and acts by inhibiting CNS neuronal uptake of serotonin. Also indicated in the treatment of obsessive-compulsive disorder and bulimia nervosa.

Warnings: Adverse reactions include anxiety, nervousness, insomnia, nausea, diarrhea, and rash and/or urticaria. Dizziness and other CNS effects may develop and patients should be cautioned regarding activities such as driving and operating machinery, as well as interactions with other CNS-acting drugs including alcohol. Concurrent use with tryptophan has resulted in the development of agitation and restlessness in some patients. Use in combination with a monoamine oxidase inhibitor should be avoided and at least 14 days should elapse between discontinuation of a MAO inhibitor and initiation of treatment with fluoxetine. At least 5 weeks should elapse between discontinuation of fluoxetine and initiation of therapy with a MAO inhibitor.

Administration: Oral.

Preparations: Capsules, 10 and 20 mg. Liquid, 20 mg/5 ml.

FLUOXYMESTERONE—Halotestin®

Androgen indicated in male patients for replacement therapy in conditions associated with symptoms of deficiency or absence of endogenous testosterone (e.g., primary hypogonadism—testicular failure), and delayed puberty. Also indicated in the treatment of recurrent mammary cancer in selected female patients.

Preparations: Tablets, 2, 5, and 10 mg.

FLUPHENAZINE DECANOATE—Prolixin decanoate®

FLUPHENAZINE ENANTHATE—Prolixin enanthate®

Phenothiazine antipsychotic agent indicated for the parenteral treatment of patients requiring prolonged parenteral neuroleptic therapy (e.g., chronic schizophrenics).

Preparations: Vials and syringes, 25 mg/ml.

FLUPHENAZINE HYDROCHLORIDE—Permitil®, Prolixin®

Phenothiazine antipsychotic agent indicated for the management of manifestations of psychotic disorders.

Preparations: Tablets, 1, 2.5, 5, and 10 mg. Elixir, 2.5 mg/5 ml. Concentrate, 5 mg/ml. Vials, 2.5 mg/ml.

FLURANDRENOLIDE—Cordran®

Corticosteroid applied topically for the relief of inflammatory and pruritic manifestations of corticosteroid-responsive dermatoses.

Preparations: Cream and ointment, 0.025% and 0.05%. Lotion, 0.05%. Tape, 4 μg/sq. cm. Patch, 2 x 3 inches.

FLURAZEPAM HYDROCHLORIDE—Dalmane®

Benzodiazepine hypnotic.

Actions and Uses: A CNS depressant indicated for the management of insomnia.

Warnings: Contraindicated during pregnancy. Adverse reactions include residual sedation and other CNS effects upon awakening; patients should be cautioned regarding activities such as driving and operating machinery, as well as interactions with other CNS-acting drugs including alcohol. Can cause dependence and is included in Schedule IV.

Administration: Oral.

Preparations: Capsules, 15 and 30 mg.

FLURBIPROFEN—Ansaid®

Nonsteroidal anti-inflammatory drug.

Actions and Uses: Inhibits prostaglandin synthesis and is indicated for the treatment of rheumatoid arthritis and osteoarthritis.

Warnings: Should not be given to patients in whom aspirin or another NSAID causes asthma, rhinitis, urticaria, or other allergic-type reactions. May cause GI effects and use should be avoided in patients with active GI tract disease and closely monitored in patients with a previous history of such disorders.

Administration: Oral.

Preparations: Tablets, 50 and 100 mg.

FLURBIPROFEN SODIUM—Ocufen®

Nonsteroidal anti-inflammatory drug for ophthalmic use.

Actions and Uses: Indicated for the inhibition of intraoperative miosis to reduce the risk of complications associated with procedures such as cataract surgery.

Warnings: Contraindicated in epithelial herpes simplex keratitis. Adverse reactions include transient burning and stinging upon instillation; the drug may also delay wound healing. Caution should be exercised in the treatment of patients having a history of sensitivity to aspirin or another nonsteroidal anti-inflammatory drug.

Administration: Ophthalmic.

Preparation: Ophthalmic solution, 0.03%.

FLUTAMIDE—Eulexin®

Antineoplastic agent.

Actions and Uses: An antiandrogen that inhibits the uptake and binding of androgen. Is rapidly converted to hydroxyflutamide which is the major active metabolite. Indicated in the treatment of locally confined stage

A_2-C or metastatic prostatic carcinoma (stage D_2) in combination with an analog of luteinizing hormone-releasing hormone (LHRH) such as leuprolide.

Warnings: Adverse reactions include diarrhea, nausea, vomiting, hot flashes, loss of libido, impotence, and gynecomastia. Has caused elevations of hepatic enzyme levels, as well as clinically evident hepatitis, and periodic liver function tests should be considered in patients on long-term therapy.

Administration: Oral. It is recommended that treatment be started simultaneously with both flutamide and leuprolide. Patients should be informed that the two drugs are to be administered concurrently, and that they should not discontinue taking either medication without consulting their physician.

Preparation: Capsules, 125 mg.

FLUTICASONE PROPIONATE—Cutivate®, Flonase®, Flovent®

Corticosteroid.

Actions and Uses: Indicated (Cutivate®) for the relief of the inflammatory and pruritic manifestations of corticosteroid-responsive dermatoses. Also administered (Zlonase®) by nasal inhalation for the managment of seasonal and perennial allergic rhinitis.

Warnings: Adverse reactions include pruritus, dryness, burning, increased erythema, hypertrichosis, and numbness of fingers.

Administration: Topical, nasal, and inhalation.

Preparations: Cream, 0.05%; ointment, 0.005%. Nasal spray, 44 µg, 50 µg, 110 µg, 220 µg per actuation. Metered dose inhaler, 44, 110, and 220 µg/inh. Rotadisk, 50, 100, and 250 µg/inh. via dry powder.

FLUVASTATIN SODIUM—Lescol®

Agent for hypercholesterolemia.

Actions and Uses: Produces a significant reduction in total and low-density lipoprotein (LDL) cholesterol concentrations, a modest reduction in triglyceride concentrations, and an increase in high-density lipoprotein (HDL) cholesterol concentrations. Indicated as an adjunct to diet in the treatment of elevated total cholesterol and low-density lipoprotein cholesterol in patients with primary hypercholesterolemia whose response to dietary restriction of saturated fat and cholesterol and other nonpharmacological measures has not been adequate. Also indicated to slow the progression of coronary atherasclerosis in patients with coronary heart disease.

Warnings: Contraindicated in patients with active liver disease or unexplained, persistent elevations of serum transaminases. Is also contraindicated in pregnant women and nursing mothers. Increases in serum transaminases may occur and it is recommended that liver function tests be performed before the initiation of treatment, at 6 and 12 weeks after initiation of therapy or elevation in dose, and periodically thereafter (e.g., every 6 months). Should be used with caution in patients with a history of liver disease or heavy alcohol ingestion. Adverse reactions include dyspepsia, abdominal pain, arthropathy, and exercise-related muscle pain. Patients should be advised to promptly report unexplained muscle pain, tenderness or weakness. The concurrent use of clofibrate or gemfibrozil is best avoided, and caution should be exercised if cyclosporine or erythromycin is used concurrently. When used concomitantly with a bile acid-binding resin, it should be administered at least 4 hours after the resin.

Administration: Oral. Should be administered at bedtime.

Preparations: Capsules, 20 and 40 mg.

FLUVOXAMINE MALEATE—Luvox®

Actions and Uses: Selective serotonin reuptake inhibitor indicated for the treatment of obsessive–compulsive disorder.

Warnings: Concurrent administration of terfenadine or astemizole is contraindicated. Adverse reactions include somnolence, insomnia, nervousness, dizziness, and tremor. Advise patients to avoid driving or operating machinery until response is ascertained. Alcohol should be avoided. It is recommended that fluvoxamine not be used in combination with MAO inhibitors or within 14 days of discontinuing an MAO inhibitor.

Administration: Oral.

Preparations: Tablets, 50 and 100 mg.

FML®, see Fluorometholone

FOLIC ACID—Folvite®

Agent for anemias that is indicated in the prevention and treatment of megaloblastic anemias due to a deficiency of folic acid as may be seen in sprue, anemias of nutritional origin, pregnancy, infancy, or childhood.

Preparations: Tablets, 0.1, 0.4, 0.8, and 1 mg. Vials 5 mg/ml and 10 mg/ml.

FOLINIC ACID, see Leucovorin

FOLLUTEIN®, see Chorionic gonadotropin

FOLVITE®, see Folic Acid

FORTAZ®, see Ceftazidime

FORTOVASE®, see Saquinavir

FOSAMAX®, see Alendronate

FOSCARNET SODIUM—Foscavir®

Antiviral agent.

Actions and Uses: Inhibits replication of herpesviruses including cytomegalovirus (CMV). Indicated for the treatment of cytomegalovirus retinitis in patients with AIDS. Also indicated for the treatment of acyclovir-resistant mucocutaneous herpes simplex virus infections in immunocompromised patients.

Warnings: May cause renal impairment and creatinine clearance should be determined at baseline, 2–3 times per week during induction therapy, and at least once every 1 or 2 weeks during maintenance therapy. Concurrent use with other potentially nephrotoxic drugs (e.g., aminoglycosides) should be avoided when possible.

Has the potential to chelate divalent metal ions such as calcium and has been associated with changes in serum electrolytes including hypocalcemia and hypomagnesemia, as well as hypokalemia, hypophosphatemia, and hyperphospha- temia. Serum calcium, magnesium, potassium, and phosphorus should be monitored on a schedule similar to that recommended for serum creatinine. Patients should be advised to report symptoms such as perioral tingling, numbness in the extremities, and paresthesias which may be associated with electrolyte ab- normalities. The concomitant use with intravenous pentamidine may increase the risk of severe hypocalcemia. Other adverse reactions include seizures, anemia, granulocytopenia, fever, nausea, vomiting, diarrhea, and headache.

Administration: Intravenous infusion. Must not be administered by rapid or bolus injection because of the increased risk of toxicity.

Preparations: Bottles, 250 and 500 ml containing the drug in a concentration of 24 mg/ml.

FOSCAVIR®, see Foscarnet

FOSFOMYCIN—Monurol®

Actions and Uses: Synthetic, broad spectrum antibiotic that has bactericidal activity in the urine at therapeutic doses. Indicated in the treatment of uncomplicated susceptible UTIs in women.

Warnings: Adverse reactions include diarrhea, vaginitis, nausea, headache, dizziness, asthenia, and dyspepsia.

Usual adult dose (oral) for UTIs: Female: single dose of 3 g in 4 oz. of water; male: 3 g once daily for 2–3 days for complicated UTIs. Dissolve granules in 3–4 oz. of water (not hot), stir to dissolve, and drink immediately. Follow manufacturer's guidelines for dosing for each episode of acute cystitis, since repeated daily doses do not improve clinical success but increase the incidence of adverse events. If bacteria persist or reappear after treatment with fosfomycin, other therapeutic agents should be selected. Urine specimen should be obtained for culture and sensitivity testing before and after completion of therapy.

Preparation: Single dose sachet packets of 3 g.

FOSINOPRIL SODIUM—Monopril®

Antihypertensive agent.

Actions and Uses: An angiotensin-converting enzyme (ACE) inhibitor that is a prodrug. Following oral administration, is converted to its active metabolite, fosinoprilat. Indicated for the treatment of hypertension and may be used alone or in combination with a thiazide diuretic. Also indicated in the management of congestive heart failure.

Warnings: Adverse reactions include headache, dizziness, fatigue, cough, diarrhea, and nausea/vomiting. May cause an elevation in serum potassium levels; the risk of hyperkalemia is increased in patients also taking a potassium-sparing diuretic, a potassium supplement, and/or a potassium-con- taining salt substitute. May cause symptomatic postural hypotension. There have been infrequent reports of angioedema of the face, extremities, lips, tongue, glottis, and larynx, especially following the first dose. Patients should be told to report immediately any symptoms suggesting angioedema and to stop taking the drug. When used during the second and third trimesters of pregnancy, ACE inhibitors have been reported to be associated with the development of neonatal hypertension, renal failure, and skull hypoplasia; use during pregnancy should be avoided. May increase serum lithium levels and concurrent therapy should be closely monitored.

Administration: Oral.

Preparations: Tablets, 10 and 20 mg.

FOSPHENYTOIN SODIUM—Cerebyx®

For short-term (up to 5 days) IV/IM administration when other forms of phytoin administration are unavailable or deemed less advantageous. See phytoin.

FRAGMIN®, see Dalteparin

FRUCTOSE—Levulose

Carbohydrate administered parenterally as a source of calories.

Preparations: Solution, 10%.

FUDR®, see Floxuridine

FULVICIN®, see Griseofulvin

FUNGIZONE®, see Amphotericin B

FURACIN®, see Nitrofurazone

FURADANTIN®, see Nitrofurantoin

FURAZOLIDONE—Furoxone®

Anti-infective agent indicated in the treatment of bacterial or protozoal diarrhea and enteritis caused by susceptible organisms.

Preparations: Tablets, 100 mg. Liquid, 50 mg/15 ml.

FUROSEMIDE—Lasix®

Diuretic and antihypertensive agent.

Actions and Uses: Is a loop diuretic indicated

(1) for the treatment of edema associated with congestive heart failure, cirrhosis of the liver, and renal diseases and (2) hypertension. Is also indicated via intravenous use as adjunctive therapy in acute pulmonary edema.

Warnings: Is contraindicated in anuria. May cause volume and electrolyte depletion. Potential for hypokalemia warrants periodic measurement of serum potassium levels. Reduction in potassium levels may increase the action and toxicity of digoxin and related glycosides. Parenteral therapy is best avoided in patients receiving aminoglycoside antibiotics because of an increased risk of ototoxicity.

Administration: Oral, intravenous, and intramuscular.

Preparations: Tablets, 20, 40, and 80 mg. Oral solution, 10 mg/ml. Ampules, vials, and syringes, 10 mg/ml.

FUROXONE®, see Furazolidone

G

GABAPENTIN—Neurontin®

Antiepileptic agent.

Actions and Uses: Indicated as adjunctive therapy in the treatment of partial seizures with and without secondary generalization in patients over 12 years of age with epilepsy.

Warnings: Adverse reactions include somnolence, dizziness, ataxia, nystagmus, and tremor. Patients should be cautioned not to drive or operate machinery until they have gained sufficient experience with the use of the drug to determine whether it affects their mental and/or motor performance adversely. Bioavailability is reduced by the administration of aluminum/magnesiun-containing antacids and it should be administered at least 2 hours following the antacid.

Administration: Oral. If treatment is to be discontinued and/or an alternative anticonvulsant is added to the therapy, this should be done gradually over a minimum of 1 week.

Preparations: Capsules, 100, 300, and 400 mg.

GALLAMINE TRIETHIODIDE—Flaxedil®

Neuromuscular blocking agent indicated as an adjunct to anesthesia to induce skeletal muscle relaxation. Also used to manage patients undergoing mechanical ventilation.

Preparation: Vials, 20 mg/ml.

GALLIUM NITRATE—Ganite®

Agent for hypercalcemia.

Actions and Uses: Exerts a hypocalcemic effect by inhibiting calcium resorption from bone. Indicated for the treatment of symptomatic cancer-related hypercalcemia that has not responded to adequate hydration.

Warnings: Contraindicated in patients with severe renal impairment. May cause renal effects and serum creatinine levels should be monitored. Concurrent use with other potentially nephrotoxic drugs (e.g., aminoglycosides, amphotericin B) may increase the risk of developing severe renal insufficiency. Other adverse reactions include hypocalcemia, transient hypophosphatemia, decreased sodium bicarbonate, anemia, decreased blood pressure, and nausea and/or vomiting.

Administration: Intravenous. The daily dose must be administered as an IV infusion over 24 hours. Adequate hydration must be maintained throughout the treatment period.

Preparations: Vials, 500 mg.

GAMMA BENZENE HEXACHLORIDE, see Lindane

GANCICLOVIR SODIUM—Cytovene®

Antiviral agent.

Actions and Uses: Inhibits replication of herpes viruses including cytomegalovirus (CMV). Indicated for the treatment of cytomegalovirus retinitis in immunocompromised individuals, including patients with AIDS. Also indicated in transplant patients at risk for CMV disease.

Warnings: May cause granulocytopenia and thrombocytopenia and it is recommended that neutrophil counts and platelet counts be performed every 2 days during the period in which ganciclovir is dosed twice daily and at least weekly thereafter. Other adverse reactions include anemia, fever, rash, and abnormalliver function values. Has been reported to be teratogenic in animals and it should be used during pregnancy only if the benefits outweigh the risks. Because of the mutagenic potential of ganciclovir, women of childbearing potential should be advised to use effective contraception during treatment, and male patients should be advised to practice barrier contraception during and for at least 90 days following treatment with the drug. The concurrent use of ganciclovir and zidovudine is associated with an increased risk of granulocytopenia. Seizures have been reported in some patients receiving ganciclovir and imipenem-cilastatin concurrently and the use of these agents in combination should be avoided if possible. Probenecid may reduce the renal clearance and increase the action of ganciclovir.

Administration: Intravenous infusion (at a constant rate over a period of 1 hour) and oral which should be taken with food.

Preparation: Vials, containing ganciclovir sodium equivalent to 500 mg ganciclovir. Capsules, 250 mg.

GANITE®, see Gallium nitrate

GANTANOL®, see Sulfamethoxazole

GANTRISIN®, see Sulfisoxazole

GANTRISIN ACETYL®, see Sulfisoxazole acetyl

GARAMYCIN®, see Gentamicin

GASTROCROM®, see Cromolyn

G-CSF, see Filgrastim

GEMCITABINE HYDROCHLORIDE—Gemzar®

Antineoplastic.

Actions and Uses: Antineoplastic agent used in the treatment of adenocarcinoma of the pancreas and as a first-line treatment for patients with locally advanced (nonresectable stage II or III) or metastatic (stage IV) disease in patients previously treated with 5-FU.

Warnings: Prolongation of infusion time beyond 30 minutes and more frequent administration than weekly dosing have been shown to increase toxicity. Side effects include myelosuppression, fever, rash, pruritis, transient elevations in serum transaminases, mild hematuria, and proteinuria. Monitor patients prior to each dose with a CBC including differential and platelet count.

Administration: 1,000mg/m^2 IV over 30 minutes once weekly for up to 7 weeks or until toxicity necessitates holding or reducing the dose. Follow with 1 week of rest and then begin subsequent cycles of infusions once weekly for 3 consecutive weeks out of every 4 weeks.

GEMFIBROZIL—Lopid®

Antihyperlipidemic agent indicated as adjunctive therapy to diet for (1) the treatment of patients with very high serum triglyceride levels (type IV or type V hyperlipoproteinemia) who present a risk of abdominal pain and pancreatitis and who do not respond adequately to dietary measures, and (2) reducing the risk of coronary heart disease.

Preparation: Capsules, 300 and 600 mg.

GEMZAR®—see Gemcitabine

GENOTROPIN®—see somatropin

GENTAMICIN SULFATE—Garamycin®

Aminoglycoside antibiotic.

Actions and Uses: Indicated for the parenteral treatment of serious infections caused by gram-negative bacteria including *Pseudomonas aerugino-sa.* Is also effective in the treatment of staphylococcal infections. Has also been used topically in the treatment of dermatologic and ocular infections.

Warnings: May cause nephrotoxicity, ototoxicity and neurotoxicity, and the concurrent or serial use of other nephrotoxic or ototoxic agents should be avoided.

Administration: Intravenous, intramuscular, intrathecal, topical, and ophthalmic.

Preparations: Vials, 40 mg/ml. Vials, syringes, and piggyback units, 60, 70, 80, 90, 100, 120, 160, and 180 mg. Vials (for intrathecal use), 2 mg/ml. Cream and ointment, 0.1%. Ophthalmic solution and ointment, 0.3%.

GENTIAN VIOLET—Methylrosaniline chloride

Anti-infective agent used topically in the treatment of dermatologic and vaginal infections.

Preparations: Solutions, 1% and 2%.

GENTRAN®, see Dextran

GEOCILLIN®, see Carbenicillin indanyl sodium

GLIMEPIRIDE—Amaryl®

Oral antidiabetic sulfonylurea.

Action and Uses: Used as an adjunct to diet and exercise in non-insulin dependent diabetes mellitus (NIDDM) in indivuals who are unable to maintain glycemic control by diet and exercise alone. Also indicated for secondary failure in combination with insulin.

Warnings: Contraindicated in Ketoacidosis as this condition should be treated with insulin. Administration of oral hypoglycemic drugs has been reported to be associated with increased cardiovascular mortality as compared to treatment with diet alone or diet plus insulin. May cause hypoglycemia, dizziness, asthenia, headache, nausea, allergic skin reactions, and blood dyscrasias.

Administration: Oral once daily with breakfast or first main meal.

Preparation: Scored tablets, 1, 2, and 4 mg.

GLIPIZIDE—Glucotrol®, Glucotrol XL

Sulfonylurea hypoglycemic agent.

Actions and Uses: Indicated as an adjunct to diet for the control of hyperglycemia and its associated symptomatology in patients with non-insulin-dependent diabetes mellitus, after an adequate trial of dietary therapy has proved unsatisfactory.

Warnings: May cause hypoglycemia and patients should be advised to contact their physician if symptoms of hypoglycemia develop. Adverse reactions include nausea, diarrhea, pruritus, and erythema. Oral hypoglycemic agents have been suggested to be associated with increased cardiovascular mortality as compared to treatment with diet alone or diet plus insulin. Corticosteroids and thiazide and other diuretics may increase blood glucose levels and necessitate an increase in dosage of glipizide. Therapy in patients also receiving a beta-adrenergic blocking agent should be monitored closely.

Administration: Oral.

Preparations: Tablets, 5 and 10 mg. Controlled-release tablet (Glucotrol XL), 5 and 10 mg.

GLUCAGON

Agent to increase blood glucose levels. Indicated for parenteral use in counteracting severe hypoglycemic reactions in diabetic patients or during insulin shock therapy in psychiatric patients. Used to facilitate radiographic examination of the GI tract.

Preparations: Vials, 1 and 10 mg.

GLUCOPHAGE® see Metformin hydrochloride

GLUCOSE, see Dextrose

GLUCOTROL®, see Glipizide

GLUCOTROL XL®, *see Glipizide*

GLUTAMIC ACID HYDROCHLORIDE

Gastric acidifier used in the treatment of conditions associated with a deficiency of hydrochloric acid in the gastric juice.

Preparation: Capsules, 340 mg.

GLUTETHIMIDE—Doriglute®

Hypnotic indicated for the short-term treatment of insomnia, sedative effect preoperatively and during the first stage of labor.

Preparations: Tablets, 250 mg.

GLYBURIDE—DiaBeta®, Micronase®, Glynase®

Sulfonylurea hypoglycemic agent.

Actions and Uses: Indicated as an adjunct to diet to lower the blood glucose in patients with non-insulin-dependent diabetes mellitus whose hyperglycemia cannot be controlled by diet alone.

Warnings: May cause hypoglycemia and patients should be advised to contact their physician if symptoms of hypoglycemia develop. Adverse reactions include nausea, heartburn, epigastric fullness, pruritus, erythema, urticaria, and rash. Oral hypoglycemic agents have been suggested to be associated with increased cardiovascular mortality as compared to treatment with diet alone or diet plus insulin. Corticosteroids and thiazide and other diuretics may increase blood glucose levels and necessitate an increase in dosage of glyburide. Therapy in patients also receiving a beta-adrenergic blocking agent should be monitored closely.

Administration: Oral.

Preparations: Tablets, 1.25, 2.5, and 5 mg. Tablets, micronized, 1.5, 3, and 6 mg (Glynase PresTab).

GLYCERYL TRIACETATE, see Triacetin

GLYCERYL TRINITRATE—Former name for Nitroglycerin

GLYCINE, see Aminoacetic Acid

GLYCOPYRROLATE—Robinul®

Anticholinergic agent used as adjunctive therapy in the treatment of peptic ulcer. Is also used parenterally as a preoperative antimuscarinic, intraoperatively to counteract drug induced or vagal traction reflexes with the associated arrhythmias, or to protect against the peripheral muscarinic effects of cholinergic agents given to reverse the neuromuscular blockade due to nondepolarizing muscle relaxants.

Preparations: Tablets, 1 and 2 mg. Vials, 0.2 mg/ml.

GLYNASE®, see Glyburide

GLY-OXIDE®, see Carbamide peroxide

GM-CSF, see Sargramostim

GOLD SODIUM THIOMALATE—Myochrysine®

Gold formulation indicated for the intramuscular.

treatment of rheumatoid arthritis.

Preparations: Ampules, 10, 25, and 50 mg.

GoLYTELY®, see Polyethylene glycol 3350

GONADORELIN HYDROCHLORIDE—Factrel®

Synthetic luteinizing hormone releasing hormone indicated for diagnostic use in evaluating the functional capacity and response of the gonadotropes of the anterior pituitary.

Preparation: Vials, 100 mg.

GONADOTROPIN, CHORIONIC see Chorionic gonadotropin

GOSERELIN ACETATE—Zoladex®

Antineoplastic agent.

Actions and Uses: Is a synthetic analog of gonadotropin releasing hormone. Chronic administration leads to a sustained suppression of pituitary gonadotropins, resulting in a fall in serum testosterone levels. Indicated in the palliative treatment of advanced carcinoma of the prostate, treatment of endometriosis, and palliative treatment of advanced breast cancer in peri- and post-menopausal women.

Warnings: Is contraindicated during pregnancy. Adverse reactions include hot flashes, sexual dysfunction, decreased erections, lower urinary tract symptoms, pain, lethargy, dizziness, insomnia, anorexia, nausea, upper respiratory infection, chronic obstructive pulmonary disease, edema, congestive heart failure, rash, and sweating. When treatment is initiated, there is a transient increase in serum testosterone levels which may cause a temporary worsening of signs and symptoms during the first few weeks of therapy.

Administration: Subcutaneous. The formulation is implanted into the upper abdominal wall and provides a continuous release of the drug over a 28-day period.

Preparations: Implant, 3.6 mg.

GRANISETRON HYDROCHLORIDE—Kytril®

Antiemetic.

Actions and Uses: Is a selective blocking agent of the serotonin 5-HT_3 receptor type. Indicated for intravenous administration for the prevention of nausea and vomiting associated with initial and repeat courses of emetogenic cancer therapy, including high-dose cisplatin.

Warnings: Adverse reactions include headache, asthenia, somnolence, diarrhea, and constipation.

Administration: Oral and intravenous. When administered intravenously, is given as a single dose infused over 5 minutes, beginning within 30 minutes before initiation of chemotherapy, and only on the day(s) chemotherapy is given. Should not be mixed in solution with other drugs. Oral doses are administered up to 1 hour before chemotherapy and second dose 12 hours after the first.

Preparations: Tablets, 1 mg. Vials, 1 mg.

GRANULOCYTE COLONY STIMULATING FACTOR, see Filgrastim

GRANULOCYTE-MACROPHAGE COLONY STIMULATING FACTOR, see Sargramostim

GRIFULVIN®, see Griseofulvin

GRISACTIN®, See Griseofulvin

GRISEOFULVIN MICROSIZE—Fulvicin-U/F®, Grifulvin V®, Grisactin®

GRISEOFULVIN ULTRAMICROSIZE—Fulvicin P/G®, Grisactin Ultra®, Gris-PEG®.

Antifungal agent administered orally for tinea (ringworm) infections of the skin, hair, and nails. Should not be used for superficial infection that may respond to topical antifungals.

Preparations: Microsize—Capsules and tablets, 125, 250, and 500 mg. Suspension, 125 mg/5 ml. Ultramicrosize—Tablets, 125, 165, 250, and 330 mg.

GRIS-PEG®, see Griseofulvin

GUAIFENESIN—Humabid LA®, Humabid Sprinkle®, Robitussin®, Sinumist SR Caplets®

Expectorant indicated for the symptomatic relief of respiratory conditions characterized by dry, nonproductive cough and in the presence of mucus in the respiratory tract.

Preparations: Capsules and tablets, 100 and 200 mg. Syrup, 67 mg/5 ml, 100 mg/5 ml, and 200 mg/5 ml. Extended release capsules/tablets, 300 and 600 mg.

GUANABENZ ACETATE—Wytensin®

Antihypertensive agent which exhibits a central alpha-2 adrenergic agonist action.

Preparations: Tablets, 4, and 8 mg.

GUANADREL SULFATE—Hylorel®

Antihypertensive agent indicated in the treatment of hypertension in patients who have not responded adequately to a thiazide-type diuretic.

Preparations: Tablets, 10 and 25 mg.

GUANETHIDINE MONOSULFATE—Ismelin®

Antihypertensive agent indicated for the treatment of moderate and severe hypertension, and for the management of renal hypertension.

Preparations: Tablets, 10 and 25 mg.

GUANFACINE HYDROCHLORIDE—Tenex®

Antihypertensive agent.

Actions and Uses: Is a centrally acting alpha-2 adrenergic receptor agonist. Indicated in the management of hypertension.

Warnings: Adverse reactions include sedation, weakness, dizziness, dry mouth, constipation, and impotence. Patients should be advised to exercise caution when operating machinery or driving motor vehicles until it is determined that they do not become drowsy or dizzy from the medication. A potential exists for interactions with other drugs that have a central nervous system depressant action, and patients should be warned that their tolerance for alcohol and other CNS depressants may be decreased. The abrupt discontinuation of therapy may be associated with symptoms of nervousness and anxiety as well as increases in blood pressure (rebound hypertension).

Administration: Oral.

Preparation: Tablets, 1 mg.

GYNE-LOTRIMIN®, see Clotrimazole

H

HABITROL®, see Nicotine

HALAZEPAM—Paxipam®

Benzodiazepine antianxiety agent indicated for the management of anxiety disorders or the short-term relief of the symptoms of anxiety.

Preparations: Tablets, 20 and 40 mg.

HALCINONIDE—Halog®

Corticosteroid applied topically for the relief of the inflammatory and pruritic manifestations of corticosteroid-responsive dermatoses.

Preparations: Cream, 0.025% and 0.1%. Ointment and solution, 0.1%.

HALCION®, see Triazolam

HALDOL®, see Haloperidol

HALOBETASOL PROPIONATE—Ultravate®

Topical corticosteroid.

Actions and Uses: A high to super-high potency topical corticosteroid indicated for the relief of the inflammatory and pruritic manifestations of corticosteroid-responsive dermatoses.

Warnings: Adverse reactions include stinging, burning, itching, dry skin, erythema, and skin atrophy. May cause suppression of the hypothalamic-pituitary-adrenal (HPA) axis and appropriate precautions should be taken (e.g., regarding the extent and duration of treatment).

Administration: Topical. Should not be used with occlusive dressings. Because of its high potency, treatment should be limited to 2 weeks, and amounts greater than 50 grams/week should not be used.

Preparations: Cream and ointment, 0.05%.

HALOG®, see Halcinonide

HALOPERIDOL—Haldol®

Antipsychotic agent.

Actions and Uses: A butyrophenone derivative indicated for (1) the management of manifestations of psychotic disorders; (2) the control of tics and vocal utterances of Tourette's disorder; and, in children who have not responded to psychotherapy or medications other than neuroleptics; (3) the treatment of severe behavior problems in children of combative, explosive hyperexcitability; and (4) the short-term treatment of hyperactive children who show excessive motor activity with accompanying conduct disorders.

Warnings: Contraindicated in patients with parkinsonism or severe CNS depression. Adverse reactions include drowsiness and other CNS effects;

patients should be cautioned regarding activities such as driving and operating machinery, as well as interactions with other CNS-acting drugs including alcohol. Other adverse reactions include extrapyramidal reactions, tardive dyskinesia, neuroleptic malignant syndrome, and hypotension. Concomitant therapy with lithium must be closely monitored because there have been reports of an encephalopathic syndrome in some patients receiving both medications.

Administration: Oral and intramuscular.

Preparations: Tablets, 0.5, 1, 2, 5, 10, and 20 mg. Solution concentrate (as the lactate), 2 mg/ml. Ampules and vials (as the lactate), 5 mg/ml.

HALOPERIDOL DECANOATE—Haldol decanoate®

Antipsychotic agent.

Actions and Uses: Is a long-acting parenterally administered form of haloperidol indicated in the management of patients requiring prolonged parenteral neuroleptic therapy.

Warnings: See discussion of haloperidol.

Administration: Intramuscular. The recommended interval between doses is 4 weeks.

Preparations: Ampules, 50 and 100 mg per ml.

HALOPROGIN—Halotex®

Antifungal agent indicated for the topical treatment of superficial tinea (ringworm) infections and tinea versicolor.

Preparations: Cream and solution, 1%.

HALOTESTIN®, see Fluoxymesterone

HALOTEX®, see Haloprogin

HALOTHANE—Fluothane®

Inhalation general anesthetic indicated for the induction and maintenance of general anesthesia.

Preparations: Liquid, 125 and 250 ml.

HELIDAC®

Combination agent used in treatment of active duodenal ulcer associated with H.pylori. Bismuth subsalicylate, metronidazole, tetracyline.

HEMABATE®, see Carboprost tromethamine

HEPARIN SODIUM—Liquaemin sodium®

Anticoagulant.

Actions and Uses: Exhibits an anti-coagulant action, in part, by inhibiting the conversion of fibrinogen to fibrin. Indicated in the prophylaxis and treatment of venous thrombosis and its extension, pulmonary embolism, peripheral arterial embolism, and atrial fibrillation with embolization. Also used in the diagnosis and treatment of acute and chronic consumptive coagulopathies, in a low-dose regimen for prevention of postoperative deep vein thrombosis and pulmonary embolism in patients undergoing major surgery, as an adjunct in the treatment of coronary occlusion with acute myocardial infarction, in the prevention of clotting in arterial and heart surgery, and in blood transfusions, extracorporeal circulation, and dialysis procedures. Used in very low doses to maintain patency of IV catheters (heparin flush).

Warnings: May cause hemorrhage and therapy must be closely monitored. Action may be increased by agents such as aspirin and nonsteroidal anti-inflammatory drugs.

Administration: Intravenous or deep subcutaneous. Intramuscular use should be avoided because of the danger of hematoma formation.

Preparations: Ampules and vials, 10, 100, 1,000, 5,000, 10,000, 20,000, and 40,000 units/ml.

HEROIN—Diacetylmorphine

Narcotic analgesic not legally available in the United States.

HERPLEX®, see Idoxuridine

HESPAN®, see Hetastarch

HETASTARCH—Hespan®

Plasma expander with colloidal properties approximating those of human albumin. Indicated for intravenous infusion when plasma volume expansion is desired as an adjunct in the treatment of shock due to hemorrhage, burns, surgery, sepsis, or other trauma.

Preparation: Solution, 6% in 250- and 500-cc bottles.

HEXACHLOROPHENE—pHisoHex®

Anti-infective agent indicated for topical use as a surgical scrub and a bacteriostatic skin cleanser.

Preparation: Emulsion, 3%.

HEXADROL®, see Dexamethasone

HEXALEN®, see Altretamine

HEXAVITAMIN

Vitamin mixture that includes Vitamins A, D, B_1, B_2, and C, and nicotinic acid. Used in the prevention and treatment of deficiencies of these vitamins.

Preparations: Capsules and Tablets.

HIBICLENS®, see Chlorhexidine gluconate

HIBISTAT®, see Chlorhexidine gluconate.

HIPREX®, see Methenamine hippurate

HISMANAL®, see Astemizole

HISTAMINE PHOSPHATE

Diagnostic agent used to test the ability of the gastric mucosa to produce hydrochloric acid, and in the diagnosis of pheochromocytoma.

Preparations: Ampules containing the equivalent of 0.1 and 0.2 mg histamine base/ml.

HISTRELIN ACETATE—Supprelin®

Agent for precocious puberty.

Actions and Uses: Is an analog of naturally occurring gonadotropin releasing hormone (GnRH), and is a potent inhibitor of gonadotropin secretion when administered daily in therapeutic doses. Chronic daily administration inhibits the secretion of pituitary gonadotropin which, in turn, causes a reduction in ovarian and testicular steroid production. Indicated for the control of the manifestations of centrally mediated precocious puberty occurring before the age of 8 years in girls or 9.5 years in boys.

Warnings: Also contraindicated in women who are or may become pregnant while receiving the drug, and in nursing mothers. Adverse reactions include skin reactions at the injection site (e.g., redness, swelling, itching), vaginal bleeding, and hypersensitivity reactions.

Administration: Subcutaneous. Daily injection should be rotated through different body sites (upper arms, thighs, abdomen). Patients and their families should be informed of the need to give injections at approximately the same time each day; otherwise the pubertal process may be reactivated. Treatment should be discontinued when the onset of puberty is desired.

Preparations: Vials (and syringes with needles) that deliver 0.6 ml of a solution containing 200 ug/ml (120 ug/vial), 500 ug/ml (300 ug/vial), or 1,000 ug/ml (600 ug/vial).

HIVID®, see Zalcitabine

HOMATROPINE HYDROBROMIDE

Anticholinergic agent for ophthalmic use. Indicated for use as a mydriatic and cycloplegic for refraction, and in the management of certain ocular inflammatory conditions. Also used orally for anticholinergic action in combination with other agents.

Preparations: Ophthalmic solutions, 2% and 5%.

HUMABID LA®, see Guaifenesin

HUMABID SPRINKLE®, see Guaifenesin

HUMALOG®, see Insulin

HUMATIN®, see Paromomycin

HUMATROPE®, see Somatropin

HUMORSOL®, see Demecarium

HUMULIN®, see Insulin

HYALURONIDASE—Wydase®

Enzyme indicated as an adjuvant to increase the absorption and dispersion of other injected drugs, for hypodermoclysis, and as an adjunct in subcutaneous urography for improving resorption of radiopaque agents.

Preparations: Vials, 150 and 1500 units.

HYCAMTIN®, see Topotecan Hydrochloride

HYCODAN®, Combination of hydrocodone and homatropine

HYDELTRA®, see Prednisolone tebutate

HYDELTRASOL®, see Prednisolone sodium phosphate

HYDERGINE®, see Ergoloid mesylates

HYDRALAZINE HYDROCHLORIDE—Apresoline®

Antihypertensive agent.

Preparations: Tablets, 10, 25, 50, and 100 mg. Injection, 20 mg/ml.

HYDREA®, see Hydroxyurea

HYDROCHLOROTHIAZIDE—Esidrix®, HydroDIURIL®, MIcrozide®, Oretic®

Thiazide diuretic.

Actions and Uses: Indicated in the management of hypertension, and as adjunctive therapy in edema associated with congestive heart failure, hepatic cirrhosis, and corticosteroid and estrogen therapy. Is also useful in edema due to various forms of renal dysfunction such as nephrotic syndrome.

Warnings: May cause hypokalemia, and serum potassium levels should be determined periodically. Reduction in potassium levels may increase the action and toxicity of digoxin and related glycosides. Concurrent use with lithium is best avoided because of an increased risk of lithium toxicity. May cause hyperglycemia and hyperuricemia, and therapy in patients having diabetes or gout should be closely monitored.

Administration: Oral.

Preparations: Tablets, 25, 50, and 100 mg. Capsules, 12.5 mg. Oral solution, 50 mg/5 ml. Concentrated oral solution, 100 mg/ml.

HYDROCODONE BITARTRATE—Hycodan®

Opioid analgesic and antitussive indicated for the relief of moderate to moderately severe pain, and for the relief of cough. Used in combination with other agents.

HYDROCODONE BITARTATE WITH ACETAMINOPHEN—Norco®

HYDROCORTISONE—Cortisol, Cortef®, Hydrocortone®, Pandel®

Corticosteroid indicated in a wide range of endocrine, rheumatic, allergic, dermatologic, respiratory, hematologic, neoplastic, and other disorders.

Preparations: Tablets, 5, 10, and 20 mg. Oral suspension (as the cypionate), 10 mg/5 ml. Vials, (as the sodium phosphate), 50 mg/ml. Vials (as the sodium succinate), 100, 250, 500, and 1000 mg. Vials (as the acetate for intralesional, intra-articular, or soft tissue injection), 25 mg/ml and 50 mg/ml. Retention enema, 100 mg. Cream, ointment, lotion, gel, aerosol for topical use (some for mulations contain the acetate salt), 0.25%, 0.5%, 1%, and 2.5%. Cream and ointment (as the butyrate), 0.1%. Cream (as buteprate) and ointment (as the valerate), 0.2%.

HYDROCORTONE®, see Hydrocortisone

HYDRODIURIL®, see Hydrochlorothiazide

HYDROFLUMETHIAZIDE—Diucardin®, Saluron®

Thiazide diuretic indicated as adjunctive therapy in the treatment of edema. Is also indicated in the management of hypertension.

Preparation: Tablets, 50 mg.

HYDROGEN PEROXIDE

Antiseptic/cleansing agent applied to the skin and certain mucous membranes.

Preparation: Solution, 3%.

HYDROMORPHONE HYDROCHLORIDE—Dilaudid®

Opioid analgesic indicated for the relief of moderate to severe pain. Has also been used to suppress cough.

Preparations: Tablets, 1, 2, 4, and 8 mg. Suppositories, 3 mg. Ampules, vials, and syringes, 1 mg/ml, 2 mg/ml, 3 mg/ml, 4 mg/ml, and 10 mg/ml.

HYDROMOX®, see Quinethazone

HYDROPHILIC OINTMENT

Ointment base that is "water removable" and into which medications are often incorporated and applied.

HYDROPHILIC PETROLATUM

Ointment base capable of absorbing quantities of water or aqueous solutions containing medications.

HYDROQUINONE—Eldoquin®

Skin bleaching agent indicated for the gradual bleaching of hyperpigmented skin conditions such as freckles, chloasma, and melasma.

Preparations: Cream, 2% and 4%.

HYDROXOCOBALAMIN

Vitamin B12 analog indicated in the parenteral treatment of pernicious anemia, dietary deficiency of Vitamin B12, malabsorption of vitamin B12, and other situations in which there is inadequate utilization of vitamin B12. Also used for the Schilling test.

Preparations: Vials, 1000 µg/ml.

HYDROXYAMPHETAMINE HYDROBROMIDE

Sympathomimetic amine indicated for ophthalmic use to dilate the pupil.

Preparation: Ophthalmic solution, in combination with other agents.

HYDROXYCHLOROQUINE SULFATE—Plaquenil®

Antimalarial agent indicated for the treatment of acute attacks and suppression of malaria. Also used in the management of rheumatoid arthritis and lupus erythematosus in patients who have not responded satisfactorily to drugs having a lesser potential to cause serious adverse effects.

Preparation: Tablets, 200 mg.

HYDROXYPROGESTERONE CAPROATE—Duralutin®

Progestin administered intramuscularly in the management of amenorrhea, abnormal uterine bleeding due to hormonal imbalance, production of secretory endometrium and desquamation, and adenocarcinoma of uterine corpus in advanced stage.

Preparations: Vials, 125 mg/ml and 250 mg/ml.

HYDROXYUREA—Hydrea®

Antineoplastic agent indicated in the treatment of melanoma, chronic myelocytic leukemia, and carcinoma of the ovary. Has also been of benefit in reducing the frequency and severity of painful sickle cell crises.

Preparation: Capsules, 500 mg.

HYDROXYZINE—Atarax®, Vistaril

Antianxiety agent.

Actions and Uses: Exhibits sedative and antihistaminic actions. Indicated (1) for symptomatic relief of anxiety and tension associated with psychoneurosis and as an adjunct in organic disease states in which anxiety is manifested; (2) in the management of pruritus due to allergic conditions such as chronic urticaria and atopic and contact dermatoses, and in histamine-mediated pruritus; and (3) as a sedative when used as premedication and following general anesthesia.

Warnings: Contraindicated in early pregnancy. Adverse reactions include drowsiness and other CNS effects; patients should be cautioned regarding activities such as driving and operating machinery, as well as interactions with other CNS-acting drugs including alcohol. When other CNS-depressant drugs are administered concurrently, their dosage should be appropriately reduced.

Administration: Oral and intramuscular.

Preparations: Tablets and capsules, 10, 25, 50, and 100 mg. Syrup, 10 mg/5 ml, oral suspension, 25 mg/5 ml. Vials, 25 and 50 mg/ml.

HYGROTON®, see Chlorthalidone

HYLOREL®, see Guanadrel

HYOSCINE, see Scopolamine

HYOSCYAMINE SULFATE—Anaspaz, Cystospaz®, Levbid®, Levsin®, Levsinex®

Anticholinergic agent used as adjunctive therapy in the treatment of peptic ulcer. Also used in other gastrointestinal disorders, biliary and renal conditions, as a drying agent in acute rhinitis, and in the management of parkinsonism.

Preparations: Tablets, 0.125 and 0.15 mg. Controlled-release capsules, 0.375 mg. Elixir, 0.125 mg/5 ml. Drops, 0.125 mg/ml. Vials, 0.5 mg/ml.

HYPERSTAT®, see Diazoxide

HYTAKEROL®, see Dihydrotachysterol

HYTRIN®, see Terazosin

HYZAAR®, see Lorsartan potassium and Hydrochlorothiazide

I

IBUPROFEN—Advil®, Children's Advil®, Motrin®, Children's Motrin®, Nuprin®, Rufen®

Nonsteroidal anti-inflammatory drug.

Actions and Uses: Inhibits prostaglandin synthesis and is indicated for the relief of mild to moderate pain, primary dysmenorrhea, rheumatoid arthritis, osteoarthritis, and reduction of fever.

Warnings: Should not be given to patients in whom aspirin or another NSAID causes asthma, rhinitis, urticaria, or other allergic-type reactions. May cause GI effects, and use should be avoided in patients with active GI tract disease and closely monitored in patients with a previous history of such disorders. Other adverse reactions include dizziness and rash.

Administration: Oral.

Preparations: Caplets and tablets, 100, 200, 300, 400, 600, and 800 mg. Chewable tablets, 50 and 100 mg. Suspension, 100 mg/5 ml, oral drops 40 mg/ml.

IBUTILIDE FUMARATE—Corvert®

Antiarrhythmic.

Actions and Uses: Predominantly Class III antiarrhythmic used in the Rapid Conversion of atrial fibrillation or atrial flutter of recent onset to sinus rhythm. Patients with atrial arrhythmias of longer duration are less likely to respond to ibutilide. The effectiveness of ibutilide has not been determined in patients with arrhythmias of > 90 days duration.

Warnings: Administer in appropriate treatment environment as this drug may cause life-threatening arrhythmias such as sustained polymorphic ventricular tachycardia, usually in association with QT prolongation (torsades de pointes) but sometimes without QT prolongation. These arrhythmias can be reversed if treated promptly with cardioversion. An appropriate environment should include continuous ECG monitoring, personnel skilled in arrhythmia recognition, and life-support equipment. Reports of reversible heart block have been associated with ibutilide administration.

Administration: Intravenous with an initial dose over 10 minutes with a second 10-minute infusion if arrhythmia does not terminate within 10 minutes after the end of the initial infusion. Maintain continuous ECG monitoring for 4 hours following the infusion or until QT has returned to baseline.

Preparations: Solution, 0.1mg/ml in 10 ml vials.

ICHTHAMMOL

Antibacterial agent and astringent applied topically in certain dermatologic disorders.

Preparations: Ointment, 10% and 20%.

IDAMYCIN®, see Idarubicin hydrochloride

IDARUBICIN HYDROCHLORIDE —Idamycin®

Antineoplastic agent.

Actions and Uses: Is an anthracycline derivative that is indicated for use in combination with other antileukemic drugs (usually cytarabine) for the treatment of acute myeloid leukemia in adults.

Warnings: May cause severe myelosuppression and should not be given to patients with preexisting bone marrow suppression induced by previous drug therapy or radiotherapy unless the benefit warrants the risk. Other adverse reactions include myocardial toxicity (e.g., congestive heart failure, arrhythmias), GI effects (e.g., nausea, vomiting, mucositis, abdominal pain, diarrhea), alopecia, dermatologic effects (e.g., rash, urticaria), pulmonary effects, mental status effects, fever, headache, neurologic effects, hyperuricemia secondary to rapid lysis of leukemic cells, and extravasation. Should not be used in pregnant women unless the benefit out-weighs the risk. In patients with hepatic or renal impairment, a reduction in dosage should be considered and treatment should be closely monitored.

Administration. Intravenous. Follow vesicant procedures.

Preparations: Vials, 5 and 10 mg.

IDOXURIDINE—IDU, Herplex®, Stoxil®

Antiviral agent indicated for ophthalmic use in the treatment of herpes simplex keratitis.

Preparations: Ophthalmic solution, 0.1%. Ophthalmic ointment, 0.5%

IDU, see Idoxuridine

IFEX® see Ifosfamide

IFOSFAMIDE—Ifex®

Antineoplastic agent.

Actions and Uses: Is an analog of cyclophosphamide and requires metabolic activation by liver microsomal enzymes to produce biologically active metabolites. Indicated for use in combination with other antineoplastic agents, for third line chemotherapy of germ cell testicular cancer. Should be used in combination with mesna to reduce the risk of hemorrhagic cystitis.

Warnings: May cause leukopenia, thrombocytopenia, and urotoxic effects, especially hemorrhagic cystitis. Other adverse reactions include sedation confusion, hallucinations, alopecia, nausea, and vomiting.

Administration: Intravenous infusion (lasting a minimum of 30 minutes). Should be given with extensive hydration consisting of at least 2 liters of oral or intravenous fluid per day, and with the uroprotective agent, mesna.

Preparation: Vials, 1 and 3 g.

ILETIN®, see Insulin

ILOPAN®, see Dexpanthenol

ILOSONE®, see Erythromycin estolate.

ILOTYCIN®, see Erythromycin base and gluceptate

IMDUR®, see Isosorbide mononitrate

IMIGLUCERASE—Cerezyme®

Agent for Gaucher disease.

Actions and Uses: Is an analog of the human enzyme, beta-glucocerebrosidase produced by recombinant technology. Indicated for long-term enzyme replacement therapy for patients with a confirmed diagnoses of Type I Gaucher disese that results in one or more of the following conditions: anemia; thrombocytopenia; bone disease; hepatomegaly or splenomegaly.

Warnings: Adverse reactions include headache, nausea, abdominal discomfort, dizziness, pruritus, and rash. Caution should be exercised in patients previously treated with alglucerase and who have developed antibody to alglucerase or who have exhibited symptoms of hypersensitivity to alglucerase.

Administration: Intravenous. Is administered by IV infusion over 1-2 hours.

Preparation: Vials, 200 units.

IMIPENEM-CILASTATIN SODIUM—Primaxin IV®, Primaxin IM®

Carbapenem antibiotic.

Actions and Uses: Imipenem has a very broad spectrum of action that includes almost all gram-positive and gram-negative bacteria. Cilastatin is an enzyme inhibitor which significantly reduces the renal metabolism of imipenem, resulting in a much greater urinary recovery of the antibiotic. Indicated for intravenous use for the treatment of lower respiratory tract infections, urinary tract infections, intra- abdominal infections, gynecologic infections, bacterial septicemia, bone and joint infections, skin and skin-structure infections, endocarditis, and polymicrobic infections caused by susceptible organisms. Indicated for intramuscular use in the treatment of serious infections of mild to moderate severity for which IM therapy is appropriate.

Warnings: Must be used cautiously, if at all, in patients who have experienced hypersensitivity reactions to a penicillin or cephalosporin. Seizures have been reported although infrequently, and therapy must be closely supervised in patients with predisposing factors such as a history of seizures.

Administration: Intravenous and intramuscular.

Preparations: Vials and infusion bottles for intravenous use, 250 mg imipenem equivalent with 250 mg cilastatin equivalent, and 500 mg of each agent. Vials for intramuscular use, 500 mg imipenem equivalent with 500 mg cilastatin equivalent, and 750 mg of each agent.

IMIPRAMINE HYDROCHLORIDE—Tofranil®

IMIPRAMINE PAMOATE—Tofranil-PM®

Tricyclic antidepressant indicated for the relief of symptoms of depression. Oral formulation of imipramine hydrochloride is also used in the management of childhood enuresis.

Preparations: Tablets, 10, 25, and 50 mg. Capsules (pamoate), 75, 100, 125, and 150 mg. Ampules, 25 mg.

IMIQUIMOD—Aldara®

Actions and Uses:

Immune Response Modifier indicated in the treatment of external genital and perianal warts (condyloma acuminata). The effect of imiquimod cream in the transmission of genital/perianal warts is unknown. Other therapies used to treat genital warts can cause damage to tissue and surrounding areas and imiquimod should not be applied until these areas have healed.

Warnings: Not for use in treating urethral, intravaginal, cervical, rectal, or intra-anal human papilloma viral disease. Not for use on lesions that have not healed from other therapies (drug or surgical). Avoid sexual contact while cream is applied to skin. Avoid eyes. Do not occlude. May exacerbate inflammatory skin conditions. Concomitant use of diaphragms or condoms not recommended. Adverse reactions include local and remote reactions (e.g., erythema, erosion, itching, burning, soreness), headache, flulike symptoms and myalgia.

Administration: Apply a thin layer to warts and rub in 3 times per week at bedtime (e.g., Mon-Wed-Fri or Tues-Thurs-Sat). Maximum usage not to exceed 16 weeks. Remove with soap and water after 6–10 hours. If local reactions occur, suspend therapy until reaction subsides. When treating warts under foreskin of uncircumcised males, the foreskin should be retracted and cleansed daily. New warts may develop during therapy. Wash hands before and after application. Notify prescriber of severe skin reactions.

Preparation: Single-use packets of 5% cream (250 mg each).

IMITREX®, see Sumatriptan succinate

IMODIUM®, see Loperamide

IMODIUM ADVARCED®—Combination agent lopermide and simethicone (opiod and antiflatulert)

IMODIUM A-D®, see Loperamide

IMURAN®, see Azathioprine

INAPSINE®, see Droperidol

INDAPAMIDE—Lozol®

Diuretic indicated for the treatment of hypertension and for the treatment of salt and fluid retention associated with congestive heart failure.

Preparation: Tablets, 1.25 and 2.5 mg.

INDERAL®, see Propranolol

INDINAVIR—Crixivan®

Antiviral, protease inhibitor.

Action and Uses: Used in treatment of H.I.V. infection.

Warnings: Contraindicated with concurrent use of terfenadine, astemizole, cisapride, triazolam and midazolam. Adverse reactions include nephrolithiasis, aymptomatic hyperbilirubinemia, GI upset, abdominal pain, kidney stones, headache, fatigue, insomnia, flank pain, and dysguesia. Maintain adequate hydration (1.5 L/day). Discontinue or suspend therapy (e.g., 1–3 days) during acute nephrolithiasis or impaired hepatic function.

Administration: Oral with water on an empty stomach or with a light meal. Usual dose is 800 mg every 8 hours. Reduce dose of indinavir sulfate to 600 mg every 8 hours in hepatic insufficiency or with concomitant use of Ketoconazole.

Preparations: Capsules, 200 and 400 mg.

INDOCIN®, see Indomethacin

INDOMETHACIN—Indocin®, Indocin SR®

Nonsteroidal anti-inflammatory drug.

Actions and Uses: Inhibits prostaglandin synthesis and is indicated in the treatment of rheumatoid arthritis, osteoarthritis, ankylosing spondylitis, acute painful shoulder, and acute gouty arthritis. Used as an alternative to surgery in the management of patent ductus arteriosus in premature neonates.

Warnings: Should not be given to patients in whom aspirin or another NSAID causes asthma, rhinitis, urticaria, or other allergic-type reactions. Suppositories are contraindicated in patients with a history of proctitis or recent rectal bleeding. May cause GI effects and use should be avoided in patients with active GI tract disease and closely monitored in patients with a previous history of such disorders. Other reactions include headache and dizziness.

Administration: Oral, rectal, and intravenous. Should be administered with food or antacids, or immediately after meals, to reduce GI effects.

Preparations: Capsules, 25 and 50 mg. Sustained-release capsules, 75 mg. Oral suspension, 25 mg/5 ml. Suppositories, 50 mg. Injection, 1 mg vials.

InFeD®, see Iron dextran

INH, see Isoniazid

INOCOR®, see Amrinone

INSULATARD®, see Insulin

INSULIN INJECTION—Regular Iletin I and II®, Humalog®, Humulin R®, Novolin R®, Velosulin®
INSULIN ZINC SUSPENSION, PROMPT (Semilente)
ISOPHANE INSULIN SUSPENSION (NPH)—NPH Iletin I and II®, Insulatard NPH®, Humulin N®, Novolin N®
INSULIN ZINC SUSPENSION (Lente)—Lente Iletin I and II®, Humulin L®, Novolin L®
PROTAMINE ZINC INSULIN SUSPENSION (PZI)
INSULIN ZINC SUSPENSION, EXTENDED (Ultralente)

Hypoglycemic agent.

Actions and Uses: Is the principal hormone required for proper glucose use in normal metabolic processes. Indicated in the treatment of diabetes mellitus that cannot be properly controlled by diet alone. Also used in severe ketoacidosis or diabetic coma.

Warnings: Hypoglycemia may result from excessive dosage. Adverse reactions include allergic responses and lipodystrophy. Corticosteroids and thiazide and other diuretics may increase blood glucose levels and necessitate an increase in insulin dosage.

Administration: Subcutaneous. Insulin injection (regular insulin) has been administered intravenously or intramuscularly in certain situations (e.g., severe ketoacidosis, diabetic coma).

Preparations: Preparations are classified as rapid-acting (Regular, Semilente), intermediate-acting (NPH, Lente), and long-acting (PZI, Ultralente), based on the promptness, duration, and intensity of action following subcutaneous administration. Some preparations contain human insulin prepared using recombinant DNA technology (Humu- lin) or semisynthetically (Novolin, Insulatard, Velosulin); other preparations are derived from beef and pork sources. Vials, 100 units/ml. A concentrated solution of regular insulin containing 500 units per ml is available for the treatment of patients with insulin resistance.

INTAL®, see Cromolyn

INTERFERON ALFA-2a RECOMBINANT—Roferon-A®

INTERFERON ALFA-2b RECOMBINANT—Intron A®

Antineoplastic agent/antiviral agent.

Actions and Uses: Prepared using recombinant DNA technology. Indicated for the treatment of hairy-cell leukemia in patients 18 years of age or older and in the treatment of AIDS-related Kaposi's sarcoma in patients 18 years of age or older. Interferon alfa-2b is also indicated for the treatment of chronic hepatitis non-A, non-B/C, chronic hepatitis B, and for the intralesional treatment of condylomata acuminata (venereal or genital warts). Interferon Alfa 2a is indicated in the treatment of chronic hepatitis C in patients with compensated liver disease.

Warnings: Most patients experience flulike symptoms (e.g., fever, headache, myalgia, chills) at the beginning of therapy; these effects can often be effectively managed with an analgesic-antipyretic such as acetaminophen. Fatigue, dizziness, and other CNS effects may occur, and patients should be cautioned about the risks of engaging in activities in which full mental and physical alertness and coordination are required.

Administration: Intramuscular and subcutaneous for hairy-cell leukemia, AIDS-related Kaposi's sarcoma, and chronic hepatitis non-A, non-B/C. Intralesion- al for condylomata acuminata.

Interferon alfa-2a- Vials, 3, 9, 18, and 36 million IU, and a powder formulation in vials containing 18 million IU. Interferon alfa-2b-Vials containing 3, 5, 10, 18, 25, and 50 million IU of lyophilized powder.

INTERFERON ALFA-N3 (HUMAN LEUKOCYTE DERIVED)—Alferon N®

Antiviral agent.

Actions and Uses: Is manufactured from pooled units of human leukocytes and is designated as a natural interferon. Indicated for the intralesional treatment of refractory or recurring external condylomata acuminata (genital warts) in patients 18 years of age or older.

Warnings: Adverse reactions include flu-like symptoms (e.g., fever, headache, myalgia, chills, back pain, and insomnia).

Administration: Intralesional. The drug should be injected into the base of each wart.

Preparations: Vials, 5 million international units.

INTERFERON BETA-1A—Avonex®

Actions and Uses: For the treatment of relapsing forms of multiple sclerosis to slow the accumulation of physical disability and decrease the frequency of clinical exacerbations.

Preparations: Powder for injection, 33 mg.

INTERFERON BETA-1B—Betaseron®

Agent for multiple sclerosis.

Actions and Uses: Produced by recombinant DNA technology and exhibits antiviral and immunoregulatory activities. Indicated for use in ambulatory patients with relapsing-remitting multiple sclerosis to reduce the frequency of clinical exacerbations and slow the accumulation of physical disability.

Warnings: Adverse reactions include injection site reactions, flu-like symptoms, menstrual disorders, reduction in neutrophil and white blood cell counts, and elevation in SGPT levels. Use has been associated with depression and suicide attempts and patients should be advised to immediately report symptoms of depression. Has been reported in animal studies to have abortifacient activity.

Administration: Subcutaneous, administered every other day. Sites for self-injection include arms, abdomen, hips, and thighs.

Preparations: Vials, 0.3 mg Betaseron (9.6 million IU), 33 mg Avonex, plus a separate vial containing diluent.

INTERFERON GAMMA-1B - Actimmune®

Biologic response modifier.

Actions and Uses: Prepared by recombinant DNA technology. Exhibits immunomodulatory properties and a phagocyte-activating effect which mediates the killing of microorganisms. Indicated for reducing the frequency and severity of serious infections associated with chronic granulomatous disease.

Warnings: Adverse reactions include flulike symptoms (e.g., fever, headache, chills, myalgia, fatigue) which may decrease in severity as treatment continues. Some symptoms may be minimized by bedtime administration. Acetaminophen may be useful in alleviating fever and headache. May cause CNS effects (e.g., dizziness, decreased mental status) and caution should be exercised in patients with known seizure disorders and/or compromised CNS function. May cause hematologic effects (e.g., neutropenia) and caution should be exercised when used in patients with myelosuppression or when used in combination with other potentially myelosuppressive agents.

Administration: Subcutaneous. Optimum sites of injection are the right deltoid and anterior thigh. Vials should not be shaken.

Preparations: Vials, 100 ug (3 million units).

INTERLEUKIN-2, see Aldesleukin

INTRON A®, see Interferon alfa-2b recombinant

INTROPIN®, see Dopamine

INVERSINE®, see Mecamylamine

INVERT SUGAR—Travert®

Mixture of dextrose and fructose used intravenously for fluid and caloric replacement.

Preparation: Solution, 10%.

INVIRASE®, see Saquinavir

IODINATED GLYCEROL

Mucolytic/expectorant indicated as adjunctive treatment in respiratory conditions such as bronchitis and asthma.

Preparations: Tablets, 30 mg. Elixir, 1.2%. Solution, 5%.

IODINE

Antiseptic applied topically to prevent or treat dermatologic infections. Also used to disinfect the skin preoperatively. Has also been used (often as sodium iodide or potassium iodide) orally and parenterally in the management of certain thyroid conditions.

Preparations: Solution (with sodium or potassium iodide), 2% and 5% (Lugol's solution). Tincture (with sodium or potassium iodide), 2% and 5%.

IODOCHLORHYDROXYQUIN—former name of Clioquinol

IODOQUINOL—Diiodohydroxyquin, Yodoxin®

Amebicide indicated in the treatment of intestinal amebiasis.

Preparations: Tablets, 210 and 650 mg.

IOPIDINE®, see Apraclonidine

IPECAC

Emetic used in the management of drug overdose and in certain other poisonings.

Preparation: Syrup.

IPRATROPIUM BROMIDE—Atrovent®

Bronchodilator, anticholinergic.

Actions and Uses: Is an anticholinergic agent administered by inhalation for the maintenance treatment of bronchospasm associated with chronic obstructive pulmonary disease, including chronic bronchitis and emphysema. Nasal spray is used for rhinorrhea associated with allergic and nonallergic perennial rhinitis and rhinorrhea associated with the common cold.

Warnings: Adverse reactions include cough, exacerbation of symptoms, nervousness, dizziness, headache, nausea, gastrointestinal distress, and palpitations. Nasal spray may cause epistaxis, pharyngitis, nasal dryness or irritation. Systemic anticholinergic effects are uncommon, but caution should be exercised in patients with narrow-angle glaucoma, prostatic hypertrophy, or bladder-neck obstruction. Teach patients to avoid use during acute bronchospasm. Patients should be warned against spraying the aerosol into their eyes, because temporary blurring of vision may result.

Administration: Oral inhalation, nasal spray.

Preparation: Metered-dose inhaler. Inhalation solution, 0.02%. Nasal spray, 0.03% aqueous solution.

IRON DEXTRAN—InFeD®

Iron formulation indicated for the parenteral treatment of iron deficiency anemia.

Preparations: Ampules and vials, 50 mg iron/ml.

ISMELIN®, see Guanethidine

ISMO®, see Isosorbide mononitrate

ISOETHARINE—Bronkometer®, Bronkosol®

Bronchodilator administered by inhalation and indicated for bronchial asthma and for reversible bronchospasm that may occur in association with bronchitis and emphysema.

Preparations: Solution for nebulization (as the hydrochloride), numerous concentrations ranging from 0.062% to 1%. Metered dose inhaler (as the mesylate), 340 µg/metered dose.

ISOFLUROPHATE—Floropryl®

Cholinesterase inhibitor indicated for ophthalmic use in the treatment of open-angle glaucoma, conditions obstructing aqueous outflow, following iridectomy, and accommodative esotropia.

Preparation: Ophthalmic ointment, 0.025%

ISOMETHEPTENE MUCATE

Sympathomimetic agent used in combination with other agents in the treatment of tension and vascular headaches.

ISONIAZID—INH, Nydrazid®

Antitubercular agent used in the treatment of tuberculosis and as preventive therapy in selected patients who are at risk of tubercular infection.

Preparations: Tablets, 50, 100, and 300 mg. Syrup, 50 mg/ml. Vials, 100 mg/ml.

ISOPROPYL ALCOHOL

Antiseptic that is applied to the skin as isopropyl rubbing alcohol and in other formulations.

Preparations: Solutions, 70%, 91%, and 100%.

ISOPROTERENOL HYDROCHLORIDE—Isuprel®

Bronchodilator indicated for the treatment of bronchospasm associated with bronchial asthma, pulmonary emphysema, bronchitis, and bronchiectasis. Also used as an adjunct in the management of shock and in the treatment of cardiac standstill or arrest, in the management of certain ventricular arrhythmias and other serious cardiac complications. May also be used in the management of bronchospasm during anesthesia.

Preparations: Solution for nebulization, 0.25% (1:400), 0.5% (1:200), and 1% (1:100). Aerosol solution and metered dose inhalers. Sublingual tablets, 10 and 15 mg. Ampules, vials, and syringes, 0.2 mg/ml. (1:5000).

ISOPTIN®, see Verapamil

ISOPTIN SR®, see Verapamil

ISOPTO-CARBACHOL®, see Carbachol

ISORDIL®, see Isosorbide dinitrate

ISOSORBIDE DINITRATE—Isordil®, Sorbitrate®

Antianginal agent.

Actions and Uses: An organic nitrate indicated

for the treatment and prevention of angina pectoris.

Warnings: Adverse reactions include headache, dizziness, hypotension, and cutaneous vasodilation with flushing.

Administration: Oral and sublingual.

Preparations: Sublingual tablets, 2.5, 5, and 10 mg. Tablets, 2.5, 5, 10, 20, 30, and 40 mg. Controlled-release tablets, 40 mg. Chewable tablets, 5 and 10 mg.

ISOSORBIDE MONONITRATE—Imdur®, Ismo®, Monoket®

Antianginal agent.

Actions and Uses: An organic nitrate that has a primary action of relaxation of vascular smooth muscle. Is the major active metabolite of isosorbide dinitrate. Indicated for the prevention of angina pectoris due to coronary artery disease.

Warnings: Adverse reactions include headache, dizziness, and nausea/vomiting. May cause hypotension and should be used with caution in patients who are volume depleted or who are already hypotensive.

Symptomatic hypotension may occur when used concurrently with a calcium channel blocking agent and dosage adjustments may be necessary.

Administration: Oral. When administered twice a day, is given in an "asymmetric" dosing schedule (2 doses a day given 7 hours apart) which has been designed to avoid tolerance. The controlled-release formulation is administered once a day.

Preparation: Tablets, 10 and 20 mg. Controlled-release tablets (Imdur®), 30 and 60 mg.

ISOTRETINOIN—Accutane®

Retinoid (vitamin A analog) indicated for the treatment of severe recalcitrant cystic acne.

Warnings: May cause fetal abnormalities and must not be taken during pregnancy.

Preparations: Capsules, 10, 20, and 40 mg.

ISOVEX®, see Ethaverine

ISOXSUPRINE HYDROCHLORIDE—Vasodilan®

Peripheral vasodilator used for relief of symptoms associated with cerebral vascular insufficiency, in peripheral vascular disease of arteriosclerosis obliterans, thromboangiitis obliterans, and Raynaud's disease. Has been utilized investigationally in threatened premature labor.

Preparations: Tablets, 10 and 20 mg.

ISRADIPINE—DynaCirc®

Antihypertensive agent.

Actions and Uses: A calcium channel blocking agent that is indicated in the management of hypertension. May be used alone or concurrently with a thiazide-type diuretic.

Warnings: Adverse reactions include dizziness, edema, palpitations, flushing, tachycardia, fatigue and headache. Caution should be exercised when the drug is used in patients with congestive heart failure. Concurrent use with a beta-adrenergic blocking agent may be employed advantageously in some patients but may be associated with risks such as an excessive reduction in blood pressure.

Administration: Oral.

Preparations: Capsules, 2.5 and 5 mg, controlled release tablets 5 and 10 mg.

ISUPREL®, see Isoproterenol

ITRACONAZOLE—Sporanox®

Triazole antifungal agent.

Actions and Uses: Inhibits the cytochrome P-450-dependent synthesis of ergosterol, which is a vital component of fungal cell membranes. Indicated for the treatment of blastomycosis (pulmonary and extrapulmonary) and histoplasmosis, including chronic cavitary pulmonary disease (and disseminated, nonmeningeal histoplasmosis. Is indicated for these infections in both immunocompromised and non-immunocompromised patients. Also indicated for the treatment of pulmonary aspergillosis in patients who are intolerant of or who are refractory to amphotericin B therapy. Indicated the onchomycosis of the toenail with or without fingernail involvement and in onchomycosis of the fingernail.

Warnings: Caution must be exercised in patients who are hypersensitive to other azole antifungal agents. Concurrent use with terfenadine astemizole or cisapride, is contraindicated. Adverse reactions include nausea, vomiting, diarrhea, edema, fatigue, fever, rash, headache, and hypertension. Abnormal hepatic function, including rare reports of reversible idiosyncratic hepatitis, has been experienced and patients should be advised to report any signs or symptoms that may suggest liver dysfunction.

Administration: Oral. Should be administered with food.

Preparations: Capsules, 100 mg. Oral solution, 10 mg/ml.

K

KADIAN®, see Morphine Sulfate

KANAMYCIN SULFATE—Kantrex®

Aminoglycoside antibiotic primarily used in the parenteral treatment of infections caused by gram-negative bacteria. Has been used orally for the suppression of intestinal bacteria in the management of hepatic coma and in com- bination with other drugs to treat tuberculosis in patients resistant to conventional therapy.

Administration: IV, IM, intraperitoneal, inhalation, and irrigation.

Preparations: Vials and syringes, 75 and 500 mg and 1 gram. Capsules, 500 mg.

KANTREX®, see Kanamycin

KAOLIN

Adsorbent used in combination with other agents in the management of diarrhea.

KAON®, see Potassium gluconate

KAY CIEL®, see Potassium chloride

KAYEXALATE®, see Sodium polystyrene sulfonate

KEFLEX®, see Cephalexin

KEFLIN®, see Cephalothin

KEFTAB®, see Cephalexin hydrochloride

KEFUROX®, see Cefuroxime sodium

KEFZOL®, see Cefazolin

KEMADRIN®, see Procyclidine

KENACORT®, see Triamcinolone

KENALOG®, see Triamcinolone

KERLONE®, see Betaxolol

KETALAR®, see Ketamine

KETAMINE HYDROCHLORIDE—Ketalar®

General anesthetic administered parenterally as the sole anesthetic in certain procedures, for the induction of anesthesia prior to the administration of other general anesthetic agents, and to supplement lowpotency agents such as nitrous oxide.

Preparations: Vials, 10 mg/ml, 50 mg/ml, and 100 mg/ml.

KETOCONAZOLE—Nizoral®

Antifungal agent.

Actions and Uses: Indicated for oral use in the treatment of systemic fungal infections and for the treatment of severe recalcitrant cutaneous dermatophytic infections which have not responded to topical therapy or oral griseofulvin, or in patients who are unable to take griseofulvin. Also used topically in the treatment of tinea corporis, tinea cruris, and tinea versicolor, cutaneous candidiasis, and seborrheic dermatitis. Used as a shampoo in the reduction of scaling due to dandruff.

Warnings: Should not be used concurrently with terfenadine, astemizole, or cisapride.

Administration: Oral and topical.

Preparations: Tablets, 200 mg. Cream, 2%. Shampoo, 2%.

KETOPROFEN—Actron®,Orudis®, Oruvail®

Nonsteroidal anti-inflammatory drug.

Actions and Uses: Inhibits prostaglandin synthesis and is indicated for the treatment of rheumatoid arthritis and osteoarthritis, mild to moderate pain, and dysmenorrhea.

Warnings: Should not be given to patients in whom aspirin or another NSAID causes asthma, rhinitis, urticaria, or other allergic-type reactions. May cause GI effects and use should be avoided in patients with active GI tract disease and closely supervised in patients with a previous history of such disorders. Other adverse reactions include headache, malaise, nervousness, and edema.

Administration: Oral.

Preparations: Tablets, 12.5 mg. Capsules, 25, 50, and 75 mg. Controlled-release capsules (Oruvail), 200 mg.

KETOROLAC TROMETHAMINE—Acular®, Acalar PF®, Toradol®

Analgesic.

Actions and Uses: A nonsteroidal anti-inflammatory drug (NSAID) that inhibits prostaglandin synthesis. Indicated for intramuscular or intravenous use for the short-term (up to 5 days) management of moderately severe, acute pain, usually in a postoperative setting. Therapy should be initiated by the IM or IV route and is to be used orally only as a continuation treatment. Treatment by any route (or combination of routes) of administration should not exceed 5 days. Indicated for ophthalmic use for the relief of itching due to seasonal allergic conjunctivitis and post-op inflammation after cataract extraction.

Warnings: Should not be given to patients in whom aspirin or another NSAID causes asthma, rhinitis, urticaria, or other allergic-type reactions. Use is contraindicated in patients at risk of GI bleeding or other bleeding reactions, and in patients with advanced renal impairment. Adverse reactions include nausea, dyspepsia, gastrointestinal pain, and drowsiness.

Administration: Oral, intravenous, intramuscular, and ophthalmic.

Preparations: Tablets, 10 mg. Single-dose syringes, 15, 30, and 60 mg. Ophthalmic solution, 0.5% and as persative free.

KLARON®, see Sulfacetamide sodium

K-LOR®, see Potassium chloride

KLORVESS®, see Potassium chloride

KLOTRIX®, see Potassium chloride

KONAKION®, see Phytonadione

K-TAB®, see Potassium chloride

KWELL®, see Lindane

KYTRIL® , see Granisetron hydrochloride

L

LABETALOL HYDROCHLORIDE—Normodyne®, Trandate®

Antihypertensive agent.

Actions and Uses: Exhibits nonselective beta-adrenergic and selective alpha 1-adrenergic blocking actions. Indicated in the management of hypertension and, when administered intravenously, is also indicated for the treatment of severe hypertension.

Warnings: Contraindicated in patients with bronchial asthma, overt cardiac failure, greater than first-degree heart block, cardiogenic shock, or severe bradycardia. Adverse reactions include fatigue, dizziness, nausea, and nasal stuffiness. Use is best avoided in patients with bronchospastic diseases and therapy in diabetic patients must be closely monitored.

Administration: Orral and intravenous. Patientsshould be cautioned about the interruption or discontinuation of therapy; exacerbation of angina pectoris may occur following the abrupt cessation of therapy and, when therapy is to be discontinued, the dosage should be gradually reduced over a period of 1 to 2 weeks.

Preparations: Tablets, 100, 200, and 300 mg. Ampules and vials, 5 mg/ml.

LAC-HYDRIN®, see Ammonium lactate

LACTATED RINGER'S INJECTION

Intravenous electrolyte replenishment solution containing sodium, potassium, calium, chloride, and lactate.

Preparations: Solutions, 250, 500, and 1000 ml.

LACTULOSE—Cephulac®, Chronulac®

Disaccharide used orally in the treatment of constipation, and orally or rectally in the prevention and treatment of portal-systemic encephalopathy, including the states of hepatic pre-coma and coma.

Preparation: Syrup, 10 g/15 ml.

LAMISIL®, see Terbinafine hydrochloride

LAMIVUDINE—Epivir®, 3TC®

Actions and Uses: Antiretroviral indicated in the management of HIV infection (AIDS) in combination with zidovudine.

Warnings: Use cautiously in patients with renal dysfunction and children with a history of, or other risk factors for, pancreatitis. Adverse reactions in adults include headache, malaise, fever, GI upset, neuropathy, dizziness, sleep or depressive disorders, rash, respiratory effects, and musculoskeletal pain. Adverse reactions in children include pancreatitis, paresthesias, and peripheral neuropathy.

Administration: Oral without regard to food.

Preparation: Tablets, 150 mg. Oral solution, 10 mg/ml.

LAMOTRIGINE—Lamictal®

Actions and Uses: Antiepileptic drug indicated as an adjunctive therapy in the treatment of partial seizures in patients with epilepsy.

Warnings: Use cautiously in patients with reduced renal function, impaired cardiac or hepatic function. Adverse reactions include ataxia, dizziness, headache, somnolence, nausea, vomiting, rash, and photosensitivity.

Administration: Oral without regard to meals. Abrupt discontinuation may result in an increase in seizure activity so gradual withdrawal over two weeks is recommended unless safety concerns require more rapid withdrawal.

Preparations: Tablets, 25, 100, 150, and 200 mg.

LAMPRENE®, see Clofazimine

LANOLIN—Wool fat

Ointment base used topically in the management of certain dermatological conditions associated with dry skin, and as a vehicle into which other medications are incorporated.

LANOXICAPS®, see Digoxin

LANOXIN®, see Digoxin

LANSOPRAZOLE—Prevacid®

Actions and Uses: Acid (proton) pump inhibitor that blocks the final step of gastric acid production. Indicated for short-term treatment (up to 4 weeks) of active duodenal ulcer, short-term treatment (up to 8 weeks) of erosive esophagitis, and long-term treatment of pathological hypersecretory states (e.g., Zollinger-Ellison syndrome). In combination with clarithromgcin and/or amoxilillin for H. Pylori eradication in duoderal ulcer disease, to reduce the risk of duodenal ulcer recurrence.

Warnings: Adverse reactions include diarrhea, abdominal pain, and nausea. Because it is a potent acid inhibitor, those drugs which require an acidic environment may not be as well absorbed.

Administration: Oral or may open capsules and mix intact granule with 40 ml of spple juice and inject via nasogastric tube.

Preparations: Delayed release capsules, 15 and 30 mg.

LARGON®, see Propiomazine

LARIAM®, see Mefloquine

LARODOPA®, see Levodopa

LASIX®, see Furosemide

LATANOPROST—Xalatan®

Latanoprost is indicated in the treatmennt of open angle glaucoma or ocular hypertension in patients intolerant of, or who have failed to respond to, other agents.

Warnings: Use cautiously in renal or hepatic impairment. Adverse reactions include blurred vision, burning, stinging, increased pigmentation of the iris, punctate epithelial keratopathy, photophobia, upper respiratory tract infection, pain, angina, and rash.

Administration: 1 drop once daily in the pm. Do not exceed the once daily dosage because it has been shown that more frequent administration may decrease the IOP lowering effect. Remove contact lenses before use and do not reinsert for 15 minutes afterwards. Allow at least 5 minutes between application of other topical ophthalmic agents.

Preparations: 0.005% ophthalmic solution containing benzalkonium chloride.

LEDERCILLIN VK®, see Penicillin V potassium

LENTE INSULIN, see Insulin

LESCOL®, see Fluvastatin sodium

LEUCOVORIN CALCIUM—Citrovorum factor, folinic acid, Wellcovorin®

Folic acid analog indicated to prevent and treat the hematologic and other undesired effects of folic acid antagonists (e.g., methotrexate), and to counteract the effect of overdosage of these agents. Has also been used in the treatment of certain megaloblastic anemias. Is also indicated for parenteral use in combination with 5-fluorouracil to prolong survival in the palliative treatment of patients with advanced colorectal cancer.

Preparations: Tablets, 5, 10, 15, and 25 mg. Ampules, 3 mg/ml and 5 mg/ml. Vials, 50, 100, and 350 mg.

LEUKERAN®, see Chlorambucil

LEUKINE®, see Sargramostim

LEUPROLIDE ACETATE—Lupron®, Lupron Depot®, Lupron Depot-Ped®

Gonadotropin-releasing hormone analog administered parenterally in the treatment of advanced prostatic cancer, endometriosis, and central precocious puberty. Also indicated for the treatment of uterine leimyomata in women who fail iron therapy. Solution is injected daily by the subcutaneous route and the depot suspension is injected monthly by the intramuscular route.

Preparations: Powder for injection, 3.75 mg, 7.5

mg, 11.25 mg, and 15 mg. Solution for injection, 5 mg/ml.

LEUSTATIN®, see Cladribine

LEVAMISOLE—Ergamisol®

Antineoplastic agent.

Actions and Uses: An immunomodulator that appears to restore depressed immune function. Indicated as adjunct treatment in combination with fluorouracil after surgical resection in patients with Dukes' stage C colon cancer.

Warnings: May cause agranulocytosis. Use in combination with fluorouracil has been associated with neutropenia, anemia, and thrombocytopenia. Adverse reactions include nausea, vomiting, diarrhea, stomatitis, anorexia, rash and/or pruritus, flu-like symptoms, dizziness, ataxia, depression and confusion. Disulfiram-like reactions may occur following the consumption of alcoholic beverages.

Administration: Oral. Treatment should be initiated no earlier than 7 days and no later than 30 days after surgery.

Preparations: Tablets, 50 mg.

LEVAQUIN®, see Levofloxacin

LEVARTERENOL, see Norepinephrine

LEVATOL®, see Penbutolol

LEVBID®, see Hyoscyamine sulfate

LEVOBUNOLOL HYDROCHLORIDE—Betagan®

Agent for glaucoma.

Actions and Uses: A noncardioselective beta-adrenergic blocking agent indicated for ophthalmic use in the treatment of chronic open-angle glaucoma and ocular hypertension.

Warnings: Contraindicated in patients with bronchial asthma or severe chronic obstructive pulmonaryy disease, sinus bradycardia,second-and third-degree AV block, overt cardiac failure, or cardiogenic shock. Adverse reactions include transient ocular burning and stinging, and systemic effects such as decrease in heart rate and blood pressure. Caution must be exercised in patients who are also taking another beta-blocker orally for another indication.

Administration: Ophthalmic.

Preparation: Ophthalmic solution, 0.25% and 0.5%.

LEVOCABASTINE HYDROCHLORIDE—Livostin®

Antihistamine.

Actions and Uses: Indicated for topical ophthalmic use for the temporary relief of the signs and symptoms of seasonal allergic conjunctivitis.

Warnings: Adverse reactions include mild, transient stinging and burning, and headache. Contains benzalkonium chloride and patients should be instructed not to wear soft contact lenses during treatment.

Administration: Ophthalmic.

Preparation: Ophthalmic suspension, 0.05%.

LEVODOPA—Dopar®, Larodopa®

Antiparkinson agent.

Actions and Uses: Is converted to dopamine, which is the active pharmacologic agent. Indicated in the treatment of parkinsonism.

Warnings: Should not be given concomitantly with a monoamine oxidase inhibitor or in patients with narrow-angle glaucoma. Should be administered cautiously in patients with severe cardiovascular or pulmonary disease, bronchial asthma, renal, hepatic, or endocrine disease. Adverse reactions include choreiform and/or dystonic movements, palpitations, orthostatic hypotension, mental changes, headache, dizziness, nausea, and vomiting. Effect may be reduced by pyridoxine, and preparations containing this vitamin should be avoided unless carbidopa is being given concomitantly with levodopa (i.e., in the combination product, Sinemet® and Sinemet CR®). Not useful for treatment of drug-induced extra-pyramidal reactions.

Administration: Oral.

Preparations: Capsules and tablets, 100, 250, and 500 mg. Sinemet tablets, 10 mg/100 mg, 25 mg/100 mg, and 25 mg/250 mg carbidopa/levodopa. Sinemet CR (controlled release) tablets, 50 mg/200 mg carbidopa/levodopa.

LEVO-DROMORAN®, see Levorphanol

LEVOFLOXACIN—Levaquin®

Fluoroquinolone

Anti-infective agent indicated in treatment of susceptible infections. Maintain adequate hydration. Use cautiously in patients with renal impairment, severe cerebral arterioslcerosis, epilepsy, and other seizure risks. Discontinue if rash, other signs of hypersensitivity, hypoglycemic reactions, phototoxicity, or tendon pain with inflammation or rupture, occurs. Monitor blood, renal, hepatic and hematopoetic function in prolonged use. Adverse reactions include nausea and diarrhea. Not recommended for children < 18 years of age.

Administration: 500 mg once daily. Take tabs with full glass of water. Infuse IV over 60 minutes.

Preparations: Tablets, 250 and 500 mg. Solution for I.V. infusion, 25 mg/ml.

LEVOMETHADYL ACETATE HYDROCHLORIDE—ORLAAM®

Agent for opiate dependence.

Actions and Uses: Is an opiate agonist indicated for the management of opiate dependence as part of a comprehensive treatment plan that also includes appropriate medical evaluation, treatment planning, and counseling. Is approved for use only when dispensed by a licensed facility.

Warnings: May cause CNS effects and impair the mental and physical abilities required for such potentially hazardous tasks as driving a car. May cause dependence and is classified in Schedule II. Other adverse reactions include abdominal pain, constipation, diarrhea, dry mouth, nausea, vomiting, cough, rhinitis, rash, sweating, difficult ejaculation, impotence, bradycardia, arthralgia, blurred vision, flu syndrome, and malaise. Withdrawal symptoms are likely to occur if a narcotic antagonist (e.g., naloxone) or a mixed agonist/antagonist analgesic (e.g., pentozocine) is used concurrently. Should not be used concurrently with meperidine or propoxyphene. Is not recommended for use during pregnancy and monthly pregnancy tests are required in patients of child-bearing potential.

Administration: Oral. Is usually administered 3 times a week. Doses must not be given on consecutive days.

Preparation: Oral solution, 10 mg/ml. Should always be diluted before administration.

LEVONORGESTREL

Progestin component in certain oral contraceptive formulations.

LEVONORGESTREL IMPLANT—Norplant®

Progestin implant system used as a contraceptive and which is effective for up to 5 years.

Preparations: Kit containing 6 capsules (each containing 36 mg) and the equipment needed to implant all 6 capsules subdermally in the mid-portion of the upper arm.

LEVOPHED®, see Norepinephrine

LEVOPROME®, see Methotrimeprazine

LEVORPHANOL TARTRATE—Levo-Dromoran®

Opioid analgesic indicated for the relief of moderate to severe pain.

Preparations: Tablets, 2 mg. Ampules and vials, 2 mg/ml.

LEVOTHYROXINE SODIUM—Eltroxin®, Levoxyl®, Synthroid®

Agent for thyroid replacement.

Actions and Uses: Is the principal hormone secreted by the normal thyroid gland. Indicated as replacement therapy for reduced or absent thyroid function.

Warnings: Use is best avoided in patients with acute myocardial infarction, uncorrected adrenal insufficiency, and thyrotoxicosis. Must be used cautiously in patients with cardiovascular disorders and endocrine disorders such as diabetes. Adverse reactions include headache, nervousness, palpitations, tachycardia, and nausea. May increase the action of anticoagulants.

Administration: Oral, intravenous, and intramuscular.

Preparations: Tablets, 0.025, 0.05, 0.075, 0.088, 0.1, 0.112, 0.125, 0.137, 0.15, 0.175, 0.2, and 0.3 mg. Vials, 0.2 and 0.5 mg.

LEVOXYL®, see Levothyroxine sodium

LEVSIN®, see Hyoscyamine

LEVSINEX®, see Hyoscyamine

LEVULOSE, see Fructose

LEXXEL®—Combination of Enalapril maleate extended release tablets, 5 mg and felodipine, 5 mg.

LIBRAX®, Combination of chlordiazepoxide and clidinium

LIBRITABS®, see Chlordiazepoxide

LIBRIUM®, see Chlordiazepoxide

LIDEX®, see Fluocinonide

LIDOCAINE HYDROCHLORIDE—Xylocaine®

Local anesthetic and antiarrhythmic agent. Used by the intravenous and intramuscular routes in the management of ventricular arrhythmias. Also administered parenterally as a local anesthetic for infiltration and nerve block, and by transtracheal and retrobulbar injection. Is also used topically during certain procedures (e.g., urological) and for dermatologic conditions. Several formulations are intended for application to the mucous membranes of the mouth and pharynx.

Preparations: Vials (for IV infusion), 0.2%, 0.4%, and 0.8%. Vials and syringes (for IV admixtures), 4%, 10%, and 20%. Ampules, vials, and syringes (for direct IV administration), 1%, and 2%. Ampules and automatic injection device (for IM administration), 10%. Ampules, vials, and syringes (for infiltration and nerve block), 0.5%, 1%, 1.5%, 2%, 4%, and in combination with epinephrine. Premixed IV solutions for infusion, 2 mg/ml (0.2%), 4 mg/ml (0.4%), and 8 mg/ml (0.8%) in 250- and 500-ml containers. Ointment, 2.5% and 5%. Solution (for topical application to mucous membranes), 2%, 4%, and 10%. Jelly, 2% and ointment, 5%, both for topical application to mucous membranes.

LIME SULFUR SOLUTION, see Sulfurated lime

LINCOCIN®, see Lincomycin

LINCOMYCIN HYDROCHLORIDE—Lincocin®

Antibiotic indicated for the treatment of infections caused by susceptible gram-positive bacteria. Infrequently used drug as it has been replaced by safer, more effective agents.

Preparations: Capsules, 250 and 500 mg. Vials and syringes, 300 mg/ml.

LINDANE—Gamma benzene hexachloride, Kwell®

Parasiticide indicated in the treatment of patients with scabies and lice infestations. Contraindicated in neonates. Adverse reactions include seizures.

Children are at increased risk of systemic absorption and CNS side effects. Instruct parents and/or patients to follow application instructions carefully to minimize systemic absorption and toxic effects.

Preparations: Cream, lotion, and shampoo, 1%

LIORESAL®, see Baclofen

LIOTHYRONINE SODIUM—Triiodothyronine, T_3, Cytomel®, Triostat®

A thyroid hormone indicated as replacement or supplemental therapy in patients with hypothyroidism, as a pituitary thyroid-stimulating hormone suppressant in the treatment or prevention of various goiters, as a diagnostic agent, and, via parenteral use, for myxedema coma and precoma.

Preparations: Tablets, 5, 25, and 50 μg..Vials, 10μg/ml (Triostat®)

LIPITOR®, see Atrovastatin

LIQUAEMIN®, see Heparin

LIQUEFIED PHENOL, see Phenol

LIQUID PETROLATUM, see Mineral oil

LISINOPRIL—Prinivil®, Zestril®

Antihypertensive agent.

Actions and Uses: An angiotensin converting enzyme (ACE) inhibitor that is a derivative of enalaprilat, the active form of enalapril. Indicated for the treatment of hypertension and may be used alone or concomitantly with other antihypertensive agents. Also indicated as adjunctive therapy in the management of congestive heart failure in patients not responding adequately to diuretics and digitalis. Used as an adjunct to other therapies within 24 hours post MI in hemodynamically stable patients, to reduce mortality.

Warnings: Adverse reactions include dizziness, headache, fatigue, diarrhea, upper respiratory symptoms, cough, and hyperkalemia. An excessive reduction in blood pressure may occur, particularly in patients with severe salt/ volume depletion (e.g., those treated vigorously with diuretics). Angioedema has occurred infrequently, sometimes after the first dose. The concurrent use of indomethacin may reduce the effect of lisinopril.

Administration: Oral.

Preparations: Tablets, 2.5, 5, 10, 20, and 40 mg.

LITHANE®, see Lithium carbonate

LITHIUM CARBONATE—Eskalith®, Lithane®, Lithium citrate, Lithonate®

Psychotherapeutic agent indicated in the acute treatment of manic episodes of manic-depressive illnesses, and as prophylaxis against their recurrence.

Preparations: Capsules and tablets, 150, 300 and 600 mg. Controlled-release tablets, 300 and 450 mg. Syrup, 300 mg/5ml.

LITHONATE®, see Lithium carbonate

LITHOSTAT®, see Acetohydroxamic acid

LIVER

Antianemic agent used as a source of Vitamin B_{12}.

Preparations: Tablets. Vials, 2, 10, and 20 μg Vitamin B_{12}/ml.

LOBELINE

Smoking deterrent used as a temporary aid to break the habit of smoking cigarettes.

Preparation: Tablets, 2 mg.

LODINE®, see Etodolac

LODOSYN®, see Carbidopa

LODOXAMIDE TROMETHAMINE —Alomide®

Agent for ocular disorders.

Actions and Uses: Indicated for the topical treatment of vernal keratoconjunctivitis, vernal conjunctivitis, and vernal keratitis.

Warnings: Adverse reactions include transient burning, stinging, or discomfort upon instillation. Contains benzalkonium chloride and patients should be instructed not to wear soft contact lenses during treatment.

Administration: Ophthalmic.

Preparation: Ophthalmic solution, 0.1%.

LOESTRIN®—Oral contraceptive combination of ethinyl estradiol and norethindrone acetate.

LOFENE®, see Diphenoxylate

LOMANATE®, see Diphenoxylate

LOMEFLOXACIN HYDROCHLORIDE—Maxaquin®

Fluoroquinolone antiinfective agent.

Actions and Uses: Inhibits DNA gyrase and exhibits a bactericidal action against many gram-positive and gram-negative bacteria. Indicated for lower respiratory tract infections, and urinary tract infections caused by susceptible oorganisms. Also indicated forprophylaxis (preoperatively) to reduce the incidence of urinary tract infections in the early postoperative period (3–5 days postsurgery) in patients undergoing transurethral surgical procedures.

Warnings: Contraindicated in patients with a known hypersensitivity to any of the fluoroquinolones or the related quinolone antibacterial agents (i.e., nalidixic acid, cinoxacin). Fluoroquinolones have caused erosion of cartilage in weight-bearing joints and other signs of arthropathy in juvenile animals, and use in children under 18, pregnant women, and women who are nursing is best avoided. Adverse reactions include nausea, diarrhea, headache, dizziness, and photosensitivity reactions. Patients should be advised to avoid excessive sunlight and artificial ultraviolet light during the period of treatment. May cause dizziness, lightheadedness, and other central nervous system effects, and patients should know how they tolerate the drug before they engage in activities that require mental alertness and coordination.

Administration: Oral.

Preparation: Tablets, 400 mg.

LOMOTIL®, see Diphenoxylate

LOMUSTINE—CCNU®, CeeNU®

Antineoplastic agent indicated in the treatment of brain tumors and Hodgkin's disease.

Preparations: Capsules, 10, 40, and 100 mg.

LONITEN®, see Minoxidil

LONOX®, see Diphenoxylate

LO/OVRAL®, Oral contraceptive combination of ethinyl estradiol and norgestrel

LOPERAMIDE HYDROCHLORIDE—Imodium®, Imodium A-D®

Antidiarrheal.

Actions and Uses: Indicated for the control and symptomatic relief of acute nonspecific diarrhea and of chronic diarrhea associated with inflammatory bowel disease. Also indicated for reducing the volume of discharge from ileostomies.

Warnings: Adverse reactions include abdominal pain, nausea, vomiting, constipation, and tiredness.

Administration: Oral.

Preparations: Capsules and caplets, 2 mg. Liquid, 1 mg/5 ml.

LOPID®, see Gemfibrozil

LOPRESSOR®, see Metroprolol

LOPROX®, see Ciclopirox olamine

LOPURIN®, see Allopurinol

LORABID®, see Loracarbef

LORACARBEF—Lorabid®

Carbacephem antibiotic.

Actions and Uses: Inhibits bacterial cell wall synthesis and exhibits a bactericidal action against many gram-positive and gram-negative bacteria. Indicated for upper respiratory tract infections, lower respiratory tract infections, acute maxillary sinusitis, uncomplicated skin and skin structure infections, and urinary tract infections caused by susceptible organisms.

Warnings: Contraindicated in patients with a known hypersensitivity to loracarbef or any of the cephalosporins. Must be used cautiously, if at all, in penicillin-sensitive patients and use should be avoided in patients with a history of immediate and/or severe reactions to penicillins. Adverse reactions include diarrhea, nausea, vomiting, abdominal pain, rash, headache, and vaginitis.

Administration: Oral. Should be administered at least one hour before or 2 hours after a meal. The rate of absorption from the suspension is faster than from the capsule; capsules should not be substituted for the oral suspension in the treatment of otitis media.

Preparations: Capsules, 200 mg. Powder for oral suspension, 100 mg/5 ml and 200 mg/5 ml.

LORATADINE—Claritin®

Antihistamine.

Actions and Uses: Selectively antagonizes peripheral histamine H_1-receptors and is designated as a nonsedating antihistamine. Indicated for the relief of symptoms of seasonal allergic rhinitis and idiopathic chronic urticaria.

Warnings: Adverse reactions include headache, somnolence, fatigue, and dry mouth although the incidence of these effects was similar in patients receiving placebo.

Administration: Oral. Should be administered on an empty stomach.

Preparations: Tablets, 10 mg. Reditabs, 10 mg. Syrup, 1 mg/ml.

LORAZEPAM—Ativan®

Benzodiazepine antianxiety agent.

Actions and Uses: A CNS depressant indicated for the management of anxiety disorders or for the short-term relief of the symptoms of anxiety and insomnia. Also indicated for parenteral use as a preanesthetic medication and in status epilepticus.

Warnings: Contraindicated in patients with acute narrow-angle glaucoma. Adverse reactions include drowsiness and other CNS effects; patients should be cautioned regarding activities such as driving and operating machinery, as well as interactions with other CNS-acting drugs including alcohol. Can cause dependence and is included in Schedule IV.

Administration: Oral, intravenous, and intramuscular.

Preparations: Tablets, 0.5, 1, and 2 mg. Vials, 2 and 4 mg/ml. Concentrated solution, 2 mg/ml.

LORTAB®, Combination opioid and analgesic.

Hydrocodone bitartrate and acetaminophen

LOSARTAN POTASSIUM—Cozaar®

Actions and Uses: Angiotensin II receptor antagonist indicated in the treatment of hypertension as monotherapy or as an adjunct to other antihypertensive agents.

Precautions: Adverse reactions include hypotension and dizziness. Contraindicated in pregnancy. May increase serum potassium levels.

Administration: Oral.

Preparations: Tablets, 25 and 50 mg. Available in combination formulation (Hyzaar) that contains 50 mg of losartan potassium and 12.5 mg of hydrochlorothiazide.

LOTEMEX®, see Loteprednol etabonate

Actions and Uses: Anti-inflammatry agent indicated in the treatment of seasonal allergic conjunctives (Alrex®) steroid responsive ocular disease, and post-op inflammation after ocular surgery (Lotemax®).

Warnings: Contraindicated in ocular fungal, viral, or mycobacterial infections. Revaluate if no improvement after 2 days. Prescribe initially and renew after 14 days only after appropriate exam. use cautiously in corneal or scleral thinning, glaucoma, or a history of herpes simplex. Monitor IOP and for secondary infections in prolonged therapy (> 10 days). Avoid abrupt cessation. Remove soft contact lenses for installation and wait 10 minutes before reinserting. Included local reactions (e.g., blurred vision, burning, itching eyes, dry eye), photophobia, headache, rhinitis, and pharyngitis. May mask or exacerbate ocular infections. Prolonged use may result in increased IOP, Optic nerve damage, visual acuity and field defects, cataract formation, and corneal perforation.

Administrations: Opthalmic.

Preparations: 2% opthalmic suspension (contains benzakonium chloride).

LOTENSIN®, see Benazepril hydrochloride

LOTEPREDNOL ETABONATE—Alrex®, Lotemax®

LOTREL®, Combination of amlodipine and benazepril

LOTRIMIN®, see Clotrimazole.

LOTRIMIN AF®, see Clotrimazole.

LOTRISONE®, Combination of clotrimazole and betamethasone dipropionate

LO-TROL®, see Diphenoxylate.

LOVASTATIN—Mevacor®

Antihyperlipidemic agent.

Actions and Uses: Results in a reduction of low-density lipoprotein (LDL) cholesterol and total plasma cholesterol, while high-density lipoprotein (HDL) concentrations increase. Indicated as an adjunct to diet for the reduction of elevated total and LDL cholesterol levels in patients with primary hypercholesterolemia (Types IIa and IIb), when the response to diet and other nonpharmacologic measures alone has been inadequate. Also indicated to slow the progression of coronary atherosclerosis in patients with coronary heart disease.

Warnings: Contraindicated during pregnancy and lactation because lovastatin has been reported to exhibit teratogenic effects in some animal studies. It is also contraindicated in patients with active liver disease or unexplained persistent elevations of serum transaminases. Marked persistent increases in serum transaminases may occur and it is recommended that liver function tests be performed every 4 to 6 weeks during the first 15 months of therapy and periodically thereafter. Adverse reactions include headache, rash, pruritus, nausea, diarrhea, constipation, abdominal pain, and myalgia. Some individuals experience myositis and patients should be advised to report unexplained muscle pain or tenderness. Although it is not known whether lovastatin causes ocular problems, it is recommended that ophthalmologic exams be conducted before or shortly after starting therapy, and annually thereafter.

Administration: Oral.

Preparations: Tablets, 10, 20, and 40 mg.

LOVENOX®, see Enoxaparin

LOXAPINE—Loxitane®

Antipsychotic agent indicated for the management of the manifestations of psychotic disorders.

Preparations: Capsules (as the succinate), 5, 10, 25, and 50 mg. Oral concentrate (as the hydrochloride), 25 mg/ml. Ampules and vials (as the hydrochloride and for IM use), 50 mg/ml.

LOW-QUEL®, see Diphenoxylate

LOXITANE®, see Loxapine

LOZOL®, see Indapamide

LUDIOMIL®, see Maprotiline

LUFYLLIN®, see Dyphylline

LUGOL'S SOLUTION, see Iodine

LUMINAL®, see Phenobarbital

LUPRON®, see Leuprolide

LUPRON DEPOT®, see Leuprolide

LUPRON DEPOT-PED®, see Leuprolide

LURIDE®, see Sodium fluoride

LUTREPULSE®, see Gonadorelin acetate

LUVOX®, see Fluvoxamine maleate

LYPHOCIN®, see Vancomycin

LYSODREN®, see Mitotane

M

MAALOX®, see Aluminum and magnesium hydroxides

MACROBID®, see Nitrofurantoin

MACRODANTIN®, see Nitrofurantoin macrocrystals

MACRODEX®, see Dextran

MAFENIDE ACETATE—Sulfamylon®

Sulfonamide anti-infective agent indicated for topical use as adjunctive therapy of patients with second- and third-degree burns.

Preparation: Cream, 8.5%.

MAGALDRATE—Riopan®

Antacid indicated for the relief of hyperacidity and related symptoms.

Preparations: Tablets and chewable tablets, 480 mg. Suspension, 540 mg/5 ml.

MAGAN®, see Magnesium salicylate

MAGNESIUM CARBONATE

Antacid used in combination with other agents.

MAGNESIUM CHLORIDE—Slow-Mag®

Magnesium supplement.

Preparations: Controlled-release tablets, 64 mg magnesium (as chloride).

MAGNESIUM CITRATE—Citrate of magnesia

Laxative used in the treatment of constipation and with other agents as a bowel evacuant in the preparation of the colon for radiologic examinations.

Preparation: Solution.

MAGNESIUM HYDROXIDE—Milk of magnesia

Antacid and laxative used alone or in combination with other agents.

Preparations: Tablets, 325 mg. Suspension.

MAGNESIUM OXIDE

Antacid.

Preparations: Capsules and tablets, 140 and 420 mg.

MAGNESIUM SALICYLATE—Doan's Pills®, Magan®

Salicylate analgesic/anti-inflammatory agent indicated for the relief of pain and the signs and symptoms of arthritic disorders.

Preparations: Tablets, 325, 545, and 600 mg.

MAGNESIUM SULFATE

Laxative, anticonvulsant, and electrolyte. Used orally in the treatment of constipation, and parenterally to prevent or control convulsions. Also used parenterally as replacement therapy in the treatment of hypomagnesemia.

Preparations: Granules (to prepare solution for oral administration). Ampules and vials, 10%, 12.5%, 25%, and 50%.

MAGNESIUM TRISILICATE

Antacid used in combination with other agents.

MANDELAMINE®, see Methenamine mandelate

MANDOL®, see Cefamandole

MANNITOL—Osmitrol®

Osmotic diuretic indicated in the prevention and treatment of the oliguric phase of acute renal failure following cardiovascular surgery, severe traumatic injury, surgery in the presence of severe jaundice, hemolytic transfusion reaction, to reduce intraocular pressure (IOP) and intracranial pressure (ICP). Most common adverse reaction is electrolyte imbalance, especially hyponatremia.

Administration: Intravenous, GU irrigant.

Preparations: IV injection, 5, 10, 15, and 20%. GU irrigant, 5%. Also in combination with sorbitol for GU irrigation.

MAOLATE®, see Chlorphenesin carbamate

MAPROTILINE HYDROCHLORIDE—Ludiomil®

Tetracyclic antidepressant indicated in the treatment of depression and for the relief of anxiety associated with depression.

Preparations: Tablets, 25, 50, and 75 mg.

MARCAINE®, see Bupivacaine

MAREZINE®, see Cyclizine

MARIJUANA—See Dronabinol

MARINOL®, see Dronabinol

MASOPROCOL—Actinex®

Agent for actinic keratoses.

Actions and Uses: Indicated for the topical treatment of actinic (solar) keratoses.

Warnings: Adverse reactions include erythema, flaking, itching, dryness, edema, burning, and soreness. May induce sensitization (allergic contact dermatitis) and, if such reactions occur, the drug should be discontinued.

Administration: Topical. Patients may experience a transient local burning sensation after applying the cream. May stain clothing or fabrics.

Preparations: Cream, 10%.

MATULANE®, see Procarbazine

MAVIK®, see Trandolapril

MAXAIR®, see Pirbuterol

MAXAQUIN®, see Lomefloxacin

MAXIFLOR®, see Diflorasone

MAXIPIME®, see Cefepime

MAXIVATE®, see Betamethasone dipropionate

MAXZIDE®, combination of triamterene and hydrochlorothiazide

MAZANOR®, see Mazindol

MAZICON®, trade name formerly used for Flumazenil

MAZINDOL—Mazanor®, Sanorex®

Anorexiant indicated in the management of exogenous obesity as a short-term adjunct in a regimen of weight reduction based on caloric restriction.

Preparations: Tablets, 1 and 2 mg.

MEBARAL®, see Mephobarbital

MEBENDAZOLE—Vermox®

Anthelmintic indicated for the treatment of pinworm, whipworm, roundworm, and hookworm infections.

Preparation: Chewable tablets, 100 mg.

MECAMYLAMINE HYDROCHLORIDE—Inversine®

Antihypertensive agent indicated in the management of moderately severe to severe hypertension.

Preparation: Tablets, 2.5 mg.

MECHLORETHAMINE HYDROCHLORIDE—Mustargen®, Nitrogen Mustard

Antineoplastic agent indicated for the parenteral treatment of Hodgkin's disease, lymphosarcoma, chronic myelocytic or chronic lymphocytic leukemia, polycythemia vera, mycosis fungoides, and bronchogenic carcinoma. Also administered intrapleurally, intraperitoneally, or intrapericardially for the palliative treatment of metastatic carcinoma resulting in effusion.

Preparation: Vials, 10 mg.

MECLAN®, see Meclocycline

MECLIZINE HYDROCHLORIDE—Antivert®, Bonine®

Antihistamine.

Actions and Uses: Exhibits antihistaminic and anticholinergic activity. Indicated for the management of nausea, vomiting, and dizziness associated with motion sickness, and in vertigo associated with diseases affecting the vestibular system.

Warnings: Must be used with caution in patients with asthma, glaucoma, or enlargement of the prostate. Adverse reactions include drowsiness, and patients should be cautioned regarding activities such as driving and operating machinery, as well as interactions with other CNS-acting drugs including alcohol. Other adverse reactions include dry mouth.

Administration: Oral.

Preparations: Tablets, 12.5, 25, and 50 mg. Chewable tablets, 25 mg. Capsules, 15, 25, and 30 mg.

MECLOCYCLINE SULFOSALICYLATE—Meclan®

Tetracycline antibiotic indicated for topical use in the treatment of inflammatory acne vulgaris.

Preparation: Cream, 1%

MEDROL®, see Methylprednisolone

MEDROXYPROGESTERONE ACETATE—Cycrin®, Depo-Provera®, Provera®

Progestational agent.

Actions and Uses: Is a derivative of progesterone and is indicated in the treatment of secondary amenorrhea, and abnormal uterine bleeding due to hormonal imbalance in the absence of organic pathology, such as fibroids or uterine cancer. Also indicated for intramuscular use as adjunctive therapy and palliative treatment of inoperable, recurrent, and metastatic endometrial carcinoma or renal carcinoma. Also indicated for intramuscular use as a long-term injectable contraceptive when administered at 3-month intervals.

Warnings: Contraindicated in patients with hepatic dysfunction, undiagnosed vaginal bleeding, and known or suspected malignancy of breast or genital organs. May cause thromboembolic phenomena including thrombophlebitis and pulmonary embolism, and use is contraindicated in patients with a history of such disorders. May cause adverse effects in the fetus, and use during the first 4 months of pregnancy is not recommended. Other adverse reactions include rash, pruritus, edema, nausea, insomnia, depression, somnolence, and breakthrough bleeding.

Administration: Oral and intramuscular.

Preparations: Tablets, 2.5, 5, and 10 mg. Vials (Depo-Provera), 100 mg/ml, 150 mg/ml, and 400 mg/ml. Prefilled syringe, 150 mg/ml.

MEFENAMIC ACID—Ponstel®

Nonsteroidal anti-inflammatory drug indicated for the relief of moderate pain and the treatment of primary dysmenorrhea.

Preparation: Capsules, 250 mg.

MEFLOQUINE HYDROCHLORIDE
—Lariam®

Antimalarial agent

Actions and Uses: Acts as a blood schizonticide, but does not eliminate exoerythrocytic (hepatic phase) parasites. Indicated for the treatment of moderate acute malaria caused by susceptible strains of *Plasmodium falciparum or Plasmodium vivax.* Is also indicated for the prophylaxis of *Plasmodium falciparum* and *Plasmodium vivax* malaria infections.

Warnings: The drug should not be used during pregnancy and women of childbearing potential should use reliable contraceptive measures for the duration of mefloquine use and for 2 months after the last dose. Adverse reactions include CNS effects and patients should be cautioned regarding activities such as driving and operating machinery, as well as interactions with other CNS-acting drugs including alcohol. Other adverse reactions include nausea, vomiting, diarrhea, abdominal pain, loss of appetite, headache, tinnitus, fever, chills, myalgia, and rash. Concomitant use with chloroquine may increase the risk of convulsions.

Administration: Oral. For malaria prophylaxis, therapy should be initiated one week prior to departure to an endemic area and the drug should be administered on the same day of the week. Prophylaxis should be continued for 4 additional weeks following return. Doses of mefloquine should not be taken on an empty stomach and should be administered with at least 8 ounces of water.

Preparation: Tablets, 250 mg.

MEFOXIN®, see Cefoxitin

MEGACE®, see Megestrol

MEGESTROL ACETATE—
Megace®

Antineoplastic agent indicated for the treatment of advanced carcinoma of the breast or endometrium. Also indicated for the treatment of anorexia, cachexia, or significant weight loss in patients with AIDS.

Preparations: Tablets, 20 and 40 mg. Suspension, 40 mg/ml.

MELLARIL®, see Thioridazine

MELPHALAN—Alkeran®

Antineoplastic agent indicated for the treatment of multiple myeloma and for the palliation of nonresectable carcinoma of the ovary. Administered by intravenous infusion for the palliative treatment of multiple myeloma when oral therapy is not appropriate.

Preparations: Tablets, 2 mg. Vials, 50 mg.

MENEST®, see Estrogens, esterified

MENOTROPINS—Pergonal®

Gonadotropins [follicle stimulating hormone (FSH) and luteinizing hormone (LH)] administered intramuscularly for the induction of ovulation and pregnancy in anovulatory women, and to stimulate spermatogenesis in men with infertility.

Preparations: Ampules, 75 IU each of FSH and LH and 150 IU each of FSH and LH.

MENTAX®, see Butenafine
Hydrochloride

MENTHOL

Analgesic/cooling agent included with other agents in formulations that are applied topically to the skin or throat (e.g., lozenges).

MEPERIDINE HYDROCHLORIDE—Demerol®

Opioid analgesic.

Actions and Uses: Indicated for the relief of moderate to severe pain, for preoperative medication, for support of anesthesia, and for obstetrical analgesia.

Warnings: Adverse reactions include sedation and other CNS effects; patients should be cautioned regarding activities such as driving and operating machinery, as well as interactions with other CNS-acting drugs including alcohol. Other adverse reactions include flushing of the face, hypotension, and pain at the injection site. Is contraindicated in patients receiving a monoamine oxidase inhibitor. Can cause dependence, and formulations are covered under the provisions of the Controlled Substances Act.

Administration: Oral, intramuscular, intravenous, and subcutaneous.

Preparations: Tablets, 50 and 100 mg. Syrup, 50 mg/5 ml. Ampules, vials, and syringes, 10 mg/ml, 25 mg/ml, 50 mg/ml, 75 mg/ml, and 100 mg/ml.

MEPHENTERMINE SULFATE—Wyamine®

Sympathomimetic agent indicated for the parenteral treatment of hypotension secondary to ganglionic blockade and that occurring with spinal anesthesia.

Preparations: Ampules and vials, 15 mg/ml and 30 mg/ml.

MEPHENYTOIN—Mesantoin®

Anticonvulsant indicated for the control of grand mal, focal, Jacksonian, and psychomotor seizures in those patients who are refractory to less toxic anticonvulsants.

Preparation: Tablets, 100 mg.

MEPHOBARBITAL—Mebaral®

Barbiturate indicated as a sedative for the relief of anxiety and tension, and as an anticonvulsant for the treatment of grand mal and petit mal epilepsy.

Preparations: Tablets 32, 50, and 100 mg.

MEPHYTON®, see Phytonadione

MEPIVACAINE HYDROCHLORIDE—Carbocaine®

Local anesthetic used to produce local anesthesia by infiltration injection, peripheral nerve block, and central neural blocks by the lumbar or caudal epidural route. Also indicated for use in dental procedures.

Preparations: Vials, 1%, 1.5%, and 2%. Dental cartridges, 3%.

MEPROBAMATE—Equanil®, Meprospan®, Miltown®

Antianxiety agent indicated for the management of anxiety disorders or for the short-term relief of the symptoms of anxiety.

Preparations: Tablets, 200, 400, and 600 mg. Controlled-release capsules, 200 and 400 mg.

MEPRON®, see Atovaquone

MEPROSPAN®, see Meprobamate

MERBROMIN—Mercurochrome

Antiseptic which is applied topically.

Preparation: Solution, 2%.

MERCAPTOPURINE—Purinethol®

Antineoplastic agent indicated in the management of leukemias.

Preparation: Tablets, 50 mg.

MERCUROCHROME®, see Merbromin

MERCURY, AMMONIATED, see Ammoniated mercury

MERREM®, see Meropenem

MEROPENEM—Merrem®

Action and Uses: Synthetic, broad spectrum carbapenem antibiotic. Bactericidal activity results from the inhibition of cell wall synthesis.

Warnings: Contraindicated in patients who have experienced anaphylactic reactions to other carbopenems (imipenem) or to beta-lactam antibiotics. Use cautiously in patients with CNS disorders, history of seizures or renal impairment. Monitor renal, hepatic, and hematopoietic function in long-term use. Adverse reactions include local reactions, GI upset, headache, rash, pruritis, apnea, seizures, constipation, superinfection, and pseudomembraneous colitis.

Administration: IV infusion or bolus with dosages adjusted to renal function (see manufacturer's guidelines).

Preparations: Powder for reconstitution, 500 mg and 1 g.

MERTHIOLATE®, see Thimerosal

MESALAMINE—Asacol®, Pentasa®, Rowasa®

Agent for ulcerative colitis.

Actions and Uses: Also known as 5-aminosalicylic acid (5-ASA) and is a metabolite of sulfasalazine. Indicated in the treatment of active mild to moderate distal ulcerative colitis.

Warnings: Contraindicated in patients who are hypersensitive to the drug or to any component (e.g., sulfite) of the formulation. Adverse reactions include an acute intolerance syndrome characterized by cramping, acute abdominal pain, bloody diarrhea, and sometimes fever, headache, and a rash. Some patients experience mild hair loss.

Administration: Oral and rectal.

Preparations: Tablets, delayed release, 400 mg (Asacol®). Capsules, controlled release, 250 mg (Pentasa®). Suspension enema, 4 grams/60ml (Rowasa). Suppositories, 500 mg (Rowasa).

MESANTOIN®, see Mephenytoin

MESNA—Mesnex®

Uroprotective agent.

Actions and Uses: Reacts with the urotoxic metabolites (e.g., acrolein) of ifosfamide. Indicated as a prophylactic agent in reducing the incidence of hemorrhagic cystitis caused by ifosfamide.

Warnings: Adverse reactions include nausea, vomiting, and diarrhea.

Administration: Intravenous bolus injection. The total daily dose of mesna is 60% of the ifosfamide dose. It is given as intravenous bolus injections in a dosage equal to 20% of the ifosfamide dosage at the time of ifosfamide administration and 4 and 8 hours after each dose of ifosfamide.

Preparations: Ampules, 200 and 400 mg; 1 gram.

MESNEX®, see Mesna

MESORIDAZINE BESYLATE—Serentil®

Phenothiazine antipsychotic agent indicated in the treatment of schizophrenia, behavioral problems in mental deficiency and chronic brain syndrome, alcoholism, and psychoneurotic manifestations.

Preparations: Tablets, 10, 25, 50, and 100 mg. Oral concentrate, 25 mg/ml. Ampules, 25 mg.

MESTINON®, see Pyridostigmine

MESTRANOL

Estrogen included in combination with a progestin in various oral contraceptive formulations.

METAHYDRIN®, see Trichlormethiazide

METAMUCIL®, see Psyllium

METAPROTERENOL SULFATE—Alupent®, Metaprel®

Bronchodilator.

Actions and Uses: Stimulates beta-adrenergic receptors. Indicated for bronchial asthma and for reversible bronchospasm that may occur in association with bronchitis and emphysema.

Warnings: Contraindicated in patients with cardiac arrhythmias associated with tachycardia, and should be used with caution in patients with other cardiovascular disorders. Adverse reactions include nervousness, tremor, tachycardia, palpitations, hypertension, nausea, and vomiting. Other sympathomimetic agents should not be used concurrently. Beta-adrenergic blocking agents and metaproterenol may inhibit the effect of each other.

Administration: Oral and oral inhalation.

Preparations: Tablets, 10 and 20 mg. Syrup, 10 mg/5 ml. Metered dose inhaler. Inhalant solution, 0.4%, 0.6%, and 5%.

METARAMINOL BITARTRATE—Aramine®

Sympathomimetic agent indicated for parenteral administration in the prevention and treatment of the acute hypotensive state occurring with spinal anesthesia. Also used for the adjunctive treatment of hypotension due to other causes.

Preparation: Vials, 1%

METASTRON®, see Strontium-89 Chloride

METAXALONE—Skelaxin®

Skeletal muscle relaxant indicated as an adjunct to rest, physical therapy, and other measures for the relief of discomfort associated with acute, painful musculoskeletal conditions.

Preparation: Tablets, 400 mg.

METFORMIN HYDROCHLORIDE—Glucophage®

Antihyperglycemic agent.

Actions and Uses: Indicated as monotherapy or as an adjunct to sulfonylureas in combination with diet to lower blood glucose in patients with non-insulin-dependent diabetes mellitus (NIDDM) whose diet or sulfonylurea does not result in adequate glycemic control.

Warnings: Contraindicated in patients with renal disease and acute or chronic metabolic acidosis, CHF requiring drug treatment and concomitant intravascular iodinated radiocontrast agent. Withhold the drug in patients undergoing radiologic studies involving iodinated contrast materials as such products may result in an acute alteration of renal function. Adverse reactions include lactic acidosis, diarrhea, nausea, vomiting, abdominal bloating, flatulence, anorexia, metallic taste and asymptotic subnormal serum Vitamin B_{12} concentrations.

Administration: Oral with meals to reduce the incidence of GI effects.

Preparations: Tablets, 500 and 850 mg.

METHADONE HYDROCHLORIDE—Dolophine®

Opioid analgesic indicated for relief of severe pain, for detoxification treatment of narcotic addiction, and for temporary maintenance treatment of narcotic addiction.

Preparations: Tablets, 5, 10, and 40 mg. Oral solution, 5 mg/5 ml, and 10 mg/5 ml. Ampules and vials, 10 mg/ml.

METHAMPHETAMINE HYDROCHLORIDE—Desoxyn®

Anorexiant indicated as a short-term adjunct in a regimen of weight reduction based on caloric restriction. Also used in attention deficit disorder with hyperactivity, narcolepsy, epilepsy, post-encephalitic parkinsonism and in treatment of certain depressive reactions.

Preparations: Tablets, 5 mg. Long-acting tablets, 5, 10, and 15 mg.

METHAZOLAMIDE—Neptazane®

Carbonic anhydrase inhibitor indicated for adjunctive treatment of open-angle glaucoma, secondary glaucoma, and preoperatively in acute angle-closure glaucoma where delay of surgery is desired in order to lower intraocular pressure.

Preparation: Tablets, 25 and 50 mg.

METHENAMINE HIPPURATE—Hiprex®

METHENAMINE MANDELATE—Mandelamine®

Urinary tract antibacterial indicated for prophylactic or suppressive treatment of frequently recurring urinary tract infections.

Preparations: Tablets, 500 mg and 1 g.

METHERGINE®, see Methylergonovine

METHICILLIN SODIUM—Staphcillin®

Penicillin antibiotic indicated for the parenteral treatment of staphylococcal infections.

Preparations: Vials, 1, 4, 6, and 10 g.

METHIMAZOLE—Tapazole®

Antithyroid agent indicated for the treatment of hyperthyroidism.

Preparations: Tablets, 5 and 10 mg.

METHIONINE—Pedameth®

Indicated for the treatment of diaper rash in infants, and for control of odor, dermatitis and ulceration caused by ammoniacal urine in incontinent adults.

Preparations: Capsules, 200 mg. Liquid, 75 mg/5 ml.

METHOCARBAMOL—Robaxin®

Skeletal muscle relaxant indicated as an adjunct to rest, physical therapy, and other measures for the relief of discomfort associated with acute, painful musculoskeletal conditions.

Preparations: Tablets, 500 and 750 mg. Vials, 100 mg/ml.

METHOHEXITAL SODIUM—Brevital sodium®

Barbiturate general anesthetic indicated for intravenous use for induction of anesthesia, for supplementing other anesthetic agents, as anesthesia for short surgical procedures with minimum painful stimuli, or as an agent for inducing a hypnotic state.

Preparations: Vials, 500 mg, 2.5 and 5 g.

METHOTREXATE—Rheumatrex®

Antineoplastic agent indicated for the treatment of gestational choriocarcinoma, in patients with chorioadenoma destruens and hydatiform mole, acute lymphocytic leukemia, meningeal leukemia, breast cancer, epidermoid cancers of the head and neck, lung cancer, lymphosarcoma, and mycosis fungoides. Also used in the symptomatic control of severe, recalcitrant disabling psoriasis, and in the treatment of severe, active, classical or definite rheumatoid arthritis in selected adults who have had an insufficient therapeutic response to, or are intolerant of an adequate trial of first line therapy, including full dose NSAIDs.

Preparations: Tablets, 2.5 mg. Dose Pack, 2.5 mg tablets (Rheumatrex). Vials, 20, 50, 100, and 250 mg. Vials, 2.5 mg/ml and 25 mg/ml.

METHOTRIMEPRAZINE—Levoprome®

Analgesic administered parenterally for the treatment of moderate to severe pain in nonambulatory patients.

Preparation: Vials, 20 mg/ml.

METHOXAMINE HYDROCHLORIDE—Vasoxyl®

Sympathomimetic amine indicated for parenteral use for restoring or maintaining blood pressure during anesthesia. Also used to terminate some episodes of supraventricular tachycardia.

Preparation: Ampules, 20 mg.

METHOXSALEN—Oxsoralen®, Oxsoralen-Ultra®

Photoactive agent indicated for topical use with long wave ultraviolet radiation for the repigmentation of vitiligo, and for oral use with long-wave UVA radiation for the symptomaticcontrol of severe, recalcitrant disabling psoriasis.

Preparations: Capsules (Oxsoralen-Ultra), 10 mg. Lotion (to be applied by a physician and not to be dispensed to patients), 1%.

METHOXYFLURANE—Penthrane®

Inhalation general anesthetic usually indicated in combination with oxygen and nitrous oxide. Also used to provide analgesia in obstetrics and in minor surgical procedures.

Preparations: Bottles, 15 and 125 ml.

METHSUXIMIDE—Celontin®

Anticonvulsant indicated for the control of absence (petit mal) seizures that are refractory to other drugs.

Preparations: Capsules, 150 and 300 mg.

METHYL SALICYLATE—Oil of Wintergreen

Salicylate analgesic used in combination with other agents and applied topically in the management of certain dermatologic and muscular conditions.

Preparations: Lotion, liniment, and cream formulations.

METHYLCELLULOSE—Citrucel®

Laxative used in the treatment of constipation.

Preparations: Powder and liquid.

METHYCLOTHIAZIDE—Enduron®

Thiazide diuretic indicated as adjunctive therapy in edema, and in the management of hypertension.

Preparations: Tablets, 2.5 and 5 mg.

METHYLDOPA, METHYLDOPATE HYDROCHLORIDE—Aldomet®

Antihypertensive agent.

Actions and Uses: Indicated in the treatment of hypertension.

Warnings: Contraindicated in patients with active hepatic disease because liver disorders have been associated with therapy. Other adverse reactions include sedation, headache, orthostatic hypotension, edema, bradycardia, nausea, vomiting, positive Coombs' test, and hemolytic anemia.

Administration: Oral and intravenous.

Preparations: Tablets, 125, 250, and

500 mg. Suspension, 250 mg/5 ml. Vials, 250 mg/5 ml.

METHYLENE BLUE

Antiseptic and antidote. Has been used as a genitourinary antiseptic and in the management of patients with oxalate urinary tract calculi. Has also been used in the management of methemoglobinemia and as an antidote for cyanide poisoning.

Preparations: Tablets, 65 mg. Ampules, 10 mg/ml.

METHYLERGONOVINE MALEATE—Methergine®

Oxytocic indicated for routine management after delivery of the placenta; postpartum atony and hemorrhage; subinvolution. Under full obstetric supervision, may be given in the second stage of labor following delivery of the anterior shoulder.

Preparations: Tablets, 0.2 mg. Ampules, 0.2 mg/ml.

METHYLPHENIDATE HYDROCHLORIDE—Ritalin®, Ritalin-SR®

Central nervous system stimulant indicated in the management of attention-deficit disorder and narcolepsy.

Preparations: Tablets, 5, 10, and 20 mg. Controlled-release tablets, 20 mg.

METHYLPREDNISOLONE—Medrol®

Corticosteroid.

Actions and Uses: Indicated in a wide range of endocrine, rheumatic, allergic, dermatologic, respiratory, hematologic, neoplastic, and other disorders. Use has been reported to improve neurologic recovery in patients with acute spinal-cord injury when the medication (as methylprednisolone sodium succinate) is given in the first 8 hours.

Warnings: Contraindicated in patients with systemic fungal infections. Adverse reactions include sodium and fluid retention, potassium depletion, muscle weakness, osteoporosis, peptic ulcer, thin fragile skin, development of Cushingoid state, glaucoma, cataracts, and negative nitrogen balance. May mask signs of infection and new infections may appear during use. May increase requirements for hypoglycemic agents in diabetic patients.

Administration: Oral.

Preparations: Tablets, 2, 4, 8, 16, 24, and 32 mg.

METHYLPREDNISOLONE ACETATE—Depo-Medrol®, Medrol acetate topical®

See discussion of methylprednisolone.

Administration: Intramuscular, intra-articular,

intralesional, and soft tissue administration. Topical.

Preparations: Vials, 20, 40, and 80 mg/ml. Ointment, 0.25% and 1%.

METHYLPREDNISOLONE SODIUM SUCCINATE—Solu-Medrol® See discussion of methylprednisolone.

Administration: Intravenous and intramuscular.

Preparations: Vials, 40, 125, and 500 mg, 1 and 2 g.

METHYLROSANILINE CHLORIDE, see Gentian violet

METHYLTESTOSTERONE—Oreton methyl®

Androgen indicated for replacement therapy in conditions associated with a deficiency or absence of endogenous testosterone including primary hypogonadism (e.g., testicular failure due to cryptorchidism) and hypogonadotropic hypogonadism.

May be used to stimulate puberty in carefully selected males with clearly delayed puberty, and for the treatment of impotence and male climacteric symptoms when these are secondary to androgen deficiency. May also be used in women with advanced inoperable metastatic mammary cancer who are 1 to 5 years postmenopausal, and for the management of postpartum breast pain and engorgement.

Preparations: Tablets, 10 and 25 mg. Buccal tablets, 5 and 10 mg.

METHYSERGIDE MALEATE—Sansert®

Indicated for the prevention or reduction of intensity and frequency of vascular headaches in patients who experience frequent and/or severe head- aches. Observe for development of retroperitoneal fibrosis during long-term therapy.

Preparation: Tablets, 2 mg.

METICORTEN®, see Prednisone

METIPRANOLOL HYDROCHLORIDE—OptiPranolol®

Agent for glaucoma.

Actions and Uses: A nonselective beta-adrenergic

blocking agent indicated for ophthalmic use in the treatment of ocular conditions like chronic open angle glaucoma and ocular hypertension.

Warnings: Contraindicated in patients with a history of bronchial asthma, severe chronic obstructive pulmonary disease, symptomatic sinus bradycardia, greater than a first degree atrioventricular block, cardiogenic shock, or overt cardiac failure. Adverse reactions include transient local discomfort, conjunctivitis, abnormal vision, and occasional systemic effects. Caution must be exercised in patients taking another beta-blocker orally for another indication.

Administration: Ophthalmic.

Preparations: Ophthalmic solution, 0.3%.

METOCLOPRAMIDE HYDROCHLORIDE—Reglan®

Agent to increase GI tract motility.

Actions and Uses: Stimulates motility of the upper GI tract. Indicated (1) as short-term therapy for patients with symptomatic, gastroesophageal reflux who fail to respond to conventional therapy; (2) for the relief of symptoms associated with diabetic gastric stasis; (3) for the prophylaxis of vomiting associated with cancer chemotherapy; (4) to facilitate small bowel intubation; and (5) to stimulate gastric emptying and intestinal transit of barium in radiological examinations.

Warnings: Contraindicated in patients in whom the stimulation of GI motility may be dangerous (e.g., in the presence of GI hemorrhage), and in patients with epilepsy or pheochromocytoma. May cause extrapyramidal reactions and should not be used in patients receiving other drugs likely to cause such reactions. Adverse reactions include drowsiness and other CNS effects; patients should be cautioned regarding activities such as driving and operating machinery, as well as interactions with other CNS-acting drugs including alcohol. Other adverse reactions include nausea, diarrhea, visual disturbances, fluid retention, amenorrhea, gynecomastia, and impotence.

Administration: Oral, intravenous, and intramuscular. Oral administration should be 30 minutes before meals and at bedtime.

Preparations: Tablets, 5 and 10 mg. Syrup, 5 mg/5 ml. Ampules and vials, 5 mg/ml.

METOCURINE IODIDE—Metubine iodide®

Muscle relaxant administered intravenously as an adjunct to anesthesia to induce skeletal muscle relaxation.

Preparation: Vials, 2 mg/ml.

METOLAZONE—Zaroxolyn®

METOLAZONE (rapidly available formulation)—Mykrox®

Diuretic indicated in the management of hypertension and in the treatment of edema.

Preparations: Tablets, 0.5 (Mykrox®), 2.5, 5, and 10 mg.

METOPROLOL TARTRATE—Lopressor®

METOPROLOL SUCCINATE—Toprol XL®

Antihypertensive and antianginal agent.

Actions and Uses: A cardioselective beta-adrenergic blocking agent indicated in the management of hypertension, angina pectoris, and hemodynamically stable patients with definite or suspected acute myocardial infarction to reduce cardiovascular mortality.

Warnings: Contraindicated in patients with sinus bradycardia, heart block greater than first degree, cardiogenic shock, and overt cardiac failure. Adverse reactions include tiredness, dizziness, depression, bradycardia, shortness of breath, diarrhea, pruritus, and rash. Use is best avoided in patients with bronchospastic diseases and therapy in diabetic patients must be closely monitored.

Administration: Oral and intravenous. When administered orally should be taken with or immediately following meals. Patients should be cautioned about the interruption or discontinuation of therapy; exacerbation of angina pectoris has occurred following the abrupt cessation of therapy and, when therapy is to be discontinued, the dosage should be gradually reduced over a period of 1 to 2 weeks.

Preparations: Tablets, 50 and 100 mg. Controlled-release tablets (Toprol XL), 50, 100, and 200 mg. Ampules and syringes, 5 mg/5 ml.

METRODIN®, see Urofollitropin

METROGEL®, see Metronidazole

METRAGEL-VAGINAL®, see Metronidazole

METRONIDAZOLE—Flagyl®, MetroGel®, MetroGel-Vaginal®, Noritate®

Anti-infective agent indicated in the treatment of trichomoniasis, amebiasis, and anaerobic bacterial infections, and in the topical treatment of rosacea. Vaginal gel is indicated in the treatment of bacterial vaginosis.

Preparations: Tablets, 250 and 500 mg. Capsules, 375 mg. Extended release tablets, 750 mg. Vials (for intravenous administration), 500 mg and 500 mg/100 ml. Gel, 0.75%. Vaginal gel, 0.75%. Cream, 1%.

METUBINE®, see Metocurine

METYRAPONE

Diagnostic test of pituitary adrenocorticotropic function.

Preparation: Tablets, 250 mg.

METYROSINE—Demser®

Agent for pheochromocytoma. Indicated in the treatment of patients with pheochromocytoma for preoperative preparation of patients for surgery, management of patients when surgery is contraindicated, and the chronic treatment of patients with malignant pheochromocytoma.

Preparation: Tablets, 250 mg.

MEVACOR®, see Lovastatin

MEXILETINE HYDROCHLORIDE —Mexitil®

Antiarrhythmic agent.

Actions and Uses: A class IB antiarrhythmic agent that is similar to lidocaine in its electrophysiologic properties. Indicated for the suppression of symptomatic ventricular arrhythmias, including frequent premature ventricular contractions (unifocal or multifocal), couplets, and ventricular tachycardia.

Warnings: Contraindicated in patients with cardiogenic shock or second- or third-degree AV block (unless a pacemaker is present). Adverse reactions include proarrhythmic events, GI distress, lightheadedness, tremor, and coordination difficulties.

Administration: Oral.

Preparations: Capsules, 150, 200, and 250 mg.

MEXITIL®, see Mexiletine

MEZLIN®, see Mezlocillin

MEZLOCILLIN SODIUM—Mezlin®

Penicillin antibiotic.

Actions and Uses: Is bactericidal and is active against many gram-positive and gram-negative bacteria, including *Pseudomonas aeruginosa.* Is usually used in conjunction with an aminoglycoside antibiotic in the treatment of *Pseudomonas* infections.

Warnings: Contraindicated in patients with a history of allergic reaction to any of the penicillins. Adverse reactions include hypersensitivity reactions, GI disturbances, and local reactions at the injection site.

Administration: Intravenous and intramuscular.

Preparations: Vials and infusion bottles, 1, 2, 3, 4, and 20 g.

MIACALCIN®, see Calcitonin-salmon

MICATIN®, see Miconazole

MICONAZOLE—Monistat IV®

MICONAZOLE NITRATE— Monistat 3®, Monistat 7®, Monistat-Derm®, Micatin®

Imidazole antifungal agent.

Actions and Uses: Indicated for (1) topical application in the treatment of tinea pedis, tinea cruris, tinea corporis, candidiasis, and tinea versicolor; (2) vaginal administration for vulvovaginal candidiasis; and (3) intravenous administration for systemic fungal infections.

Warnings: Adverse reactions associated with topical and vaginal use include local irritation and itching. Adverse reactions associated with intravenous use include phlebitis, pruritus, rash, fever, nausea, and vomiting. Base contained in the vaginal suppository formulation may interact with certain rubber or latex products, such as those used in vaginal contraceptive diaphragms; therefore, concurrent use is not recommended.

Administration: Topical, vaginal, intravenous, intrathecal, and bladder instillation.

Preparations: Cream, lotion, powder, and spray, 2%. Vaginal cream, 1%. Vaginal suppositories, 100 and 200 mg. Ampules, 10 mg/ml.

MICRO-K®, see Potassium chloride

MICRONASE®, see Glyburide

MICRONOR®, see Norethindrone

MICROZIDE®, see Hydrochlorothiazide

MIDAMOR®, see Amiloride

MIDAZOLAM HYDROCHLORIDE—Versed®

Sedative/anesthetic.

Actions and Uses: A short-acting benzodiazepine CNS depressant. Indicated (1) intramuscularly for preoperative sedation and to impair memory of perioperative events, (2) intravenously as an agent for conscious sedation prior to short diagnostic or endoscopic procedures, and in therapeutic procedures, and (3) intravenously for induction of general anesthesia, before administration of other anesthetic agents; can also be used as a component of intravenous supplementation of nitrous oxide and oxygen (balanced anesthesia) for short surgical procedures.

Warnings: Contraindicated in patients with acute narrow-angle glaucoma. Adverse reactions include apnea, decreased tidal volume and/or respiratory rate decrease, hypotension, and oversedation. Effects may be increased by the concurrent administration of other agents having CNS depressant, respiratory depressant and/or hypotensive effects, and the dosage of one or both agents should be appropriately reduced. Lower dosages should be used in elderly, debilitated, and other high-risk patients.

Administration: Intravenous and intramuscular.

Preparations: Vials, 1 mg/ml and 5 mg/ml.

MIDODRINE HYDROCHLORIDE—ProAmatine®

Alpha-adrenergic agonist, indicated in the treatment of orthostatic hypotension. Also used [investigational] in managing urinary incontinence.

Warnings: Contraindicated in patients with severe heart disease, acute renal disease, urinary retention, thyrotoxicosis, pheochromocytoma, supine hypertension. Caution must be exercised in patients with diabetes. Adverse reactions include supine hypertension, bradycardia, paresthesia, pruritis (primarily of the scalp), piloerection (goose bumps), chills, dysuria, urinary frequency and urgency, and urinary retention. Use cautiously with other medications which may reduce the heart rate. Discontinue and reevaluate if the patient develops signs or symptoms of bradycardia (e.g., pulse slowing, increased dizziness, or syncope).

Administration: 10 mg 3 times a day, during daytime hours when patient is upright. Maximum dose is 40 mg/day.

Preparations: Tablets, 2.5 and 5 mg.

MILK OF MAGNESIA, see Magnesium hydroxide

MILONTIN®, see Phensuximide

MILRINONE LACTATE—Primacor®

Agent for congestive heart failure.

Actions and Uses: Is a phosphodiesterase inhibitor and increases cardiac output by inhibiting the enzymatic hydrolysis of cAMP, resulting in both positive inotropic and vasodilating effects. Indicated for the short-term intravenous treatment of congestive heart failure.

Warnings: Adverse reactions include ventricular arrhythmias, supraventricular arrhythmias, hypotension, angina or chest pain, and headache. Should not be used in patients with severe obstructive aortic or pulmonic valvular disease in lieu of surgical relief of the obstruction. It is recommended that it not be used in patients in the acute phase after myocardial infarction. May aggravate outflow tract obstruction in hypertrophic subaortic stenosis. If hypokalemia exists, should be corrected with a potassium supplement before or during the use of milrinone.

Administration: Intravenous. Administered in a loading dose (administered slowly over 10 minutes) followed by a continuous IV infusion (as the maintenance dose).

Preparations: Vials, milrinone lactate equivalent to 1 mg of milrinone per ml. Carpuject sterile cartridge-needle unit with Interlink System Cannula (1 mg/ml).

MILTOWN®, see Meprobamate

MINERAL OIL—Liquid petrolatum

Laxative used in the form of oil or in emulsion formulations.

MINIPRESS®, see Prazosin

MINITRAN®, see Nitroglycerin

MINOCIN®, see Minocycline

MINOCYCLINE HYDROCHLORIDE —Minocin®

Tetracycline antibiotic.

Actions and Uses: Active against many gram-positive and gram-negative bacteria, mycoplasmal, chlamydial, and rickettsial organisms, and certain spirochetes. Indicated in the treatment of respiratory and urinary tract infections and a number of other types of infections. Effective in the treatment of infections caused by *Chlamydia trachomatis* and *Ureaplasma urealyticum*. Is useful as adjunctive therapy in the management of severe acne. Is also indicated in the treatment of asymptomatic carriers of *Neisseria meningitidis*.

Warnings: Use is best avoided during the last half of pregnancy and in childhood to the age of 8 years because of the risk of discoloration of the teeth. May cause lightheadedness, dizziness, and vertigo, and patients should be cautioned about activities such as driving or operating machinery. Other adverse reactions include nausea, vomiting, diarrhea, rash, photosensitivity reactions, and fungal superinfections. Must be used with caution in patients with impaired renal function. Absorption may be reduced by the simultaneous administration of antacids.

Administration: Oral and intravenous. May be administered orally without regard to meals.

Preparations: Capsules and tablets, 50 and 100 mg. Suspension, 50 mg/5 ml. Vials, 100 mg.

MINOXIDIL—Loniten®, Rogaine®

Indicated for the treatment of hypertension that is symptomatic or associated with target organ damage and is not manageable with conventional antihypertensive regimens. Also indicated for the topical treatment of male pattern baldness of the vertex of the scalp, and female androgenetic alopecia (i.e., diffuse hair loss or thinning of the frontoparietal areas).

Preparations: Tablets, 2.5 and 10 mg (Loniten). Topical solution, 2% (Rogaine).

MINTEZOL®, see Thiabendazole

MIOSTAT®, see Carbachol

MIRADON®, see Anisindione

MIRTAZAPINE—Remeron®

Antidepressant of tetracylic chemical structure indicated in the treatment of depression. Patients may begin to see improvements in one to four weeks.

Warnings: Do not administer concurrently with or within 14 days of MAOIs. Use cautiously in patients with hepatic or renal dysfunction, conditions that may be exacerbated by hypotension, disease that affects hemodynamic response, history of mania or hypomania, seizure disorders, suicidal ideation, immunocompromised patients, and elderly. Adverse reactions include somnolence, increased appetite, weight gain, dizziness, nausa, dry mouth, constipation, asthenia, flu syndrome, edema, and CNS effects.

Administrations: Initially 15 mg once daily at bedtime. Increase at intervals of at least 1–2 weeks. Usual range is 15–45 mg daily.

Preparations: Tablets, 15 and 30 mg.

MISOPROSTOL—Cytotec®

Prostaglandin.

Actions and Uses: An analog of prostaglandin E_1 that exhibits actions which protect the gastroduodenal mucosa. Indicated for the prevention of NSAID-induced gastric ulcers in patients at high risk of complications from a gastric ulcer (e.g., patients over age 60, individuals with a history of ulcer, patients taking corticosteroids).

Warnings: Contraindicated during pregnancy because the drug exhibits an abortifacient action. Adverse reactions include diarrhea, abdominal pain, nausea, flatulence, dyspepsia, and headache. Should not be used in women of childbearing potential unless the patient requires NSAID therapy and is at high risk of developing gastric ulcers and/or associated complications.

Administration: Oral. Should be taken with a meal and the last dose of the day should be at bedtime.

Preparations: Tablets, 100 and 200 μg.

MITHRACIN®, see Plicamycin

MITHRAMYCIN, see Plicamycin

MITOMYCIN—Mutamycin®

Antineoplastic agent indicated for the parenteral treatment of disseminated adenocarcinoma of the stomach or pancreas, in combination with other agents.

Preparations: Vials, 5, 20, and 40 mg.

MITOTANE—Lysodren®

Antineoplastic agent indicated in the treatment of inoperable adrenal cortical carcinoma.

Preparation: Tablets, 500 mg.

MITOXANTRONE HYDROCHLORIDE—Novantrone®

Antineoplastic agent.

Actions and Uses: Indicated in combination with other approved drug(s) (e.g., cytosine arabinoside) in the initial therapy of acute nonlymphocytic leukemia in adults.

Warnings: Severe myelosuppression occurs and complete blood counts are necessary for appropriate dose adjustments. Other adverse reactions include bleeding, infection, nausea, vomiting, diarrhea, abdominal pain, stomatitis, fever, headache, alopecia, cough, dyspnea, conjunctivitis, tachycardia, and congestive heart failure. The drug may cause fetal harm when administered during pregnancy. The drug may impart a blue-green color to the urine for 24 hours after administration and patients should be advised to expect this during the therapy.

Administration: Intravenous infusion.

Preparations: Vials, 2 mg mitoxantrone

free base per ml [10 ml (20 mg), 12.5 ml (25 mg), 15 ml (30 mg)].

MITROLAN®, see Polycarbophil

MIVACRON®, see Mivacurium

MIVACURIUM CHLORIDE—Mivacron®

Nondepolarizing neuromuscular blocking agent.

Actions and Uses: Indicated as an adjunct to general anesthesia, to facilitate tracheal intubation and to provide skeletal muscle relaxation during surgery or mechanical ventilation.

Warnings: Use from multi-dose vials is contraindicated in patients with a known allergy to benzyl alcohol. Adverse reactions include transient cutaneous flushing of the face, neck and/or chest. Must be used with caution in patients with neuromuscular disease (e.g., myasthenia gravis, myasthenic syndrome), and in patients receiving other medications that may increase and/or prolong neuromuscular block (e.g., inhalation anesthetics, aminoglycosides, quinidine, magnesium salts). May cause histamine release and caution should be exercised in patients with clinically signifficant cardiovascular diseaseand patients with any history (e.g., asthma) suggesting a greater sensitivity to the release of histamine. Is metabolized by plasma cholinesterase and duration of action may be markedly prolonged in the presence of genetic abnormalities of plasma cholinesterase.

Administration: Intravenous.

Preparations: Vials, 2 mg/ml. Premixed infusion in 5% Dextrose Injection, 0.5 mg/ml. Solutions are acidic and may not be compatible with alkaline solutions having a pH greater than 8.5 (e.g., barbiturate solutions).

MOBAN®, see Molindone

MOCTANIN®, see Monooctanoin

MODANE®, see Phenolphthalein

MODERIL®, see Rescinnamine

MODURETIC®, Combination of amiloride and hydrochlorothiazide

MOEXIPRIL HYDROCHLORIDE—Univasc®, new drug, see Part II

MOLINDONE HYDROCHLORIDE—Moban®

Antipsychotic agent indicated for the management of the manifestations of psychotic disorders.

Preparations: Tablets, 5, 10, 25, 50, and 100 mg. Oral concentrate, 20 mg/ml.

MOMETASONE FUROATE—Elocon®

Topical corticosteroid.

Actions and Uses: Indicated for the relief of the

inflammatory and pruritic manifestations of corticosteroid-responsive dermatoses.

Warnings: Adverse reactions include burning, tingling/stinging, pruritus, and signs of skin atrophy.

Administration: Topical.

Preparations: Cream, ointment, and lotion, 0.1%

MONISTAT®, see Miconazole nitrate

MONOBENZONE—Benoquin®

Depigmenting agent indicated for final depigmentation in extensive vitiligo.

Preparation: Cream, 20%.

MONODOX®, see Doxycycline monohydrate

MONOOCTANOIN—Moctanin®

Agent for gallstones.

Actions and Uses: A solubilizing agent for treatment of cholesterol gallstones retained in the biliary tract after cholecystectomy, when other means of removing cholesterol stones in the common bile duct have failed or cannot be undertaken.

Warnings: Contraindicated in patients with clinical jaundice, significant biliary tract infection, or with a history of recent duodenal ulcer or jejunitis. Adverse reactions include GI pain, nausea, vomiting, and diarrhea. Patients should have periodic liver function tests.

Administration: As a continuous perfusion through a catheter inserted directly into the common bile duct, or through a nasobiliary tube placed by endoscopy.

Preparation: Bottles containing 120 ml.

MONOPRIL®, see Fosinopril sodium

MONUROL®, see Fosfomycin

MORICIZINE HYDROCHLORIDE—Ethmozine®

Antiarrhythmic agent.

Actions and Uses: A Class I antiarrhythmic agent. Indicated for the treatment of documented life-threatening arrhythmias.

Warnings: Contraindicated in the presence of cardiogenic shock, and in patients with preexisting second or third degree atrioventricular block, and in patients with right bundle branch block when associated with left hemiblock unless a pacemaker is present. Adverse reactions include proarrhythmic effects, congestive heart failure, conduction abnormalities, chest pain, palpitations, dizziness, fatigue, sleep disorders, nervousness, headache, nausea, vomiting, dyspepsia, abdominal pain, paresthesias, musculoskeletal pain, blurred vision, and dyspnea.

Administration: Oral.

Preparations: Tablets, 200, 250, and 300 mg.

MORPHINE SULFATE—Astramorph PF®, Duramorph®, Kadian®, MS Contin®, MSIR®, Oramorph SR®, RMS®, Roxanol®, Roxanol SR®

Opiate analgesic.

Actions and Uses: Indicated for the relief of moderate to severe pain, for preoperative medication, to facilitate induction of anesthesia, and as an anesthetic or adjunct to anesthesia.

Warnings: Adverse reactions include sedation and other CNS effects; patients should be cautioned regarding activities such as driving and operating machinery, as well as interactions with other CNS-acting drugs including alcohol. Other adverse reactions include constipation and hypotension. Can cause dependence and formulations are covered under the provisions of the Controlled Substances Act.

Administration: Oral, rectal, intravenous, intramuscular, subcutaneous, epidural, intrathecal.

Preparations: Tablets, 10, 15, and 30 mg. Controlled-release tablet, 15, 30, 60, and 100 mg. (MS Contin, Oramorph SR, Roxanol SR). Sustained release pellets in cap. 20, 50 and 100 mg. Oral solution, 4 mg/ml, 20 mg/ml, 10 mg/5 ml, 20 mg/5 ml, and 100 mg/5 ml. Suppositories, 5, 10, 20, and 30 mg (RMS). Ampules, vials, and syringes, 2, 4, 5, 8, 10, 15, 25, and 50 mg/ml. Ampules and vials (preservative-free and can be used via epidural and intrathecal routes), 0.5 and 1 mg/ml. (Astramorph PF, Duramorph.

Solution for IV injection (PCA device), 1 mg/ml, 2 mg/ml, 3 mg/ml, and 5 mg/ml.

MOTOFEN®, see Difenoxin hydrochloride/atropine sulfate

MOTRIN®, see Ibuprofen

MS CONTIN®, see Morphine

MSIR®, see Morphine

MUCOMYST®, see Acetylcysteine

MUPIROCIN—Bactroban®

Topical and intranasal antibiotic.

Actions and Uses: Indicated for the topical treatment of impetigo due to *Staphylococcus aureus,* beta hemolytic Streptococcus, and *Streptococcus pyogenes.* Eradication of nasal colonization of methicillin-resistant *s. aureus* (MRSA) in adult patients and healthcare workers in certain institutional settings during outbreaks with MRSA.

Warnings: Topical adverse reactions include burning, stinging, pain, and itching. Reactions to nasal applications include headache, rhinitis, respiratory disorder, pharyngitis, taste perversion, cough, and pruritus.

Administration: Topical, nasal. Nasal application is performed twice daily by applying approximately 0.25 g to the inside of each nostril for 5 days. Spread ointment by repeatedly closing and releasing nostrils for 1 minute after application.

Preparation: Ointment, 2%.

MUROMONAB-CD3—Orthoclone OKT3®

Immunosuppressant.

Actions and Uses: Indicated for the treatment of acute allograft rejection in renal, heart, and liver transplant patients.

Warnings: Contraindicated in patients who are in fluid overload. The most severe reaction is potentially fatal pulmonary edema, which has occurred in some patients with fluid overload prior to treatment. Patients should be evaluated for fluid overload by chest x-ray or according to the criterion of weight gain. Most patients experience fever and chills during the first 2 days of therapy. Other adverse reactions commonly encountered during the first 2 days of therapy include dyspnea, chest pain, nausea, vomiting, wheezing, diarrhea, and tremor. Therapy can result in increased susceptibility to infection. The dosage of other immunosuppresants (e.g., prednisone, azathioprine) used concomitantly should be reduced. The use of cyclosporine should be reduced or discontinued to reduce the risk of nephrotoxicity.

Administration: Intravenous as an IV bolus (in less than 1 minute).

Preparation: Ampules, 5 mg.

MUSTARGEN®, see Mechlorethamine

MUTAMYCIN®, see Mitomycin.

MYAMBUTOL®, see Ethambutol

MYCELEX®, see Clotrimazole

MYCIFRADIN®, see Neomycin

MYCOBUTIN®, see Rifabutin

MYCOPHENOLATE MOFETIL—CellCept®

Actions and Uses: Immunosuppressant indicated in prophylaxis of organ rejection in patients receiving allogeneic renal transplants as an adjunct to cyclosporine and corticosteroids.

Warnings: May cause neutropenia so

complete blood counts should be performed weekly for the first month, twice monthly for the second and third months, and then monthly for the first year. If neutropenia develops (absolute neutrophil count of less than 1300/ mm_2), treatment should be interrupted or dosage reduced. Adverse reactions include sepsis, diarrhea, vomiting, and GI tract hemorrhage. Caution must be exercised in patients with active digestive system disease. Counseling of appropriate contraception to prevent pregnancy is recommended as the drug is contraindicated in pregnancy.

Administration: Oral on an empty stomach. Initiate within 72 hours following transplantation.

Preparations: Capsules, 250 mg.

MYCOSTATIN®, see Nystatin

MYDRIACYL®, see Tropicamide

MYKROX®, see Metolazone

MYLANTA AR®, See Famotidine

MYLERAN®, see Busulfan

MYLICON®, see Simethicone

MYOFLEX®, see Trolamine salicylate

MYSOLINE®, see Primidone

MYTELASE®, see Ambenonium

N

NABUMETONE—Relafen®

Nonsteroidal anti-inflammatory drug.

Actions and Uses: Exhibits analgesic, anti-inflammatory, and antipyretic actions indicated for the treatment of signs and symptoms of rheumatoid arthritis and osteoarthritis.

Warnings: Contraindicated in patients in whom aspirin or another nonsteroidal anti-inflammatory drug induces asthma, urticaria, or other allergic-type reactionss. May cause gastrointestinaleffects including diarrhea, dyspepsia, abdominal pain, constipation, flatulence, nausea, vomiting, gastritis, dry mouth, and stomatitis. Use should be avoided in patients with active gas- trointestinal tract disease and closely monitored in patients with a previous history of such disorders. Other adverse reactions include fluid retention, edema, dizziness, headache, pruritus, rash, tinnitus, fatigue, increased sweating, insomnia, nervousness, somnolence, and photosensitivity reactions. Use is not recommended during the third trimester of pregnancy or in nursing mothers.

Administration: Oral.

Preparations: Tablets, 500 and 750 mg.

NADOLOL—Corgard®

Antihypertensive and antianginal agent.

Actions and Uses: A nonselective beta-adrenergic blocking agent indicated in the management of hypertension and angina pectoris.

Warnings: Contraindicated in patients with bronchial asthma, sinus bradycardia and greater than first degree conduction block, cardiogenic shock, and overt cardiac failure. Adverse reactions include sedation, dizziness, fatigue, bradycardia, and symptoms of peripheral vascular insufficiency. Use is best avoided in patients with bronchospastic diseases, and therapy in diabetic patients must be closely monitored.

Administration: Oral. Patients should be cautioned about the interruption or discontinuation of therapy; exacerbation of angina pectoris has occurred following the abrupt cessation of therapy and, when therapy is to be discontinued, the dosage should be gradually reduced over a period of 1 to 2 weeks.

Preparations: Tablets, 20, 40, 80, 120, and 160 mg.

NAFARELIN ACETATE—Synarel®

Agent for endometriosis.

Actions and Uses: A synthetic agonistic analog of gonadotropin releasing hormone. With repeated dosing, it causes a decrease in sex hormone levels. Indicated for the management of endometriosis in women 18 years of age and older, and for the treatment of central precocious puberty in children.

Warnings: Contraindicated in pregnancy, in women who are breast feeding, and in women with undiagnosed abnormal vaginal bleeding. Adverse reactions include hot flashes, decreased libido, vaginal dryness, headaches, and emotional lability. Although the drug usually inhibits ovulation and stops menstruation, contraception is not insured, particularly if patients miss successive doses and experience breakthrough bleeding or ovulation. Patients should use a nonhormonal method of contraception.

Administration: Nasal. Treatment of endometriosis should be started between days 2 and 4 of the menstrual cycle. Patients should be advised of the importance of having their prescription refilled in a timely manner so that they do not miss a dose. The duration of treatment should be limited to 6 months, primarily because of a concern about a loss in bone density. However, if symptoms of endometriosis recur following a 6-month course of therapy and further treatment is being considered, it is recommended that bone density be assessed before retreatment begins.

Preparations: Nasal solution, 2 mg/ml.

NAFCIL®, see Nafcillin sodium

NAFCILLIN SODIUM—Nafcil®, Nallpen®, Unipen®

Penicillin antibiotic indicated in the treatment of staphylococcal infections.

Preparations: Capsules, 250 mg. Tablets, 500 mg. Vials, 500 mg, 1, 2, and 10 g.

NAFTIFINE HYDROCHLORIDE—Naftin®

Antifungal agent.

Actions and Uses: Indicated for the topical treatment of tinea pedis, tinea cruris, and tinea corporis.

Warnings: Adverse reactions include burning/stinging, dryness, erythema, itching, and local irritation.

Administration: Topical.

Preparation: Cream and gel, 1%.

NAFTIN®, see Naftifine

NALBUPHINE HYDROCHLORIDE—Nubain®

Opioid agonist-antagonist analgesic indicated for parenteral use for the relief of moderate to severe pain. Also used as a supplement to balanced anesthesia, for preoperative and postoperative analgesia, and for obstetrical analgesia during labor and delivery.

Preparations: Ampules, vials, and syringes, 10 mg/ml and 20 mg/ml.

NALFON®, see Fenoprofen

NALIDIXIC ACID—NegGram®

Anti-infective agent indicated for the treatment of urinary tract infections caused by susceptible gram-negative bacteria.

Preparations: Tablets, 250 and 500 mg., 1 g. Suspension, 250 mg/5 ml.

NALLPEN®, see Nafcillin sodium

NALMEFENE HYDROCHLORIDE—Revex®

Actions and Uses: Opioid antagonist indicated in the complete or partial reversal of effects induced by opioids and in the management of known or suspected opioid overdose. Is longer acting than naloxone.

Warnings: Adverse reactions include nausea, vomiting, tachycardia, and hypertension. Can produce acute withdrawal symptoms in patients with physical dependence on opioids or following surgery involving high doses of opioids.

Administration: Intravenous bolus, but may be given intramuscularly or subcutaneously if venous access cannot be established.

Preparations: Ampules, 100 ug/ml and 1 mg/ml.

NALOXONE HYDROCHLORIDE—Narcan®

Opioid antagonist indicated for parenteral use for the reversal of narcotic depression induced by opioids. Is also used for the diagnosis of suspected acute opioid overdosage. Is also included in tablet formulations of pentazocine to prevent the effect of the analgesic if the product is misused by injection. Can produce acute withdrawal symptoms in patients with physical dependence on opioids or following surgery involving high doses of opioids.

Preparations: Ampules, vials, and syringes, 0.02 mg/ml and 0.4 mg/ml.

NALTREXONE HYDROCHLORIDE—ReVia®

Opioid antagonist indicated to provide blockade of the pharmacologic effects of exogenously administered opioids as an adjunct to the maintenance of the opioid-free state in detoxified formerly opioid-dependent individuals. Also indicated for the treatment of alcohol dependence.

Preparation: Tablets, 50 mg.

NANDROLONE DECANOATE—Deca-Durabolin®

Anabolic steroid indicated for the parenteral management of the anemia of renal insufficiency. Adequate iron intake is required for optimal response. Should be administered deep into gluteal muscle.

Preparations: Ampules, vials, and syringes, 50 mg/ml, 100 mg/ml, and 200 mg/ml.

NANDROLONE PHENPROPIONATE—Durabolin®

Anabolic steroid indicated for the parenteral treatment of metastatic breast cancer. Administer deep into gluteal muscle.

Preparations: Vials, 25 mg/ml and 50 mg/ml.

NAPHAZOLINE HYDROCHLORIDE—Privine®

Decongestant indicated for nasal and ophthalmic use in the relief of congestion and related symptoms associated with various nasal and ocular conditions.

Preparations: Nasal drops and spray, 0.05%. Ophthalmic solution, 0.012%, 0.02%, 0.03%, 0.05%, 0.1%.

NAPRELAN, see Naproxen sodium

NAPROSYN®, see Naproxen

NAPROXEN—Naprosyn®, EC-Naprosyn®

NAPROXEN SODIUM—Aleve®, Anaprox®, Anaprox DS®, Naprelen®

Nonsteroidal anti-inflammatory drug.

Actions and Uses: Inhibits prostaglandin synthesis and is indicated for the relief of mild to moderate pain, primary dysmenorrhea, rheumatoid arthritis, osteoarthritis, juvenile arthritis, ankylosing spondylitis, tendinitis and bursitis, and acute gout. Also used in the treatment of fever.

Warnings: Should not be given to patients in whom aspirin or another NSAID causes asthma, rhinitis, urticaria, or other allergic-type reactions. May cause GI effects and use should be avoided in patients with active GI tract disease and closely monitored in patients with a previous history of such disorders. Other adverse reactions include headache, dizziness, drowsiness, itching, skin eruptions, tinnitus, edema, and dyspnea.

Administration: Oral.

Preparations: Naproxen—Tablets, 250, 375, and 500 mg. Enteric-coated tablets, 375 and 500 mg. Suspension, 125 mg/5 ml. Naproxen sodium—Tablets, 220 (Aleve), 275 and 550 mg. Controlled-release tablets (Naprelan), 375 and 500 mg.

NAROPIN®, see Ropivicaine Hydrochloride

NAQUA®, see Trichlormethiazide

NARCAN®, see Naloxone

NASACORT®, Nasacort AQ®, see Triamcinolone acetonide

NASALCROM®, see Cromolyn

NASALIDE®, see Flunisolide

NASAREL®, see Flunisolide

NASCOBAL®, see Cyanocobalamin

NATACYN®, see Natamycin

NATAMYCIN—Natacyn®

Antifungal agent indicated for ophthalmic use in the treatment of fungal blepharitis, conjunctivitis, and keratitis.

Preparation: Ophthalmic suspension, 5%.

NATURETIN®, see Bendroflumethiazide

NAVANE®, see Thiothixene

NAVELBINE®, see Vinorelbine tartrate

NEBCIN®, see Tobramycin

NEBUPENT®, see Pentamidine

NEDOCROMIL SODIUM—Tilade®

Antiasthmatic agent.

Actions and Uses: Is an anti-inflammatory agent that appears to inhibit the activation of, and release of mediators (e.g., histamine) from, various inflammatory cell types associated with asthma. Indicated for maintenance therapy in the management of patients with mild to moderate bronchial asthma. Should not be used for the reversal of acute bronchospasm.

Warnings: Adverse reactions include unpleasant taste, cough, pharyngitis, headache, upper respiratory tract infection, nausea, and vomiting.

Administration: Oral inhalation. Should be added to the patient's existing treatment regimen (e.g., bronchodilator).

Preparations: Metered-dose inhaler, at least 112 metered inhalations with each actuation delivering 1.75 mg of the drug from the mouthpiece. Nebulizer solution, 0.5%.

NEFAZODONE HYDROCHLORIDE—Serzone®

Actions and Uses: Inhibits neuronal reuptake of serotonin and norepinephrine and indicated in the treatment of depression.

Warnings: Concurrent administration of terfenadine or astemizole is contraindicated. Adverse reactions include somnolence, dizziness, lightheadedness, confusion, nausea, constipation, dry mouth, asthenia, blurred vision, abnormal vision, headache, sinus bradycardia, and orthostatic hypotension. Patients should be advised to avoid the consumption of alcoholic beverages, and cautioned about operating machinery until response is ascertained.

Administration: Oral.

Preparations: Tablets, 100, 150, 200, and 250 mg.

NEGGRAM®, see Nalidixic Acid

NELFINAVIR—Viracept®

Protease inhibitor indicated in the treatment of HIV infection when antiretroviral therapy is warranted, preferably in combination with other antiretroviral agents.

Warnings: Contraindicated with concurent use of terfenadine, astemisole, cisapride, triazolom, or midazolom. Prescribers should review patient's drug profile and adjust accordingly prior to prescribing. Use cautiously in patients with hepatic impairment and hemophilia. Avoid use of powder in patients with phenylketonuria, since it contains phenylalanine. Adverse reactions include diarrhea, nausea, flatulence, abdominal pain and rash.

Administrations: Take with meals or light snack. Powder may be mixed in a small amount of nonacidic food or beverage (e.g., water, milk, formula). 750 mg 3 times daily, with meals. Antiviral activity is enhanced when administered with nucleoside analogues.

Preparations: Tablets, 250 mg. Oral powder, 50 mg/gram (contains 11.2 mg phenylalanine).

NELOVA®

Oral contraceptive combination of mestranol and norethindrone.

NEMBUTAL®, see Pentobarbital

NEOMYCIN SULFATE—Mycifradin®

Aminoglycoside antibiotic most often used topically, alone or in combination with other anti-infective agents, in the treatment of dermatologic, ocular, and otic infections. Has also been used orally for preoperative suppression of intestinal bacteria, for GI infections, in hepatic coma, and to reduce elevated blood cholesterol levels. Has been used as a bladder irrigant (usually with polymyxin B to prevent urinary tract infections).

Preparations: Cream and ointment, 0.5%. Tablets, 500 mg. Oral solution, 125 mg/5 ml.

NEORAL®, see Cyclosporine

NEOSAR®, see Cyclophosphamide

NEOSTIGMINE BROMIDE—Prostigmin®

NEOSTIGMINE METHYLSULFATE—Prostigmin®

Anticholinesterase indicated for the symptomatic control of myasthenia gravis. Methylsulfate derivative is administered parenterally and is also indicated for the prevention and treatment of postoperative distention and urinary retention, and to reverse the effects of nondepolarizing neuromuscular blocking agents (e.g., tubocurarine).

Preparations: Tablets, 15 mg. Ampules and vials, 1:4000, 1:2000, and 1:1000.

NEO-SYNEPHRINE®, see Phenylephrine

NEOTHYLLINE®, see Dyphylline

NEPTAZANE®, see Methazolamide

NESACAINE®, see Chloroprocaine

NETILMICIN SULFATE—Netromycin®

Aminoglycoside antibiotic indicated for parenteral use, primarily in the treatment of infections caused by gram-negative bacteria.

Preparation: Vials, 100 mg/ml.

NETROMYCIN®, see Netilmicin

NEUPOGEN®, see Filgrastim

NEURONTIN®, see Gabapentin

NEUTRA-PHOS K®, see Potassium phosphate

NEUTREXIN®, see Trimetrexate glucuronate

NEVIRAPINE—Viramune®

Indicated in combination with nucleoside analogues in the treatment of HIV-1 infected adults who have experienced clinical and/or immunologic deterioration.

Warnings: Suspend therapy if severe rash or any rash accompanied by fever, blistering, oral lesions, conjunctivitis, swellling, muscle or joint aches, or general malaise occurs. Discontinue if rash reoccurs on rechallenge. Use cautiously in patients with hepatic dysfunction. Monitor and discontinue if moderate or sèvere liver dysfunction occurs. Advere reactions include rash (may be life threatening), fever, nausea, headache, and liver dysfunction.

Administrations: 200 mg once daily for 14 days and if no rash appears then 200 mg twice daily.

Preparations: Tablets, 200 mg (scored).

NIACIN, see Nicotinic Acid

NIACINAMIDE, see Nicotinamide

NIASPAN, see Nicotinic Acid

NICARDIPINE HYDROCHLORIDE—Cardene®, Cardene IV®

Antihypertensive and antianginal agent.

Actions and Uses: A calcium channel blocking agent that is indicated for the treatment of hypertension and for the management of chronic stable angina.

Warnings: Contraindicated in patients with advanced aortic stenosis. Adverse reactions include flushing, headache, edema of the feet, asthenia, palpitations, dizziness, tachycardia, and nausea. Some angina patients experience increased anginal symptoms.

Administration: Oral and intravenous.

Preparations: Capsules, 20 and 30 mg. Sustained-release capsules, 30, 45, and 60 mg. Ampules, 2.5 mg/ml.

NICLOSAMIDE—Niclocide®

Anthelmintic indicated for the treatment of tapeworm infections caused by beef, fish, and dwarf tapeworms.

Preparation: Tablets, 500 mg.

NICODERM®, see Nicotine

NICORETTE®, see Nicotine polacrilex

NICORETTE DS®, see Nicotine polacrilex

NICOTINAMIDE—Niacinamide

Vitamin analog (of nicotinic acid) used in the prophylaxis and treatment of pellagra.

Preparations: Tablets, 50, 100, 125, 250, and 500 mg. Vials, 100 mg/ml.

NICOTINE—Habitrol®, Nicoderm®, Nicoderm CQ®, Nicotrol®, Nicotrol NS®, ProStep®

Adjunct for smoking cessation.

Actions and Uses: Nicotine is contained in a multilayered transdermal system that provides systemic delivery of the drug following its application to intact skin. Indicated as an aid to smoking cessation as part of a comprehensive behavioral smoking-cessation program.

Warnings: Contraindicated during the immediate postmyocardial infarction period, and in patients with life-threatening arrhythmias or severe or worsening angina pectoris. Adverse reactions include headache, insomnia, tachycardia, erythema, pruritus and burning at application sites.

Administration: Topical, nasal spray.

Preparations: Transdermal systems, 7, 14, and 21 mg absorbed in 24 hours (Habitrol®, Nicoderm®), 11 and 22 mg absorbed in 24 hours (ProStep®), and 5, 10, and 15 mg absorbed in 16 hours (Nicotrol). Nasal spray, 0.5 mg/spray (nicotrol NS). Inhalation system, 10mg (4 mg delivered), contains menthol.

NICOTINE POLACRILEX—Nicorette®, Nicorette DS®

Adjunct for smoking cessation.

Actions and Uses: Nicotine is bound to an ion exchange resin in a chewing gum base, and is absorbed through the buccal mucosa as the gum is chewed. Indicated as a temporary aid to the cigarette smoker seeking to give up his or her smoking habit while participating in a behavioral modification program.

Warnings: Contraindicated in patients during the immediate post-myocardial infarction period, and in patients with life-threatening arrhythmias or severe or worsening angina pectoris. Should be used with caution in patients with dental problems, or with dentures, dental caps, or partial bridges to which the gum may stick and cause damage. Adverse reactions include jaw muscle ache, hiccups, nausea, vomiting, and pharyngitis.

Administration: Buccal.

Preparation: Chewing gum pieces, 2 and 4 mg.

NICOTINIC ACID—Niacin, Niaspan®, Nicobid®, Slo-Niacin®, Vitamin B_3

Vitamin used to correct nicotinic acid deficiency, and in the prevention and treatment of pellagra. Has been used as adjunctive therapy in patients with significant hyperlipidemia.

Preparations: Tablets, 25, 50, 100, 125, 250, and 500 mg. Controlled-release capsules, 125, 250, 375, 400, 500, 750, and 1,000 mg. Elixir, 50 mg/5 ml. Vials, 100 mg/ml.

NICOTROL®, Nicotrol® NS, see Nicotine

NIFEDIPINE—Adalat®, Adalat CC®, Procardia®, Procardia XL®

Antianginal and antihypertensive agent.

Actions and Uses: Is a calcium channel blocking agent that is indicated in the treatment of (1) vasospastic angina, (2) chronic stable angina in patients who remain symptomatic despite adequate doses of beta-adrenergic blocking agents and/or organic nitrates or who cannot tolerate these agents, and (3) hypertension.

Warnings: Adverse reactions include hypotension, flushing, peripheral edema, dizziness, nervousness, and muscle cramps. Although usually well tolerated, concurrent therapy with a beta-adrenergic blocking agent should be closely monitored because of an increased possibility of hypotension, congestive heart failure, or exacerbation of angina.

Administration: Oral.

Preparations: Capsules, 10 and 20 mg. Controlled-release tablets, 30, 60, and 90 mg.

NILSTAT®, see Nystatin

NIMODIPINE—Nimotop®

Agent for spasm following subarachnoid hemorrhage.

Actions and Uses: A calcium channel blocking agent that prevents or relieves the spasm following subarachnoid hemorrhage, thereby reducing the risk of severe ischemic neurologic deficits. Indicated for the improvement of neurological deficits due to spasm following subarachnoid hemorrhage from ruptured congenital intracranial aneurysms in patients who are in good neurological condition.

Warnings: Adverse reactions include decreased blood pressure, headache, nausea, and bradycardia.

Administration: Oral. Therapy should be initiated within 96 hours of the subarachnoid hemorrhage. If the capsules cannot be swallowed (e.g., at the time of surgery, or if the patient is unconscious), a hole should be made in both ends of the capsule with an 18 gauge needle, and the contents of the liquid filled capsule withdrawn into a syringe. The contents should then be emptied into the patient's *in situ* nasogastric tube and washed down the tube with 30 ml of normal saline (0.9%).

Preparation: Capsules, 30 mg.

NIMOTOP®, see Nimodipine

NIPENT®, see Pentostatin

NISOLDIPINE—Sular®

Actions and Uses: Calcium channel blocker indicated in the treatment of hypertension as monotherapy or as an adjunct to other antihypertensives.

Warnings: Use cautiously in patients with hypotension, heart failure, hepatic impairment, and coronary artery disease. Adverse reactions include peripheral edema, headache, dizziness, pharyngitis, vasodilation, sinusitis, palpitations, chest pain, nausea, rash, increased angina, and MI (rare).

Administration: Oral. Do not crush, chew, divide, or take with a high-fat meal or grapefruit juice.

Preparations: Extended-release tablets, 10, 20, 30, and 40 mg.

NITRO-BID®, see Nitroglycerin

NITRODISC®, see Nitroglycerin

NITRO-DUR®, see Nitroglycerin

NITROFURANTOIN—Furadantin®, Macrobid®

NITROFURANTOIN MACROCRYSTALS—Macrodantin®

Urinary tract antibacterial agent.

Actions and Uses: Indicated for urinary tract infections caused by susceptible strains of *E. coli, Proteus* species, *Klebsiella* species, *Enterobacter* species, *S. aureus,* and enterococci.

Warnings: Contraindicated in patients

with significantly impaired renal function, in pregnancy at term, and in infants under 1 month of age. Adverse reactions include nausea, vomiting, pulmonary reactions, dizziness, drowsiness, headache, peripheral neuropathy, anemia, pruritus, and urticaria.

Administration: Oral. Should be administered with food.

Preparations: Tablets, 50 and 100 mg. Suspension, 25 mg/5 ml. Capsules (macrocrystals), 25, 50, and 100 mg. Capsules (Macrobid), 100 mg (25 mg macrocrystals and 75 mg monohydrate).

NITROFURAZONE—Furacin®

Anti-infective agent used topically for adjunctive therapy of patients with second- and third-degree burns, and in skin grafting where bacterial contamination may cause graft rejection and/or donor site infection.

Preparations: Cream and soluble dressing, 0.2%.

NITROGARD®, see Nitroglycerin

NITROGEN MUSTARD, see Mechlorethamine

NITROGLYCERIN (see list of preparations below for trade names)

Antianginal agent.

Actions and Uses: An organic nitrate indicated for the prophylaxis and treatment of patients with angina pectoris.

Warnings: Adverse reactions include headache, dizziness, hypotension, palpitation, and cutaneous vasodilation with flushing.

Administration: Sublingual, translingual, transmucosal, oral, topical, and transdermal.

Preparations: Sublingual tablets (Nitrostat®), 0.15, 0.3, 0.4, and 0.6 mg. Translingual metered dose spray for oral use (Nitrolingual®), 0.4 mg/dose. Transmucosal (buccal) tablets (Nitrogard®), 1, 2, and 3 mg. Sustained-release capsules (Nitro-Bid®, Nitroglyn®), 2.5, 6.5, and 9 mg. Ointment (Nitro-Bid®, Nitrol®, Nitrostat®), 2%. Transdermal systems (Minitran®, Nitro-Dur®, Nitro-disc®), Transderm-Nitro®, Deponit®), 2.5, 5, 7.5, 10, and 15 mg/24 hours.

NITROGLYCERIN, INTRAVENOUS—Nitro-Bid IV®, Tridil®

Actions and Uses: Administered intravenously for (1) control of blood pressure in perioperative hypertension, (2) congestive heart failure associated with acute myocardial infarction, (3) treatment of angina pectoris, and (4) production of controlled hypotension during surgical procedures.

Preparations: Ampules and vials, 0.5, 0.8, 5, and 10 mg/ml.

NITROGLYN®, see Nitroglycerin

NITROL®, see Nitroglycerin

NITROLINGUAL®, see Nitroglycerin

NITROPRESS®, see Sodium nitroprusside

NITROSTAT®, see Nitroglycerin

NITROUS OXIDE—Laughing gas

Anesthetic gas usually used in conjunction with other anesthetics.

NIX®, see Permethrin

NIZATIDINE—Axid®

Antiulcer agent.

Actions and Uses: A histamine H_2-receptor antagonist indicated for the treatment of active duodenal ulcer, for maintenance therapy for duodenal ulcer patients, for benign gastric ulcer, and for gastroesophageal reflux disease including erosive esophagitis.

Warnings: Adverse reactions include somnolence, sweating, urticaria. Patients receiving high doses of aspirin may experience increased salicylate levels when nizatidine is given concurrently.

Administration: Oral.

Preparations: Capsules, 150 and 300 mg.

NIZORAL®, see Ketoconazole

NODOZ®, see Caffeine

NOLAHIST®, see Phenindamine

NOLVADEX®, see Tamoxifen

NONOXYNOL-9—Emko®

Spermicide used in contraceptive formulations.

Preparations: Vaginal foam, jelly, gel, cream, and suppositories.

NORCO®, see Hydrocodone bitartrate with Acetaminophen

NORCURON®, see Vecuronium

NOREPINEPHRINE BITARTRATE—Levarterenol, Levophed®

Sympathomimetic agent having inotropic stimulating and peripheral vasoconstricting actions. Indicated for the restoration of blood pressure in controlling certain acute hypotensive states, and as an adjunct in the treatment of cardiac arrest and profound hypotension.

Preparation: Ampules, 1 mg/ml.

NORETHINDRONE—Micronor®, Norlutin®, Nor-QD®

NORETHINDRONE ACETATE—Norlutate®

Progestin indicated in the treatment of amenorrhea, in abnormal uterine bleeding due to hormonal imbalance (e.g., uterine cancer), and in endometriosis. Used in combination with an estrogen in oral contraceptive formulations and also in progestin-only oral contraceptive formulations.

Preparations: Tablets, 0.35 mg norethindrone for use as an oral contraceptive. Tablets, 5 mg.

NORETHYNODREL

Progestin used in combination with an estrogen in various oral contraceptive formulations.

NORFLEX®, see Orphenadrinecitrate

NORFLOXACIN—Chibroxin®, Noroxin®

Fluoroquinolone antibacterial agent.

Actions and Uses: Indicated for the treatment of adults with complicated and uncomplicated urinary tract infections caused by susceptible strains. Also indicated for uncomplicated urethral and cervical gonorrhea, and prostatitis caused by *E. coli*. Indicated for ophthalmic use for ocular infections caused by susceptible bacteria.

Warnings: Adverse reactions include nausea, headache, and dizziness. Because the drug may cause CNS effects, patients should be cautioned about engaging in activities that require mental alertness or coordination. The drug has caused arthropathy in immature animals, and it is recommended that norfloxacin not be used in children or pregnant women.

Administration: Oral and ophthalmic.

Preparation: Tablets, 400 mg. Ophthalmic solution, 0.3%.

NORGESTIMATE/ETHINYL ESTRADIOL—Ortho-Cyclen®, Ortho Tri-Cyclen®

Oral contraceptive.

Actions and Uses: Is a progestin/estrogen combination that acts primarily by the suppression of gonadotropins and inhibition of ovulation. Norgestimate exhibits a highly selective progestational action and minimal androgenicity. Indicated for the prevention of pregnancy in women who elect to use oral contraceptives as a method of contraception.

Warnings: Contraindicated in women who have thrombophlebitis or a thromboembolic disorder, a past history of such disorders, cerebral vascular or coronary artery disease, known or suspected carcinoma of the breast, carcinoma of the endometrium or other known or suspected estrogen-dependent neoplasia, undiagnosed abnormal genital bleeding, cholestatic jaundice of pregnancy or jaundice with prior oral contraceptive use, hepatic adenomas or carcinomas, or known or suspected pregnancy. Adverse reactions include bleeding irregularities (e.g., breakthrough bleeding, spotting, changes in menstrual flow), gastrointestinal effects (e.g., nausea, vomiting, abdominal cramps), fluid retention, melasma, rash, reduced tolerance to carbohydrates, and vaginal candidiasis. Women should be strongly advised not to smoke because of the increased risk of cardiovascular effects.

Administration: Oral. Administered once a day at about the same time each day. Available in packages designed for a 21-day regimen (i.e., one tablet a day for 21 days, followed by 7 days in which medication is not taken) and a 28-day regimen (i.e., one tablet a day for 21 days, followed by one inactive "reminder" tablet a day for 7 days).

Preparations: Tablets (monophasic formulation), 0.25 mg of norgestimate and 35 ug of ethinyl estradiol in 21-day and 28-day regimens. Tablets (triphasic formulation), graduated doses of 0.18, 0.215, and 0.25 mg of norgestimate with each dosage used in 7 tablets in combination with 35 ug of ethinyl estradiol, in 21-day and 28-day regimens.

NORGESTREL—Ovrette®

Progestin used alone as an oral contraceptive and also in combination with an estrogen in various oral contraceptive formulations.

Preparation: Tablets, 0.075 mg.

NORINYL®

Oral contraceptive combination of ethinyl estradiol or mestranol with norethindrone.

NORITATE®, see Metronidazole

NORLESTRIN®

Oral contraceptive combination of ethinyl estradiol with norethindrone acetate.

NORLUTATE®, see Norethindrone acetate

NORLUTIN®, see Norethindrone

NOR-MIL®, see Diphenoxylate

NORMODYNE®, see Labetalol

NOROXIN®, see Norfloxacin

NORPACE®, see Disopyramide

NORPLANT®, see Levonorgestrel implant

NORPRAMIN®, see Desipramine

NOR-QD®, see Norethindrone

NORTRIPTYLINE HYDROCHLORIDE—Aventyl®, Pamelor®

Tricyclic antidepressant indicated for the relief of symptoms of depression.

Preparations: Capsules, 10, 25, 50, and 75 mg. Oral solution, 10 mg/5ml.

NORVASC®, see Amlodipine besylate

NORVIR®, see Ritinovir

NORZINE®, see Thiethylperazine

NOSCAPINE

Antitussive used in combination with other agents in the treatment of various respiratory conditions.

NOVAFED®, see Pseudoephedrine

NOVANTRONE®, see Mitoxantrone

NOVOBIOCIN SODIUM—Albamycin®

Antibiotic used in selected infections when primary less toxic anti-infective agents are not effective or are contraindicated.

Preparation: Capsules, 250 mg.

NOVOCAIN®, see Procaine

NOVOLIN®, see Insulin

NOVOPEN®

Insulin delivery device which uses penfill insulin cartridges.

NPH INSULIN®, see Insulin

NUBAIN®, see Nalbuphine

NUMORPHAN®, see Oxymorphone

NUPERCAINAL®, see Dibucaine

NUPRIN®, see Ibuprofen

NUROMAX®, see Doxacuriumchloride

NYDRAZID®, see Isoniazid

NUTROPRIA®, see somatropin

NYSTATIN—Mycostatin®, Nilstat®

Antifungal agent indicated in the treatment of cutaneous, mucocutaneous, vaginal, oral, and intestinal infections caused by *Candida albicans* and other *Candida* species.

Preparations: Tablets, 500,000 units. Troches, 200,000 units. Oral suspension, 100,000 units/ml. Vaginal tablets, 100,000 units. Cream, ointment, and powder, 100,000 units/g.

NYTOL®, see Diphenhydramine

O

OCTREOTIDE ACETATE—Sandostatin®

Agent for hypersecretory disorders.

Actions and Uses: Exhibits actions that are similar to those of the natural hormone somatostatin. Suppresses the secretion of growth hormone, serotonin, and the gastroenteropancreatic (GEP) peptides-gastrin, vasoactive intestinal peptide (VIP), insulin, glucagon, secretin, motilin, and pancreatic polypeptide. Indicated for the treatment of the symptoms of two types of gastroenteropancreatic carcinoma.

Suppresses or inhibits the severe diarrhea and flushing episodes associated with metastatic carcinoid tumors, and is also indicated for the treatment of profuse watery diarrhea associated with vasoactive intestinal peptide-secreting tumors. Also indicated in the treatment of acromegaly.

Warnings: Adverse reactions include nausea, diarrhea, loose stools, abdominal discomfort, vomiting, cholelithiasis, and pain at the injection site. May cause hyperglycemia or hypoglycemia and, in patients with diabetes, it may be necessary to adjust the dosage of insulin or oral hypoglycemic agent. May alter the absorption of nutrients, as well as medications that are administered orally.

Administration: Subcutaneous; intravenous bolus injections have been used under emergency conditions.

Preparations: Ampules (1-ml), 0.05, 0.1, 0.2, and

0.5 mg.

OCUCLEAR®, see Oxymetazoline

OCUFEN®, see Flurbiprofen sodium

OCUFLOX®, see Ofloxacin

OCUPRESS®, see Carteolol

OFLOXACIN—Floxin®, Floxin IV®, Floxin otic®, Ocuflox®

Fluoroquinolone antiinfective agent.

Actions and Uses: Exhibits a bactericidal action against many gram-positive and gram-negative bacteria. Indicated for the treatment of lower respiratory tract infections, acute, uncomplicated urethral and cervical gonorrhea, chlamydial urethritis and cervicitis, skin and skin structure infections, urinary tract infections, and prostatitis. Also indicated for ophthalmic use in the treatment of bacterial conjunctivitis and corneal ulcers.

Warnings: Has caused arthropathy and damage to weight-bearing joints in immature animals and its use in children under the age of 18, pregnant women, and women who are nursing is best avoided. Adverse reactions include nausea, headache, diarrhea, phototoxicity reactions and hypersensitivity reactions. May cause dizziness, lightheadedness, insomnia, and other central nervous system effects, and patients should know how they tolerate the drug before they engage in activities (e.g., driving) that require mental alertness and coordination.

Administration: Oral, intravenous, and ophthalmic. The drug should not be taken with food.

Preparations: Tablets, 200, 300, and 400 mg. Vials, 200 and 400 mg. Ophthalmic solution (Ocuflox), 0.3%.

OGEN®, see Estropipate

OLANZAPINE—Zyprexa®

Antipsychotic. Indicated in the management of the manifestations of psychotic disorders.

Warnings: Use cautiously in cardio or cerebrovascular disease, hypovolemia, dehydration, seizures, Alzheimer's disease, hepatic impairment, prostatic hypertrophy, narrow-angle glaucoma, history of paralytic ileus, breast cancer, patients at risk of aspiration pneumonia, elderly and debilitated. Adverse reactions include somnolence, dizziness, constipation, weight gain, personality disorder, akathisia, rhinitis, postural hypotension, tachycardia, headache, fever, abdominal pain, cough, pharyngitis, nervousness, joint pain, and peripheral edema. May cause tardive dyskinesia or neuroleptic malignant syndrome.

Administrations: Initially 5–10 mg once daily. Increase to 10 mg once daily within several days. Thereafter adjust by 5 mg/day at intervals of 1 week. Maximum dose is 20 mg/day.

Preparations: Tablets, 5, 7.5, and 10 mg.

OLOPATADINE HYDROCHLORIDE—Patanol®

Antiallergic agent indicated in temporary prevention of itching of the eye due to allergic conjunctivitis.

Warnings: Adverse reactions include headache, ocular effects (including burning/stinging, dry eye, foreign body sensation, hyperemia, keratitis, lid edema, pruritis), asthenia, cold syndrome, pharyngitis, rhinitis, sinusitis and taste perversion. Use proper instillation techniques being careful not to contaminate the dropper tip. Not for use with contact lenses.

Administrations: 1–2 drops in affected eye(s) twice daily at 6–8-hour intervals.

Preparations: 0.1% ophthalmic solution containing benzalkonium chloride.

OIL OF WINTERGREEN, see Methyl Salicylate

OLSALAZINE SODIUM—Dipentum®

Agent for ulcerative colitis.

Actions and Uses: Is converted in the colon into 2 molecules of 5-aminosalicylic acid (5-ASA, also known as mesalamine). Exhibits a topical anti-inflammatory action in the colon. Indicated for the maintenance of remission of ulcerative colitis in patients who are intolerant of sulfasalazine.

Warnings: Contraindicated in patients who are hypersensitive to the salicylates. Adverse reactions include diarrhea, abdominal pain or cramps, nausea, dyspepsia, bloating, headache, fatigue, depression, rash and arthralgia. Use should be monitored closely in patients with impaired renal function.

Administration: Oral. Should be administered with food to reduce the possibility of GI adverse reactions.

Preparations: Capsules, 250 mg.

OMEPRAZOLE—Prilosec®

Antisecretory agent.

Actions and Uses: Inhibits the enzyme system known as the acid or proton pump at the secretory surface of the gastric parietal cell. Blocks the final step of acid production and is a potent inhibitor of gastric acid secretion. Indicated for the short-term treatment (4-8 weeks) of symptomatic gastroesophageal reflux disease; the maintenance treatment of healed erosive esophagitis; the long-term treatment of pathological hypersecretory conditions (e.g. Zollinger-Ellison syndrome); and the short-term treatment of active duodenal ulcer. Also used in treatment of active duodenal ulcer accociated with *H. pylori* infection in combination with clarithromycin.

Warnings: Adverse reactions include headache, diarrhea, abdominal pain, and nausea.

Administration: Oral. The drug should be taken before eating and capsules should be swallowed whole and not be opened, chewed, or crushed.

Preparation: Delayed-release capsules, 10, 20, and 40 mg.

OMNIPEN®, see Ampicillin

ONCASPAR®, see Pegaspargase

ONCOVIN®, see Vincristine

ONDANSETRON HYDROCHLORIDE—Zofran®

Antiemetic.

Actions and Uses: Is a selective blocking agent of the serotonin 5-HT_3 receptor type. Indicated for the prevention of nausea and vomiting associated with initial and repeat courses of emetogenic cancer chemotherapy, including high-dose cisplatin. Also indicated for the prevention of postoperative nausea and vomiting.

Warnings: Adverse reactions include diarrhea, headache, constipation, and elevations of hepatic enzyme levels.

Administration: Oral and intravenous.

Preparations: Tablets, 4 and 8 mg. Oral solution, 4 mg/5ml. Vials, 2 mg/ml in 2 ml single-dose vials and 20 ml multidose vials; 32 mg/50 ml (premixed) in single-dose containers.

OPHTHAINE®, see Proparacaine

OPIUM

Analgesic, antitussive, and *antidiarrheal.*

Mixture of alkaloids including morphine and codeine. Various formulations are used in the management of pain, cough, and diarrhea.

Preparation: Tincture, 10% (opium tincture, deodorized).

OPTIMINE®, see Azatadine

OPTIPRANOLOL® see Metipranolol

ORALET®, see Fentanyl citrate

ORAMORPH SR®, see Morphine sulfate

ORAP®, see Pimozide

ORATROL®, see Dichlorphenamide

ORETIC®, see Hydrochlorothiazide

ORETON METHYL®, see Methyltestosterone

ORINASE®, see Tolbutamide

ORLAAM®, see Levomethadyl acetate hydrochloride

ORNADE®, Combination of chlorpheniramine and phenylpropanolamine

ORPHENADRINE CITRATE—Norflex®

Skeletal muscle relaxant indicated as an adjunct to rest, physical therapy, and other measures for the relief of discomfort associated with acute painful musculoskeletal conditions.

Preparations: Tablets, 100 mg. Ampules, 60 mg.

ORTHO-CEPT®, see Desogestrel/ethinyl estradiol

ORTHO-CYCLEN®, see Norgestimate/ethinyl estradiol

ORTHO-NOVUM®

Oral contraceptive combination of ethinyl estradiol or mestranol with norethindrone.

ORTHO TRI-CYCLEN®, see Norgestimate/ethinyl estradiol

ORTHOCLONE OKT3®, see Muromonab-CD3

ORUDIS®, see Ketoprofen

ORUVAIL®, see Ketoprofen

OS-CAL®, see Calcium carbonate

OSMITROL®, see Mannitol

OTRIVIN®, see Xylometazoline

OVRAL®

Oral contraceptive combination of ethinyl estradiol and norgestrel

OVRETTE®, see Norgestrel

OVULEN®

Oral contraceptive combination of mestranol and ethynodiol diacetate.

OXACILLIN SODIUM—Prostaphlin®

Penicillin antibiotic indicated in the treatment of staphylococcal infections.

Preparations: Capsules, 250 and 500 mg. Powder for oral solution, 250 mg/5 ml when reconstituted. Vials, 250 and 500 mg, 2, 4, and 10 g.

OXAMNIQUINE—Vansil®

Antiparasitic agent indicated in the treatment of infections caused by *Schistosoma mansoni.*

Preparation: Capsules, 250 mg.

OXANDRIN®, see Oxandrolone

OXAPROZIN—Daypro®

Nonsteroidal anti-inflammatory drug.

Actions and Uses: Inhibits prostaglandin synthesis and exhibits analgesic, anti-inflammatory, and antipyretic actions. Indicated for acute and long-term use in the management of osteoarthritis and rheumatoid arthritis.

Warnings: Contraindicated in patients with the syndrome of nasal polyps, angioedema, and bronchospastic reactivity to aspirin or another nonsteroidal anti-inflammatory drug. May cause gastrointestinal effects including nausea, dyspepsia, constipation, diarrhea, abdominal pain/distress, anorexia, flatulence, and vomiting. Use should be avoided in patients with active gastrointestinal tract disease and closely monitored in patients with a previous history of such disorders. Use is not recommended during the third trimester of pregnancy. May prolong bleeding time and concurrent use with warfarin should be closely monitored.

Administration: Oral.

Preparations: Caplets, 600 mg.

OXAZEPAM—Serax®

Benzodiazepine antianxiety agent.

Actions and Uses: A CNS depressant indicated for the management of anxiety disorders or for the short-term relief of the symptoms of anxiety. Also useful in anxiety associated with depression and in alcoholics experiencing alcohol withdrawal.

Warnings: Adverse reactions include drowsiness and other CNS effects; patients should be cautioned regarding activities such as driving and operating machinery, as well as interactions with other CNS-acting drugs including alcohol. Can cause dependence and is included in Schedule IV.

Administration: Oral.

Preparations: Capsules and tablets, 10, 15, and 30 mg.

OXICONAZOLE NITRATE—Oxistat®

Imidazole antifungal agent.

Actions and Uses: A topically-applied antifungal agent that is indicated for the topical treatment of tinea pedis, tinea cruris, and tinea corporis.

Warnings: Adverse reactions include itching, burning, and irritation.

Administration: Topical.

Preparation: Cream, 1%. Lotion, 1%.

OXISTAT®, see Oxiconazole

OXSORALEN®, see Methoxsalen

OXSORALEN-ULTRA®, see Methoxsalen

OXTRIPHYLLINE—Choline theophyllinate, Choledyl®

Bronchodilator indicated for relief of bronchial asthma and for reversible bronchospasm associated with chronic bronchitis and emphysema.

Preparations: Tablets, 100 and 200 mg. Syrup, 50 mg/5 ml. Elixir, 100 mg/5 ml.

OXYBENZONE

Sunscreen used in combination with other agents in sunscreen formulations.

OXYBUTYNIN CHLORIDE—Ditropan®

Antispasmodic indicated for the relief of symptoms associated with voiding in patients with uninhibited neurogenic and reflex neurogenic bladder. Also indicated in the treatment of nocturia, frequent urination, urgency, and incontinence.

Preparations: Tablets, 5 mg. Syrup, 5 mg/5 ml.

OXYCODONE HYDROCHLORIDE—Oxycontin®, Roxicodone®

OXYCODONE TEREPHTHALATE

Opioid analgesic.

Actions and Uses: A centrally acting analgesic indicated for the relief of moderate to moderately severe pain.

Warnings: Adverse reactions include sedation and other CNS effects; patients should be cautioned regarding activities such as driving and operating machinery, as well as interactions with other CNS-acting drugs including alcohol. Other adverse reactions include constipation, nausea, and vomiting. Can cause dependence and formulations are covered under the provisions of the Controlled Substances Act.

Administration: Oral.

Preparations: Tablets, 5 mg. Controlled-release tablets, 10, 20, 40 and 80 mg. Solution, 5 mg/5 ml. Concentrated oral solution, 20 mg/ml.

OXYGEN

Gas administered by inhalation in situations in which there is insufficient oxygen available to tissues.

Preparation: Gas

OXYMETAZOLINE HYDROCHLORIDE—Afrin®, Ocuclear®

Decongestant administered topically in the form of nose drops or a nasal spray, and as an ophthalmic solution for the relief of redness of the eye due to minor eye irritations.

Preparations: Drops, 0.025%. Drops and spray, 0.05%.

OXYMETHOLONE—Anadrol-50®

Anabolic steroid indicated in the treatment of anemias caused by deficient red cell production.

Preparation: Tablets, 50 mg.

OXYMORPHONE HYDROCHLORIDE—Numorphan®

Opioid analgesic indicated for parenteral and rectal use for the relief of moderate to severe pain.

Preparations: Ampules and vials, 1 mg/ml and 1.5 mg/ml. Suppositories, 5 mg.

OXYTETRACYCLINE HYDROCHLORIDE—Terramycin®

Tetracycline antibiotic indicated for the treatment of infections caused by susceptible organisms.

Preparations: Capsules, 250 mg. Ampules and vials (for intramuscular use), 50 mg/ml and 125 mg/ml. Formulations also including polymyxin B sulfate are used topically for the treatment of ocular, dermatologic, and vaginal infections.

OXYTOCIN—Pitocin®, Syntocinon®

Oxytocic hormone indicated for parenteral use to initiate or improve uterine contractions (e.g., when it is desirable to induce labor), and to produce uterine contractions during the third stage of labor and to control postpartum bleeding or hemorrhage. Also used in the form of a nasal spray for initial milk letdown.

Preparations: Ampules, 5 and 10 units. Vials, 10

units/ml. Syringes, 10 units. Nasal spray, 40 units/ml.

P

PABA, see Para-aminobenzoic acid

PACLITAXEL—Taxol®

Antineoplastic agent.

Actions and Uses: Indicated for the treatment of metastatic carcinoma of the ovary and metastatic carcinoma of the breast, after failure of first-line or subsequent chemotherapy.

Warnings: Contraindicated in patients who are hypersensitive to the drug or to polyoxyethylated castor oil (Cremophor EL—a solubilizing agent included in the formulation), and in patients with a history of such reactions to other drugs that are available in formulations containing polyoxyethylated castor oil. Is also contraindicated in patients with baseline neutropenia of < 1,500 cells/ mm^3. May cause myelosuppression (neutropenia, thrombocytopenia, anemia) and the resultant risks of infection and bleeding; frequent peripheral blood counts should be performed. Therapy must be closely monitored when other drugs causing myelosuppression are used concurrently or sequentially. Use has been associated with a high incidence of hypersensitivity reactions, and patients should be premedicated with a corticosteroid (e.g., dexamethasone), antihistamine (e.g., diphenhydramine), and a histamine H_2-receptor antagonist (e.g., cimetidine). Other adverse reactions include peripheral neuropathy, hypotension, bradycardia, severe conduction abnormalities, arthralgia/ myalgia, nausea, vomiting, diarrhea, mucositis, alopecia, and hepatic effects. Metabolism may be inhibited by the concurrent administration of ketoconazole. Women of childbearing potential should be advised to avoid becoming pregnant during treatment with the drug.

Administration: The concentrated solution of paclitaxel may extract the plasticizer DEHP from plasticized polyvinyl chloride (PVC) equipment or devices used to prepare solutions for infusion. Contact of the concentrate with such equipment or devices is not recommended, and diluted solutions should be stored in bottles (glass, polypropylene) or plastic bags (polypropylene, polyolefin) and administered through polyethylene-lined administration sets. The diluted solution should be administered through an in-line filter with a microporous membrane not greater than 0.22 microns. Gloves should be worn when handling and preparing the solutions.

Preparations: Vials, 30 mg/5 ml (paclitaxel concentrate).

PAMELOR®, see Nortriptyline

PAMIDRONATE DISODIUM—Aredia®

Agent for hypercalcemia of malignancy and Paget's disease.

Actions and Uses: Is a member of the bisphosphonate group of compounds and is also known as aminohydroxypropylidene diphosphonate (APD). Inhibits bone resorption; adsorbs to calcium phosphate in bone and may directly block dissolution of this mineral component of bone. Indicated in conjunction with adequate hydration (to restore the urine output to about 2 liters per day) for the treatment of moderate or severe hypercalcemia associated with malignancy, with or without bone metastases. Also indicated for the treatment of Paget's disease and management of osteolytic bone lesions associated with multiple myeloma.

Warnings: Contraindicated in patients who are hypersensitive to the drug or to etidronate. Adverse reactions include low-grade fever, infusion site reactions (redness, swelling, pain), fluid overload, generalized pain, hypertension, abdominal pain, anorexia, constipation, nausea, vomiting, urinary tract infection, bone pain, anemia, hypokalemia, hypomagnesemia, and hypophosphatemia. Serum calcium, electrolytes, phosphate, magnesium, and creatinine, and complete blood count, differential, and hematocrit/hemoglobin must be closely monitored.

Administration: Intravenous infusion. Should not be mixed with calcium-containing infusion solutions.

Preparation: Vials, 30, 60, and 90 mg.

PAMINE®, see Methscopolamine

PANADOL®, see Acetaminophen

PANCREASE®, see Pancrelipase

PANCRECARB MS-8®—
Pancreptic Enzymes—Lipase 8,000 units, amylase 4,000 units, proterse 4,500 units

PANCREATIN

Digestive enzyme often used in combination with other agents as a digestive aid.

PANCRELIPASE—
Pancrease®, Viokase®, Zymase®

Digestive enzyme representing a standardized pancreatic enzyme concentrate that is indicated as a digestive aid in the treatment of disorders associated with pancreatic insufficiency.

Preparations: Capsules, tablets, and powder.

PANCURONIUM BROMIDE—
Pavulon®

Nondepolarizing neuromuscular blocking agent indicated for parenteral use as an adjunct to general anesthesia, to facilitate tracheal intubation, and to provide skeletal muscle relaxation during surgery or mechanical ventilation.

Preparations: Ampules and vials, 1 mg/ml and 2 mg/ml.

PANDEL®, see Hydrocortisone

PANMYCIN®, see Tetracycline

PAPAVERINE HYDROCHLORIDE—Pavabid®

Vasodilator indicated for the relief of cerebral and peripheral ischemia associated with arterial spasm and myocardial ischemia complicated by arrhythmias.

Preparations: Tablets, 30, 60, 100, 200, and 300 mg. Controlled-release capsules, 150 mg. Ampules, 30 mg/ml.

PARA-AMINOBENZOIC ACID—PABA, Potaba®

Has been used orally in the treatment of conditions such as scleroderma, dermatomyositis, and Peyronie's disease, and topically as a sunscreen and protectant.

Preparations: Capsules and tablets (as the potassium salt), 500 mg. Packets (as the potassium salt), 2 g. Powder.

PARA-AMINOSALICYLIC ACID, see Aminosalicylate sodium.

PARAFLEX®, see Chlorzoxazone

PARAFON FORTE DSC®, see Chlorzoxazone

PARALDEHYDE

Sedative-hypnotic and anticonvulsant used in some patients with delirium tremens and other psychiatric states characterized by excitement. Has been used in the emergency treatment of tetanus, eclampsia, and status epilepticus.

Preparations: Liquid that has been administered orally and rectally. Ampules and vials, 1 g/ml.

PARAMETHADIONE

Anticonvulsant indicated for the control of absence (petit mal) seizures that are refractory to treatment with other drugs.

Preparations: Capsules, 150 and 300 mg. Oral solution, 300 mg/ml.

PARAPLATIN®, see Carboplatin

PAREGORIC—Camphorated opium tincture

Analgesic and antidiarrheal. Contains opium alkaloids and is used in the treatment of diarrhea and in conditions associated with pain.

Preparation: Liquid containing the equivalent of 2 mg of morphine per 5 ml.

PARLODEL®, see Bromocriptine

PARNATE®, see Tranylcypromine

PAROMOMYCIN SULFATE—Humatin®

Anti-infective agent indicated in the treatment of intestinal amebiasis. Has also been used as adjunctive therapy in the management of hepatic coma.

Preparation: Capsules, 250 mg.

PAROXETINE HYDROCHLORIDE—Paxil®

Antidepressant.

Actions and Uses: Is a selective serotonin reuptake inhibitor. Indicated for the treatment of depression and panic disorders.

Warnings: Contraindicated in patients taking a monoamine oxidase inhibitor (MAOI). Adverse reactions include nausea, dry mouth, asthenia, somnolence, dizziness, insomnia, tremor, nervousness, sweating, ejaculatory disturbance, and other male genital disorders. May decrease appetite resulting in weight loss. Should not be used concomitantly with a MAOI, or during either the 14-day period following discontinuation of treatment with a MAOI, or the 14-day period preceding initiation of treatment with a MAOI. Concomitant use with tryptophan is not recommended.

Administration: Oral, usually in the morning to reduce the possibility of insomnia.

Preparations: Tablets, 20 and 30 mg.

PARSIDOL®, see Ethopropazine

PAS, see Aminosalicylate sodium

PATANOL®—see Olopatadine Hydrochloride

PATHILON®, see Tridihexethyl chloride

PATHOCIL®, see Dicloxacillin

PAVABID®, see Papaverine

PAVULON®, see Pancuronium

PAXAREL®, see Acetylcarbromal

PAXIL®, see Paroxetine hydrochloride

PAXIPAM®, see Halazepam

PBZ®, see Tripelennamine

PCE®, see Erythromycin base

PECTIN

Adsorbent used in combination with agents such as kaolin for the treatment of diarrhea.

PEDAMETH®, see Methionine

PEDIALYTE®

Fluid and electrolyte replacement. A liter contains dextrose 25 g, (fructose 5 g, in fruit flavors), sodium 45 mEq, potassium 20 mEq, chloride 35 mEq. Citrate 30 mEq with 100 calories

Preparations: Liquid and freezer Pops

PEDIAZOLE®, Combination of erythromycin ethylsuccinate and sulfisoxazole

PEG, see Polyethylene glycol

PEGADEMASE BOVINE—Adagen®

Enzyme for replacement therapy.

Actions and Uses: Also known as PEG-ADA, is prepared by attaching numerous strands of polyethylene glycol (PEG) to adenosine deaminase (ADA) of bovine origin. Indicated for enzyme replacement therapy for ADA deficiency in patients with severe combined immunodeficiency disease (SCID) who are not suitable candidates for—or who have failed—bone marrow transplantation.

Warnings: Contraindicated in patients with severe thrombocytopenia. Adverse reactions include headache and pain at injection site.

Administration: Intramuscular.

Preparations: Vials, 250 units/ml.

PEGANONE®, see Ethotoin

PEGASPARGASE—Oncaspar®

Antineoplastic agent.

Actions and Uses: Is a modified form of L-asparaginase (derived from *E. coli*) that is produced by conjugating units of monomethoxypolyethylene glycol (PEG) to the enzyme. Causes a rapid depletion of asparagine resulting in the destruction of leukemic cells that are unable to synthesize asparagine. Indicated for patients with acute lymphoblastic leukemia who require L-asparaginase in their treatment regimen, but have developed hypersensitivity to the native forms of L-asparaginase. Is generally used in combination with other chemotherapeutic agents.

Warnings: Contraindicated in patients with a history of pancreatitis or who have had significant hemorrhagic events associated with prior asparaginase therapy. Is less likely than asparaginase to cause hypersensitivity reactions but may cause immediate and life-threatening anaphylaxis. May cause pancreatitis and frequent serum amylase determinations should be obtained to detect early evidence of pancreatitis. Thrombosis may occur and, if possible, the concurrent use of other drugs that may increase the risk of bleeding (e.g., warfarin, aspirin, NSAIDs) should be avoided. Other adverse reactions include hyperglycemia, liver function abnormalities, nausea, vomiting, fever, and malaise.

Administration: Intravenous or intramuscular. The IM route is preferred because of a lower risk of serious hypersensitivity and other adverse reactions. When administered IM, the volume of a single injection should be limited to 2 ml. When administered IV, should be given over a period of 1–2 hours in 100 ml of sodium chloride or dextrose injection 5%, through an infusion that is already running. The vials should not be shaken.

Preparation: Vials, 3,750 IU in 5 ml.

PEMOLINE—Cylert®

Central nervous system stimulant indicated in the treatment of attention-deficit disorder.

Preparations: Tablets, 18.75, 37.5, and 75 mg. Chewable tablets, 37.5 mg.

PENBUTOLOL SULFATE—Levatol®

Antihypertensive agent.

Actions and Uses: A nonselective beta-adrenergic blocking agent with mild intrinsic sympathomimetic activity. Indicated in the treatment of hypertension.

Warnings: Contraindicated in patients with bronchial asthma, cardiogenic shock, severe bradycardia, and second and third degree atrioventricular conduction block. Adverse reactions include headache, dizziness, fatigue, and nausea. Use is best avoided in patients with bronchospastic diseases and therapy in diabetic patients must be closely monitored.

Administration: Oral. Patients should be cautioned about the interruption or discontinuation of therapy; exacerbation of angina pectoris has occurred following the abrupt cessation of therapy and, when therapy is to be discontinued, the dosage should be gradually reduced over a period of 1 to 2 weeks.

Preparation: Tablets, 20 mg.

PENCICLOVIR—Denavir®

Antiviral agent indicated for the treatment of topical recurrent herpes simplex labialis (cold sores) on the lips and face in adults. Topical cream form of the active component of the oral antiviral prodrug, famciclovir.

Warnings: Contraindicated in patients with previous and significant adverse reactions to famciclovir. Do not use on mucous membranes or near eyes. Use cautiously in the immunocompromised patient. Adverse reactions include headache and mild skin irritation.

Administrations: Apply every 2 hours while awake for 4 days. Begin treatment at earliest sign or symptom (i.e., during prodrome or when lesions appear). Only to be used on lips and face.

Preparations: 1% cream.

PENETREX®, see Enoxacin

PENICILLAMINE—Cuprimine®, Depen®

Chelating agent indicated in the treatment of Wilson's disease, cystinuria, and in patients with severe, active rheumatoid arthritis who have failed to respond to an adequate trial of conventional therapy.

Preparations: Capsules and tablets, 125 and 250 mg.

PENICILLIN G POTASSIUM

Penicillin antibiotic.

Actions and Uses: Is active against gram-positive and gram-negative cocci, gram-positive and selected gram-negative bacilli, and certain spirochetes.

Warnings: Contraindicated in patients with a history of allergic reaction to any of the penicillins. Adverse reactions include hypersensitivity reactions.

Administration: Intravenous, intramuscular, and oral.

Preparations: Tablets, 200,000, 250,000 and 400,000 units. Oral solution, 400,000 units/5 ml. Vials, 200,000, 500,000, 1, 5, 10, and 20 million units.

PENICILLIN G SODIUM

Preparation: Vials, 5 million units.

PENICILLIN V POTASSIUM—Beepen VK®, Betapen VK®, Ledercillin VK®, Pen-Vee K®, V-Cillin K®, Veetids®

Penicillin antibiotic.

Actions and Uses: Is primarily active against gram-positive bacteria and is commonly used in conditions such as respiratory tract infections caused by susceptible organisms (e.g., streptococci).

Warnings: Contraindicated in patients with a history of allergic reaction to any of the penicillins. Adverse reactions include hypersensitivity reactions, rash, and nausea.

Administration: Oral. May be administered without regard to meals.

Preparations: Solution, 125 mg/5ml..

PENTAERYTHRITOL TETRANITRATE

Antianginal agent used in the prophylactic treatment of angina pectoris.

Preparations: Tablets, 10, 20, and 40 mg. Controlled-release tablets, 80 mg.

PENTAGASTRIN—Peptavlon®

Diagnostic agent for evaluation of gastric acid secretory function.

Preparation: Ampules, 0.25 mg/ml.

PENTAM 300®, see Pentamidine isethionate

PENTAMIDINE ISETHIONATE—NebuPent®, Pentam 300®

Antiprotozoal agent indicated for parenteral use in the treatment of *Pneumocystis carinii* pneumonia and for use via inhalation in the prevention of *Pneumocystis carinii* pneumonia in high-risk human immunodeficiency virus (HIV)-infected patients.

Preparations: Vials, 300 mg. Vials for aerosol use, 300 mg.

PENTASA®, see Mesalamine

PENTAZOCINE—Talwin®

Opioid agonist-antagonist analgesic indicated for the relief of moderate to severe pain, as an analgesic during labor, as a sedative prior to surgery, and as a supplement in balanced anesthesia.

Preparations: Tablets (as the hydrochloride with naloxone hydrochloride), 50 mg (Talwin Nx®). Ampules, vials, and syringes (as the lactate), 30 mg/ml.

PENTHRANE®, see Methoxyflurane

PENTOBARBITAL SODIUM—Nembutal®

Barbiturate sedative-hypnotic used in the management of anxiety and insomnia. Also used parenterally as a preanesthetic medication and for the emergency control of acute convulsive episodes.

Preparations: Capsules, 50 and 100 mg. Elixir, pentobarbital acid equivalent to 20 mg of the sodium salt/5 ml. Suppositories, 30, 60, 120, and 200 mg. Vials and syringes, 50 mg/ml.

PENTOSAN POLYSULFATE SODIUM—Elmiron®

Bladder protectant indicated in relief of bladder pain or discomfort associated with interstitial cystitis. A semisynthetic, low molecular weight, heparinlike compound which exerts both anticoagulant and fibrinolytic effects.

Warnings: Use cautiously in bleeding disorders or conditions associated with an increased risk of bleeding (e.g., surgery, coagulopathy, aneurysm, hemophilia, GI ulceration, polyps, diverticulitis), in patients with a history of heparin-induced thrombocytopenia, hepatic insufficiency, and splenic disorders. Additive effects may be expected when administered with other anticoagulant drugs, such as warfarin or heparin, and possible similar effects when administered with aspirin or thrombolytics. Adverse reactions include alopecia, GI disturbances, headache, rash, abdominal pain, liver function abnormalities, dizziness, hemorrhage or increased bleeding times.

Administrations: Take 1 hour before or 2 hours after meals with water, 100 mg three times daily. Reevaluate symptoms at 3 and 6 months.

Preparations: Capsules, 100 mg.

PENTOSTATIN—Nipent®

Antineoplastic agent.

Actions and Uses: Indicated as a single agent treatment for adult patients with alpha interferon-refractory hairy cell leukemia.

Warnings: May cause myelosuppression (e.g., neutropenia) and, in patients with infections, efforts should be made to control the infection before treatment is initiated or resumed. Other adverse reactions include gastrointestinal effects (e.g., nausea, vomiting, anorexia, diarrhea), respiratory effects (e.g., increased cough, upper respiratory infection), nervous system effects (e.g., fatigue, neurologic disorders), fever, infection, pain, elevated hepatic function tests, genitourinary disorders, headache, allergic reactions, chills, myalgia, and rash. May cause fetal harm if administered during pregnancy. Concurrent use with fludarabine phosphate is not recommended because of the risk of pulmonary toxicity.

Administration: Intravenous.

Preparation: Vials, 10 mg.

PENTOTHAL®, see Thiopental

PENTOXIFYLLINE—Trental®

Hemorrheologic agent.

Actions and Uses: A xanthine derivative that decreases the viscosity and improves the flow properties of blood. Indicated for the treatment of intermittent claudication on the basis of chronic occlusive arterial disease of the limbs.

Warnings: Contraindicated in patients who have previously exhibited intolerance to a xanthine derivative (e.g., caffeine, theophylline). Adverse reactions include nausea.

Administration: Oral.

Preparation: Controlled-release tablets, 400 mg.

PEN-VEE K®, see Penicillin V potassium

PEPCID®, see Famotidine

PEPCID AC®, see Famotidine

PEPTAVLON®, see Pentagastrin

PEPTO-BISMOL®, see Bismuth subsalicylate

PERCOCET®, Combination of oxycodone and acetaminophen

PERCODAN®, Combination of oxycodone and aspirin

PERGOLIDE MESYLATE—Permax®

Antiparkinson agent.

Actions and Uses: An ergot derivative that acts by stimulating dopamine receptors. Indicated as an adjunctive treatment to levodopa/carbidopa in the management of Parkinson's disease.

Warnings: Adverse reactions include dyskinesia, dizziness, hallucinations, fatigue, insomnia, nausea, constipation, diarrhea, dyspepsia, rhinitis, and orthostatic hypotension. Effectiveness may be decreased by dopamine antagonists (e.g., phenothiazines, haloperidol) or metoclopramide.

Administration: Oral.

Preparations: Tablets, 0.05, 0.25, and 1 mg.

PERGONAL®, see Menotropins

PERIACTIN®, see Cyproheptadine

PERIDEX®, see Chlorhexidine gluconate

PERMAPEN®, see Benzathine penicillin G

PERMAX®, see Pergolide

PERMETHRIN—Elimite®, Nix®

Pediculicide and Scabicide.

Actions and Uses: A synthetic pyrethroid that is indicated for the single-application treatment of infestation with *Pediculus humanus* var. *capitis* (the head louse) and its nits (eggs), and for the single-application treatment of scabies. Also indicated for prophylaxis during epidemic (20% of an institutional population are infected or immediate household contacts).

Warnings: Contraindicated in patients with a known hypersensitivity to any synthetic pyrethroid or pyrethrin, or to chrysanthemums. Adverse reactions include itching, mild burning or stinging, tingling, numbness, or scalp -or rash.

Administration: Topical.

Preparation: Cream, 5%. Cream rinse, 1% (for head lice infestation).

PERMITIL®, see Fluphenazine

PEROXIDE, see Hydrogen peroxide

PERPHENAZINE—Trilafon®

Phenothiazine antipsychotic agent and antiemetic.

Preparations: Tablets, 2, 4, 8, and 16 mg. Controlled-release tablets, 8 mg. Oral concentrate, 16 mg/5 ml. Ampules, 5 mg/ml.

PERSANTINE®, see Dipyridamole

PERSANTINE IV®, see Dipyridamole

PERTOFRANE®, see Desipramine

PERUVIAN BALSAM

Local irritant used topically in various dermatologic disorders.

PETROLATUM

Ointment base used as a vehicle for various topically applied medications. Sometimes used topically as a protective agent.

PHAZYME®, see Simethicone

PHENACEMIDE—Phenurone®

Anticonvulsant indicatted for the control of severeepilepsy, particularly mixed forms of complex partial (psychomotor) seizures, refractory to other drugs.

Preparation: Tablets, 500 mg.

PHENAZOPYRIDINE HYDROCHLORIDE—Azo-Standard®, Pyridium®

Urinary tract analgesic indicated for the symptomatic relief of pain, burning, urgency, frequency, and other discomforts arising from irritation of the lower urinary tract mucosa. Causes a reddish-orange discoloration of the urine and patients should be advised of this effect.

Preparations: Tablets, 100 and 200 mg.

PHENDIMETRAZINE TARTRATE—Bontril®

Anorexiant indicated in the management of exogenous obesity as a short-term adjunct in a regimen of weight reduction based on caloric restriction.

Preparations: Capsules and tablets, 35 mg. Controlled-release capsules, 105 mg.

PHENELZINE SULFATE—Nardil®

Monoamine oxidase inhibitor indicated for the treatment of depression.

Preparation: Tablets, 15 mg.

PHENERGAN®, see Promethazine

PHENINDAMINE TARTRATE—Nolahist®

Antihistamine indicated in the management of allergic disorders.

Preparation: Tablets, 25 mg.

PHENIRAMINE MALEATE

Antihistamine used in combination with other agents in the management of allergic and related disorders.

PHENOBARBITAL PHENOBARBITAL SODIUM—Luminal sodium®

Barbiturate sedative, hypnotic, and anticonvulsant.

Actions and Uses: A CNS depressant indicated (1) for anxiety-tension states, (2) for insomnia, (3) as a long-term anticonvulsant for the treatment of tonic-clonic and cortical focal seizures, (4) in the symptomatic control of acute convulsions (e.g., tetanus, status epilepticus), (5) as a preanesthetic sedative, and (6) in other situations associated with anxiety.

Warnings: Adverse reactions include drowsiness and other CNS effects; patients should be cautioned regarding activities such as driving and operating machinery, as well as interactions with other CNS-acting drugs including alcohol. Can cause dependence and is included in Schedule IV.

Administration: Oral, intravenous, and intramuscular.

Preparations: Tablets, 8, 15, 30, 60, and 100 mg. Capsules, 15 mg. Elixir, 20 mg/5 ml. Injection dosage forms (phenobarbital sodium), 30, 60, 65, and 130 mg/ml.

PHENOL—Carbolic acid

Antipruritic, topical anesthetic, antiseptic, and caustic. Used topically in the management of various dermatologic conditions, and in certain other formulations (e.g., throat lozenges, mouth- washes, and gargles) that are utilized for a local effect.

Preparations: Solutions and lotions (with other agents for dermatologic use), 0.5—1%. Liquefied phenol is phenol maintained in a liquid condition by the presence of 10% water; is used as a source of phenol for preparing various formulations.

PHENOLPHTHALEIN—Ex-Lax®, Modane®

Laxative used in the management of constipation.

Preparations: Tablets, 60, 90, 100, 120, and 130 mg. Chewable tablets, 65, 90, 97.2, and 120 mg. Liquid, 60 mg/5 ml, 65 mg/15 ml.

PHENOLSULFONPHTHALEIN

Diagnostic agent used in evaluating renal function.

Preparation: Ampules, 6 mg/ml.

PHENOXYBENZAMINE HYDROCHLORIDE—Dibenzyline®

Alpha-adrenergic receptor blocking agent indicated in the management of pheochromocytoma to control episodes of hypertension and sweating.

Preparation: Capsules, 10 mg.

PHENSUXIMIDE—Milontin®

Anticonvulsant indicated for the control of absence (petit mal) seizures in conjunction with other anticonvulsants when other forms of epilepsy coexist with petit mal.

Preparation: Capsules, 500 mg.

PHENTERMINE—Adipex®, Fastin®, Ionamin®

Anorexiant indicated in the management of exogenous obesity as a short-term adjunct in a regimen of weight reduction based on caloric restriction.

Warnings: Contraindicated in atherosclerosis, cardiovascular disease, hypertension, hyperthyroidism, glaucoma, agitation, drug or alcohol abuse, duringor within 14 days of MAOI's. Discontinue if dyspnea, angina pectoris, syncope, lower extremity edema or other symptoms of primary pulmonary hypertension occur.Discontinue after a few weeks as tolerance to anorectic effect occurs. Use cautiously in diabetes. Prescribe limited supply to prevent overdose. Pregnancy Category C. Use in nursing mother not revommended. Adverse Reactions include CNS overstimulation, dizziness, palpitation, psychosis, dry mouth, GI disturbance, urticaria, impotence, primary pulmonary hypertension and/or regurgitant cardiac valvular disease.

Preparations: Capsules and tablets (as the hydrochloride), 8, 15, 30, and 37.5 mg. Capsules (as the resin complex), 15 and 30 mg.

PHENTOLAMINE MESYLATE—Regitine®

Alpha-adrenergic blocking agent indicated for parenteral use to prevent or control hypertensive episodes in patients with pheochromocytoma, for the prevention or treatment of dermal necrosis and sloughing following intravenous administration or extravasation of norepinephrine, and for the diagnosis of pheochromocytoma.

Preparation: Vials, 5 mg.

PHENURONE®, see Phenacemide

PHENYLEPHRINE HYDROCHLORIDE—Neo-Synephrine®

Used topically in the management of nasal congestion, and in ocular conditions in which decongestant and vasoconstrictor actions are needed. Included as a decongestant in combination with other agents in orally administered formulations. Also used parenterally in the treatment of vascular failure in shock, shocklike states, drug-induced hypotension or hypersensitivity. Is also utilized parenterally to overcome paroxysmal supraventricular tachycardia, to prolong spinal anesthesia, and as a vasoconstrictor in regional analgesia.

Preparations: Nasal drops and spray, 0.125%, 0.25%, 0.5%, and 1%. Nasal jelly, 0.5%. Ophthalmic solution, 0.12%, 2.5%, and 10%. Ampules, 1%. Injection, 10 mg/ml.

PHENYLPROPANOLAMINE HYDROCHLORIDE—Acutrim®, Dexatrim®

Decongestant and anorexiant.

Actions and Uses: A sympathomimetic agent indicated (1) for the temporary relief of nasal congestion due to the common cold and allergic disorders and (2) for exogenous obesity as a short-term adjunct in a regimen of weight reduction based on caloric restriction.

Warnings: Should not be used concurrently with a monoamine oxidase inhibitor. Use is best avoided in patients with advanced arteriosclerosis, symptomatic cardiovascular disease, moderate to severe hypertension, hyperthyroidism, orr diabetes. Adverse reactionsinclude restlessness, dizziness, insomnia, palpitations, tachycardia, and blood pressure elevation.

Administration: Oral.

Preparations: Capsules and tablets, 25, 37.5, and 50 mg. Controlled-release capsules and tablets, 75 mg.

PHENYLTOLOXAMINE CITRATE

Antihistamine used in combination with other agents in the management of allergic and related disorders.

PHENYTOIN—Dilantin®

Anticonvulsant.

Actions and Uses: Indicated for the control of tonic-clonic and psychomotor (grand mal and temporal lobe) seizures, and prevention and treatment of seizures occurring during or following neurosurgery. Also indicated for parenteral administration in the control of status epilepticus of the grand mal type. Has also been used intravenously in the management of certain arrhythmias (e.g., digitalis-induced arrhythmias), and orally in the treatment of trigeminal neuralgia.

Warnings: Adverse reactions include nystagmus, ataxia, slurred speech, confusion, nausea, vomiting, rash, gingival hyperplasia, hirsutism, and hematologic effects. Effect may be reduced by chronic alcohol abuse and products containing calcium ions (e.g., antacids).

Administration: Oral, intravenous, and intramuscular. Oral formulations containing phenytoin sodium, extended may be used for once-a-day dosing. When therapy is to be discontinued, it should be done so gradually as the abrupt withdrawal of therapy in epileptic patients may precipitate status epilepticus.

Preparations: Capsules (phenytoin sodium, extended), 30 and 100 mg. Chewable infatabs, 50 mg. Oral suspension, 30 and 125 mg/5 ml.

PHISOHEX®, see Hexachlorophene

PhosLo®, see Calcium acetate

PHOSPHALGEL®, see Aluminum phosphate gel

PHOSPHOLINE IODIDE®, see Echothiophate iodide

PHOTOPLEX®, see Butyl methoxydibenzoylmethane/padimate 0

PHYLLOCONTIN®, see Aminophylline

PHYSOSTIGMINE—Eserine, Antilirium®

Cholinesterase inhibitor indicated for ophthalmic use in the treatment of glaucoma, and for parenteral use to reverse the central nervous system effects caused by excessive dosages of anticholinergic drugs including the tricyclic antidepressants.

Preparations: Ophthalmic solution (as the salicylate), 0.25% and 0.5%. Ophthalmic ointment (as the sulfate), 0.25%. Ampules and syringes (as the salicylate), 1 mg/ml.

PHYTONADIONE—Vitamin K_1, AquaMEPHYTON®, Konakion®, Mephyton®

Vitamin K analog indicated for the management of anticoagulant-induced prothrombin deficiency, and for the management of hypoprothrombinemia se- condary to other conditions or drug therapies (e.g., salicylates, antibiotics). Is also used parenterally in the prophylaxis and therapy of hemorrhagic disease of the newborn.

Preparations: Tablets, 5 mg. Ampules and vials, 2 mg/ml and 10 mg/ml.

PILOCARPINE HYDROCHLORIDE—Salagen®

Miotic indicated for ophthalmic use in the treatment of glaucoma, and to counter the effect of cycloplegics and mydriatics. Also indicated for oral use for the treatment of symptoms of xerostomia from salivary gland hypofunction caused by radiotherapy for cancer of the head and neck.

Preparations: Ophthalmic solutions, 0.25%, 0.5%, 1%, 2%, 3%, 4%, 5%, 6%, 8%, and 10%. Ophthalmic gel, 4%. Ocular therapeutic systems, release 20 or 40 μg pilocarpine per hour for one week. Tablets (Salagen), 5 mg.

PIMOZIDE—Orap®

Neuroleptic agent indicated for the suppression of motor and phonic tics in patients with Tourette's disorder who have failed to respond satisfactorily to standard treatment.

Preparation: Tablets, 2 mg.

PINDOLOL—Visken®

Antihypertensive agent.

Actions and Uses: A nonselective beta-adrenergic blocking agent with intrinsic sympathomimetic activity that is indicated in the management of hypertension.

Warnings: Contraindicated in patients with bronchial asthma, overt cardiac failure, cardiogenic shock, second- and third-degree heart block, and severe bradycardia. Adverse reactions include dizziness, fatigue, insomnia, edema, nausea, and muscle and joint pain. Use is best avoided in patients with bronchospastic diseases and therapy in diabetic patients must be closely monitored.

Administration: Oral. Patients should be cautioned about the interruption or discontinuation of therapy and, when therapy is to be discontinued, the dosage should be gradually reduced over a period of 1 to 2 weeks.

Preparations: Tablets, 5 and 10 mg.

PIPECURONIUM BROMIDE—Arduan®

Nondepolarizing neuromuscular blocking agent.

Actions and Uses: Acts by competing for cholinergic receptors at the motor end-plate, resulting in a block of neuromuscular transmission. Indicated as an adjunct to general anesthesia to provide skeletal muscle relaxation during surgery. Can also be used to provide skeletal muscle relaxation for endotracheal intubation. Has a long duration of action and is only recommended for procedures anticipated to last 90 minutes or longer.

Warnings: May cause excessive skeletal muscle weakness resulting in respiratory insufficiency and apnea. Action may be antagonized by neostigmine. Must be used with caution in patients with myasthenia gravis or myasthenic syndrome, and in patients receiving other medications that may intensify or produce neuromuscular block on their own (e.g., inhalation anesthetics, aminoglycosides, quinidine, magnesium salts). Other adverse reactions include bradycardia, hypotension, and hypertension.

Administration: Intravenous.

Preparations: Vials, 10 mg.

PIPERACILLIN SODIUM—Pipracil®

Penicillin antibiotic.

Actions and Uses: Is bactericidal and is active against many gram-positive and gram-negative bacteria, including *Pseudomonas aeruginosa.* Is often used in conjunction with an aminoglycoside antibiotic in the treatment of *Pseudomonas* infections. Is also used for surgical prophylaxis.

Warnings: Contraindicated in patients with a history of allergic reactions to any of the penicillins. Adverse reactions include hypersensitivity reactions, GI disturbances, and local reactions at the injection site.

Administration: Intravenous and intramuscular.

Preparations: Vials and infusion bottles, 2, 3, 4, and 40 g.

PIPERACILLIN SODIUM/TAZOBACTAM SODIUM—Zosyn®

Antibiotic.

Actions and Uses: Is a combination of the penicillin antibiotic piperacillin with a beta-lactamase inhibitor tazobactam. By inhibiting beta-lactamase enzymes, tazobactam extends the spectrum of action of piperacillin to include certain bacteria that are not susceptible to piperacillin alone. Indicated for the treatment of the following infections caused by piperacillin-resistant, beta-lactamase-producing strains of the bacteria designated: community-acquired pneumonia caused by *Haemophilus influenzae*; appendicitis (complicated by rupture or abscess) and peritonitis caused by *E. coli* , *Bacteroides fragilis, B. ovatus, B. thetaiomicron,* or *B. vulgatus*; postpartum endometritis or pelvic inflammatory disease caused by *E. coli*; and uncomplicated and complicated skin and skin-structure infections, including cellulitis, cutaneous abscesses, and ischemic/diabetic foot infections caused by *Staphylococcus aureus.*

Warnings: Contraindicated in patients with a history of allergic reaction to any of the penicillins, cephalosporins, or beta-lactamase inhibitors. Adverse reactions include diarrhea, constipation, nausea, dyspepsia, headache, insomnia, rash, and pruritus. Should not be administered in the same solution with an aminoglycoside antibiotic.

Administration: Intravenous. Administered as an IV infusion over a period of 30 minutes.

Preparations: Vials, 2.25, 3.375, and 4.5 grams which provide 2, 3, and 4 grams of piperacillin and 0.25, 0.375 and 0.5 grams of tazobactam, respectively.

PIPERAZINE CITRATE—Antepar®

Anthelmintic indicated in the treatment of pinworm and roundworm infections.

Preparations: Tablets, equivalent to 250 mg of piperazine hexahydrate. Syrup, equivalent to 500 mg piperazine hexahydrate/5 ml.

PIPERAZINE ESTRONE SULFATE, see Estropipate

PIPOBROMAN—Vercyte®

Antineoplastic agent indicated in the treatment of polycythemia vera and the treatment of chronic granulocytic leukemia in patients refractory to busulfan.

Preparation: Tablets, 25 mg.

PIPRACIL®, see Piperacillin

PIRBUTEROL ACETATE—Maxair®

Bronchodilator.

Actions and Uses: Stimulates beta 2-adrenergic receptors and is indicated for the prevention and reversal of bronchospasm in patients with reversible bronchospasm including asthma.

Warnings: Adverse reactions include nervousness, tremor, headache, dizziness, palpitations, tachycardia, cough, and nausea. Should be used with caution in patients with cardiovascular disorders, hyperthyroidism, diabetes mellitus, or convulsive disorders. Other beta-adrenergic aerosol bronchodilators should not be used concomitantly. It should be administered with caution to patients being treated with a tricyclic antidepressant or monoamine oxidase inhibitor.

Administration: Oral inhalation.

Preparation: Metered-dose inhaler. Each actuation delivers the equivalent of 0.2 mg pirbuterol.

PIROXICAM—Feldene®

Nonsteroidal anti-inflammatory drug.

Actions and Uses: Inhibits prostaglandin synthesis and is indicated in the treatment of rheumatoid arthritis and osteoarthritis.

Warnings: Should not be given to patients in whom aspirin or another NSAID causes asthma, rhinitis, urticaria, or other allergic-type reactions. May cause GI effects and use should be avoided in patients with active GI tract disease, and closely monitored in patients with a previous history of such disorders. Other adverse reactions include rash, edema, and decreases in hemoglobin and hematocrit. Has a long duration of action and may accumulate with continued use; particular caution should be exercised in elderly patients.

Administration: Oral.

Preparations: Capsules, 10 and 20 mg.

PITOCIN®, see Oxytocin

PITRESSIN®, see Vasopressin

PITUITARY, POSTERIOR

Hormones of the posterior pituitary administered parenterally to control postoperative ileus, to stimulate expulsion of gas prior to pyelography, as an aid to achieve hemostasis in surgery, and for treating enuresis of diabetes insipidus. Has also been used by nasal inhalation for the control of diabetes insipidus.

Preparations: Ampules, 20 units/ml. Capsules to be used for intranasal inhalation, 40 mg.

PLACIDYL®, see Ethchlorvynol

PLAQUENIL®, see Hydroxychloroquine

PLASBUMIN®, see Albumin

PLATINOL®, see Cisplatin

PLENDIL®, see Felodipine

PLICAMYCIN—Mithramycin, Mithracin®

Antineoplastic agent indicated for intravenous use in the treatment of testicular carcinoma. Also used in the treatment of symptomatic patients with hypercalcemia and hypercalciuria associated with a variety of advanced neoplasms.

Preparation: Vials, 2500 μg.

PODOFILOX—Condylox®

Antimitotic agent. An active component of podophyllum resin that is indicated for the topical treatment of external genital warts.

Preparation: Solution, 0.5%.

PODOPHYLLIN, see Podophyllum resin

PODOPHYLLUM RESIN—Podophyllin

Resin applied topically for the removal of benign epithelial growths such as common warts, and also in certain other dermatologic disorders.

Preparation: Liquid, 25%, often in tincture of benzoin.

POLARAMINE®, see Dexchlorpheniramine

POLYCARBOPHIL—Equalactin®, FiberCon®, Mitrolan®

Hydrophilic agent used in the treatment of constipation or diarrhea by regulating intestinal water and promoting well-formed stools.

Preparation: Chewable tablets, 500 mg.

POLYCILLIN®, see Ampicillin

POLYCITRA®, see Potassium citrate

POLYETHYLENE GLYCOLS—PEG, Carbowax®

Ointment and suppository bases used as vehicles for active medications.

POLYETHYLENE GLYCOL 3350—Colyte®, GoLYTELY®

Osmotic agent used with electrolytes for bowel cleansing prior to colonoscopy and barium enema x-ray examination.

Preparation: Powder for oral solution.

POLYMYXIN B SULFATE—Aerosporin®

Antibiotic used in the treatment of infections caused by gram-negative bacteria. Administered parenterally in the treatment of infections caused by bacteria such as *Pseudomonas aeruginosa* when less toxic drugs are ineffective or contraindicated. Also indicated for ophthalmic use. Is most frequently employed in combination with other antibiotics (e.g., neomycin) in the topical management of dermatologic, otic, and ophthalmic infections, and also as a genitourinary irrigant.

Preparations: Vials, 500,000 units. Powder for ophthalmic solution, 500,000 units.

POLYMIXIN E®, see Colistin sulfate

POLYTHIAZIDE—Renese®

Thiazide diuretic indicated as adjunctive therapy in edema and in the management of hypertension.

Preparations: Tablets, 1, 2, and 4 mg.

PONSTEL®, see Mefenamic Acid

PONTOCAINE®, see Tetracaine

POSTERIOR PITUITARY, see Pituitary, posterior

POSTURE®, see Calcium phosphate, tribasic

POTABA®, see Para-aminobenzoic acid

POTASSIUM ACETATE

For intravenous potassium replacement.

Preparations: Vials, 40 mEq, 120 mEq.

POTASSIUM CHLORIDE, ORAL (see list of preparations below for trade names)

Potassium supplement.

Actions and Uses: Indicated in patients with hypokalemia, in digitalis intoxication, in patients with hypokalemic familial periodic paralysis, and for the prevention of potassium depletion when the dietary intake of potassium is inadequate.

Warnings: Is contraindicated in patients with hyperkalemia; should not be used concomitantly with a potassium-sparing diuretic because of the increased risk of hyperkalemia. Solid dosage forms (e.g., tablets) have caused lesions of the small intestine and serious GI complications; these formulations should be reserved for those patients who cannot tolerate or refuse to take liquid or effervescent potassium preparations, or for patients in whom there is a problem of compliance with these preparations. Other adverse reactions include nausea and vomiting.

Administration: Oral.

Preparations: Liquid (e.g., Kay Ciel®, Klorvess®, 20 and 40 mEq/ml. Powder (e.g., Kay Ciel®, K-Lor®), 15, 20, and 25 mEq/packet. Controlled-release tablets and capsules (e.g., Slow-K®, Klotrix®, K-Tab®, Micro-K®), 8 and 10 mEq.

POTASSIUM CHLORIDE, INTRAVENOUS

Preparations: Ampules and vials, 10, 20, 30, 40, 60, and 90 mEq.

POTASSIUM CITRATE—Polycitra®, Urocit-K®

Alkalinizing agent and potassium replacement agent. Has been used to alkalinize the urine to reduce the risk of calculi in the urinary tract, as an adjunct to uricosuric agents in gout therapy, and to correct the acidosis of certain renal tubular disorders.

Preparation: Tablets, 540 mg. Syrup, 550 mg/5 ml with sodium citrate and citric acid.

POTASSIUM GLUCONATE—Kaon®

Potassium replacement agent.

Preparations: Tablets, 5 mEq. Liquid, 20 mEq/15 ml.

POTASSIUM IODIDE

Expectorant and is also used as adjunctive therapy in other respiratory conditions. Has also been used for thyroid blocking in radiation emergencies, in the treatment of thyrotoxic crisis, and as an adjunct with other antithyroid drugs in preparation for thyroidectomy.

Preparations: Enteric-coated tablets, 300 mg. Solution, 500 mg/15 ml. Saturated solution of potassium iodide (SSKI), 1 g/ml.

POTASSIUM PHOSPHATE—Neutra-Phos-K®

Phosphorus-replacement products.

Preparations: Capsules and powder concentrate are both utilized to prepare liquid for oral administration. Vials, 3 mM phosphate/ml for intravenous administration.

POVIDONE-IODINE—Betadine®

Anti-infective agent utilized for topical, vaginal, and perineal application.

Preparations: Numerous formulations including topical solution and ointment.

PRALIDOXIME CHLORIDE—Protopam®

Cholinesterase reactivator indicated as an antidote in the treatment of poisoning due to pesticides and chemicals of the organophosphate class that have anticholinesterase activity, and in the control of overdosage by anticholinesterase drugs used in the treatment of myasthenia gravis. Atropine should be administered after ventilation is established.

Preparation: Vials, 1 g.

PRAMOXINE HYDROCHLORIDE—Tronolane®, Tronothane®

Local anesthetic indicated for topical use for the temporary relief of pain and itching associated with dermatologic conditions, as well as hemorrhoids and other anorectal disorders.

Preparations: Cream, 1%. Suppositories, 1%.

PRAVACHOL®, see Pravastatin

PRAVASTATIN SODIUM—Pravachol®

Agent for hypercholesterolemia.

Actions and Uses: Reduces cholesterol biosynthesis in the liver by acting as a competitive inhibitor of 3-hydroxy-3-methylglutaryl-coenzyme A (HMG-CoA) reductase. Produces a significant reduction in total and low-density lipoprotein (LDL) cholesterol concentrations, a modest reduction in triglyceride concentrations, and an increase in high-density lipoprotein (HDL) cholesterol concentrations. Indicated as an adjunct to diet for the reduction of elevated total and LDL cholesterol concentrations in patients with primary hypercholesterolemia (type IIa and IIb) when the response to a diet restricted in saturated fat and cholesterol has not been adequate. Also indicated to reduce the risk of MI, reduce the risk of undergoing myocardial revascularization procedures and reduce the risk of cardiavascular mortality with no increase in death from non-cardiovascular causes in hypercholesterol emia without clinically evident coronary heart disease.

Warnings: Contraindicated in patients with active liver disease or unexplained persistent elevations in liver function tests. Is also contraindicated in pregnant women and nursing mothers. Increases in serum transaminases may occur and it is recommended that liver function tests be monitored before treatment begins, every 6 weeks for the first 3 months, every 8 weeks during the remainder of the first year, and periodically thereafter (at about 6-month intervals). Adverse reactions include headache, rash, influenza, myalgia, myopathy, and, rarely, rhabdo- myolysis. Patients should be advised to promptly report unexplained muscle pain, tenderness, or weakness. Because of the possibility of an increased risk of skeletal muscle reactions, the concurrent use of clofibrate, cyclosporine, erythromycin, gemfibrozil, or niacin (in lipid-lowering doses) is best avoided. When either cholestyramine or colestipol is used concomitantly, pravastatin should be administered at least one hour before or at least 4 hours after the administration of the other agent.

Administration: Oral. Should be administered at bedtime.

Preparations: Tablets, 10, 20, and 40 mg.

PRAZEPAM—Centrax®

Benzodiazepine antianxiety agent.

Actions and Uses: A CNS depressant indicated for the management of anxiety disorders or for the short-term relief

of the symptoms of anxiety.

Warnings: Contraindicated in patients

with acute narrow-angle glaucoma. Adverse reactions include drowsiness and other CNS effects; patients should be cautioned regarding activities such as driving or operating machinery, as well as interactions with other CNS-acting drugs including alcohol. Can cause dependence and is included in Schedule IV.

Administration: Oral.

Preparations: Capsules, 5, 10, and 20 mg. Tablets, 10 mg.

PRAZIQUANTEL—Biltricide®

Antiparasitic agent indicated for the treatment of schistosomiasis and other trematode infections by Chinese liver fluke.

Preparation: Tablets, 600 mg.

PRAZOSIN HYDROCHLORIDE—Minipress®

Antihypertensive agent.

Actions and Uses: Indicated in the treatment of hypertension. Investigational studies have suggested it to be useful in refractory congestive heart failure and in the management of Raynaud's vasospasm.

Warnings: May cause syncope with sudden loss of consciousness, usually attributable to an excessive postural hypotensive effect; risk may be reduced by limiting the initial dose of the drug to 1 mg, and by subsequently increasing the dosage slowly. Adverse reactions include dizziness, drowsiness, and other CNS effects; patients should be cautioned regarding activities such as driving and operating machinery, as well as interactions with other CNS-acting drugs including alcohol. Other adverse reactions include palpitations and nausea. The concurrent use of a beta-adrenergic blocking agent may increase the risk of hypotension.

Administration: Oral.

Preparations: Capsules and tablets, 1, 2, and 5 mg.

PRECOSE®, see Acarbose

PREDNICARBATE—Dermatop®

Corticosteroid applied topically for the relief of the manifestations of corticosteroid-responsive dermatoses.

Preparations: Cream, 0.1%.

PREDNISOLONE—Delta-Cortef®

Corticosteroid indicated in a wide range of endocrine, rheumatic, allergic, dermatologic, respiratory, hematologic, neoplastic, and other disorders.

Preparations: Tablets, 5 mg. Syrup, 15 mg/5 ml. Oral solution, 5 mg/ml.

PREDNISOLONE ACETATE

Preparations: Vials (for IM, intralesional, intra-articular, or soft tissue injection), 25 mg/ml, 50 mg/ml, and 100 mg/ml. Ophthalmic suspension, 0.12%, 0.125%, 1%.

PREDNISOLONE SODIUM PHOSPHATE—Hydeltrasol®

Preparations: Oral liquid, 5 mg/5 ml. Vials (for IV, IM, intralesional, intra-articular, or soft tissue injection), 20 mg/ml. Ophthalmic solution, 0.125%, 0.5%, and 1%.

PREDNISOLONE TEBUTATE—Hydeltra-TBA®

Preparations: Vials (for intralesional, intra-articular, or soft tissue injection) 20 mg/ml.

PREDNISONE—Deltasone®, Meti- corten®

Corticosteroid.

Actions and Uses: Indicated in a wide range of endocrine, rheumatic, allergic, dermatologic, respiratory, hematologic, neoplastic, and other disorders.

Warnings: Contraindicated in patients with systemic fungal infections. Adverse reactions include sodium and fluid retention, potassium depletion, muscle weakness, osteoporosis, peptic ulcer, thin fragile skin, development of cushingoid state, glaucoma, cataracts, and negative nitrogen balance. May mask signs of infection and new infections may appear during use. May increase requirements for hypoglycemic agents in diabetic patients.

Administration: Oral.

Preparations: Tablets, 1, 2.5, 5, 10, 20, and 50 mg. Oral solution, 5 mg/5 ml. Oral solution (concentrate), 5 mg/ml. Syrup, 5 mg/5 ml.

PREMARIN®, see Estrogens, conjugated.

PREMPHASE®, Combination of conjugated estrogens and medroxyprogesterone acetate

PREMPRO®, Combination of conjugated estrogens and medroxyprogesterone acetate

PREPIDIL®, see Dinoprostone

PREVACID® see Lansoprazole

PREUPAC®—Combination agent lansaprazole, amoxicillin, and claritheomycin (and pump inhibitor and antibiotics)

PRILOCAINE HYDROCHLORIDE—Citanest®

Local anesthetic administered by injection for infiltration, peripheral nerve block, central neural block, and in dental procedures.

Preparations: Ampules and vials, 1%, 2%, and 3%. Dental cartridges, 4%.

PRILOSEC®, see Omeprazole

PRIMACOR®, see Milrinone lactate

PRIMAQUINE PHOSPHATE

Antimalarial agent used to prevent relapses of infections caused by *Plasmodium vivax* and *P. ovale,* and to prevent attack after departure from areas where *P. vivax* and *P. ovale* are endemic (often administered during the last 2 weeks of chloroquine prophylaxis).

Preparation: Tablets, 26.3 mg.

PRIMATENE MIST®, see Epinephrine

PRIMAXIN IV®, see Imipenem-cilastatin sodium

PRIMAXIN IM®, see Imipenem-cilastatin sodium

PRIMIDONE—Mysoline®

Anticonvulsant indicated in the control of grand mal, psychomotor, and focal epileptic seizures.

Preparations: Tablets, 50, 125, and 250 mg. Suspension, 250 mg/5 ml.

PRINCIPEN®, see Ampicillin

PRINIVIL®, see Lisinopril

PRINZIDE®, Combination of lisinopril and hydrochlorothiazide

PRISCOLINE®, see Tolazoline

PRIVINE®, see Naphazoline

PROAMATINE®, see Midodrine Hydrochloride

PRO-BANTHINE®, see Propantheline

PROBENECID—Benemid®

Uricosuric agent indicated for the treatment of hyperuricemia associated with gout and gouty arthritis and to treat the hyperuricemia secondary to thiazide therapy. Has also been used to increase the plasma levels and activity of the penicillin derivatives.

Preparation: Tablets, 500 mg.

PROCANBID®, see Procainamide HCl

PROCAINAMIDE HYDROCHLORIDE—Procanbid®, Pronestyl®, Pronestyl-SR®, Procan SR®

Antiarrhythmic agent.

Actions and Uses: Indicated in the treatment of premature ventricular contractions and ventricular tachycardia, atrial fibrillation, and paroxysmal atrial tachycardia; also useful in preventing recurrence of certain arrhythmias after conversion to sinus rhythm by other drugs or procedures.

Warnings: Contraindicated in patients with complete heart block or lupus erythematosus, and in patients sensitive to procaine or other ester-type local anesthetics. May cause worsening of symptoms in patients with myasthenia gravis. Adverse reactions include proarrhythmic effects, hypotension (particularly after parenteral administration), nausea, vomiting, diarrhea, dizziness, weakness, pruritus, flushing, lupus erythematosus-like syndrome, and positive antinuclear antibody (ANA) test.

Administration: Oral, intravenous, and intramuscular.

Preparations: Capsules and tablets, 250, 375, and 500 mg. Sustained-release tablets, 250, 500, 750, and 1000 mg. Vials, 100 and 500 mg/ml.

PROCAINE HYDROCHLORIDE—Novocain®

Local anesthetic administered by injection for infiltration anesthesia, peripheral nerve block, spinal anesthesia, and for rectal anesthesia in proctology.

Preparations: Ampules and vials, 1% and 2%. Ampules (for spinal anesthesia), 10%.

PROCAINE PENICILLIN G—Crysticillin®, Wycillin®

Penicillin antibiotic administered intramuscularly and having an extended duration of action. Used in the treatment of streptococcal, gonococcal, and selected other infections.

Preparations: Vials and syringes, 300,000, 500,000, 600,000, 1,200,000, and 2,400,000 units.

PROCAN SR®, see Procainamide

PROCARBAZINE HYDROCHLORIDE—Matulane®

Antineoplastic agent having monoamine oxidase inhibitory activity. Indicated for use in combination with other antineoplastic drugs for the treatment of Stage III and IV Hodgkin's disease.

Preparation: Capsules, 50 mg.

PROCARDIA®, see Nifedipine

PROCARDIA XL®, see Nifedipine

PROCHLORPERAZINE—Compazine®

Phenothiazine antipsychotic agent and antiemetic.

Actions and Uses: Indicated for the control of severe nausea and vomiting, and for the management of manifestations of psychotic disorders.

Warnings: Adverse reactions include drowsiness and other CNS effects; patients should be cautioned regarding activities such as driving and operating machinery, as well as interactions withother CNS-acting drugs including alcohol. Other adverse reactions include extrapyramidal reactions, tardive dyskinesia, blurred vision, skin reactions, and hypotension. May lower the convulsive threshold necessitating dosage adjustments of anticonvulsants. May interfere with thermoregulatory mechanisms and must be used cautiously in persons who will be exposed to extreme heat; the risk of complications is increased in patients who are also taking other medications having anticholinergic activity.

Administration: Oral, rectal, intravenous, and intramuscular.

Preparations: Tablets (as the maleate), 5, 10, and 25 mg. Sustained-release capsules (as the maleate), 10, 15, and 30 mg. Syrup (as the edisylate), 5 mg/5 ml. Suppositories, 2.5, 5, and 25 mg. Ampules, vials, and syringes (as the edisylate), 5 mg/ml.

PROCRIT®, see Epoetin alfa

PROCYCLIDINE HYDROCHLORIDE—Kemadrin®

Antiparkinson agent indicated in the treatment of parkinsonism and drug-induced extrapyramidal effects.

Preparation: Tablets, 5 mg.

PRODOFILOX—Condylox®

Actions and Uses: Antimitotic indicated in the treatment of external genital warts. Not for use on mucous membrane or perianal warts. Local reactions (e.g., burning, inflammation, erosion , pain, itching, bleeding) and headache may occur.

Administration: Apply twice daily every 12 hours for 3 days then discontinue for 4 days. May repeat if needed for a maximum of 4 treatment cycles. Use applicator with solution.

Preparations: 0.5% topical solution and gel.

PROFENAL®, see Suprofen

PROGESTASERT®, see Progesterone

PROGESTERONE—Progestasert®

Progestin used intramuscularly in the management of conditions such as amenorrhea and functional uterine bleeding. Intrauterine system has been used for contraception.

Preparations: Vials (aqueous solution and in oil), 25 mg/ml, 50 mg/ml, and 100 mg/ml. Intrauterine system, 38 mg, provides contraceptive effectiveness for a period of one year.

PROGLYCEM®, see Diazoxide

PROGRAF®, see Tacrolimus

PROKINE®, see Sargramostim

PROLASTIN®, see Alpha$_1$-proteinase inhibitor (human)

PROLEUKIN®, see Aldesleukin

PROLIXIN®, see Fluphenazine

PROLOPRIM®, see Trimethoprim

PROMAZINE HYDROCHLORIDE—Sparine®

Phenothiazine antipsychotic agent indicated in the management of the manifestations of psychotic disorders.

Preparations: Tablets, 25, 50, and 100 mg. Vials and syringes, 25 mg/ml and 50 mg/ml.

PROMETHAZINE HYDROCHLORIDE—Phenergan®

Phenothiazine antihistamine indicated for allergic disorders, motion sickness, preoperative, postoperative, or obstetric sedation, postoperative pain as an adjunct to analgesics, and the prevention and control of nausea and vomiting associated with certain types of surgery.

Preparations: Tablets and suppositories, 10, 12.5, 25, and 50 mg. Syrup, 6.25 and 25 mg/5 ml. Ampules and vials, 25 and 50 mg/ml.

PRONESTYL®, see Procainamide

PROPAFENONE HYDROCHLO-RIDE—Rythmol®

Antiarrhythmic agent.

Actions and Uses: A Class IC antiarrhythmic agent that also has local anesthetic activity, beta-adrenergic blocking activity, and a weak calcium channel blocking effect. Indicated for the treatment of documented life-threatening arrhythmias or prolonged recurrence of paroxysmal atrial fibrillation/flutex or paroxysmal supraventricular tachycardia (PSVT) associated with disabling stmptoms, in patients without structural heart disease.

Warnings: Contraindicated in the presence of uncontrolled congestive heart failure, cardiogenic shock, sinoatrial, atrioventricular, and intraventricular disorders of impulse generation and/or conduction in the absence of an artificial pacemaker, bradycardia, marked hypotension, bronchospastic disorders, and electrolyte imbalance. Adverse reactions include proarrhythmic effects, congestive heart failure, conduction abnormalities, nausea and/or vomiting, unusual (e.g., metallic) taste, constipation, dizziness, fatigue and dyspnea.

Administration: Oral. If a patient misses a dose, the next dose should not be doubled because of an increased risk of adverse reactions. To help achieve a constant clinical response, the drug should be administered on a consistent basis either with food or apart from food.

Preparations: Tablets, 150, 225, and 300 mg.

PROPANTHELINE BROMIDE—Pro-Banthine®

Anticholinergic agent indicated as adjunctive therapy in the treatment of peptic ulcer.

Preparations: Tablets, 7.5 and 15 mg.

PROPARACAINE HYDROCHLO-RIDE—Ophthaine®

Local anesthetic indicated for ophthalmic use.

Preparation: Ophthalmic solution 0.5%

PROPINE®, see Dipivefrin

PROPIOMAZINE HYDROCHLO-RIDE—Largon®

Phenothiazine indicated for parenteral use for relief of restlessness and apprehension, preoperatively or during surgery or during labor.

Preparations: Ampules and syringes, 20 mg/ml.

PROPOFOL—Diprivan®

Anesthetic.

Actions and Uses: Has a rapid onset of action and the recovery from anesthesia is usually prompt. Indicated as an intravenous anesthetic agent that can be used for both induction and/or maintenance of anesthesia as part of a balanced anesthetic technique for inpatient and outpatient surgery. Also indicated for continuous sedation and control of stress responses in intubated or respiratory-controlled adult patients in intensive care units.

Warnings: Adverse reactions include excitatory reactions (e.g., spontaneous movement, twitching, tremor, myoclonus), hypotension, bradycardia, apnea, nausea, vomiting, and reactions at the injection site. Other CNS depressants can increase the depression induced by propofol and may also result in more pronounced decreases in blood pressure.

Administration: Intravenous

Preparations: Vials, 10 mg/ml. Is a white, oil-in-water emulsion that is isotonic.

PROPOXYPHENE HYDROCHLORIDE—Darvon®

PROPOXYPHENE NAPSYLATE—Darvon-N®

Analgesic.

Actions and Uses: Indicated for the relief of mild to moderate pain.

Warnings: Adverse reactions include sedation and other CNS effects; patients should be cautioned regarding activities such as driving and operating machinery, as well as interactions with other CNS-acting drugs including alcohol. Can cause dependence and is included in Schedule IV.

Administration: Oral.

Preparations: Capsules, 65 mg. Tablets (Darvon-N), 50 and 100 mg.

PROPRANOLOL HYDROCHLORIDE—Inderal®, Inderal LA®

Antihypertensive, antianginal and antiarrhythmic agent.

Actions and Uses: A nonselective beta-adrenergic blocking agent indicated in the treatment of hypertension, angina pectoris, and cardiac arrhythmias (i.e., supraventricular arrhythmias, ventricular tachycardias, tachyarrhythmias of digitalis intoxication, and resistant tachyarrhythmias due to excessive catecholamine action during anesthesia). Also indicated to reduce cardiovascular mortality in patients who have survived the acute phase of myocardial infarction, in the management of hypertrophic subaortic stenosis, in pheochromocytoma, and for the prophylaxis of common migraine headache.

Warnings: Contraindicated in patients with cardiogenic shock, sinus bradycardia and greater than first-degree block, bronchial asthma, and congestive heart failure. Adverse reactions include weakness, lightheadedness, depression, bra-dycardia, paresthesia of hands, arterial insufficiency (e.g., Raynaud type), nausea, and diarrhea. Use is best avoided in patients with bronchospastic diseases and therapy in diabetic patients must be closely monitored.

Administration: Oral and intravenous. Patients should be cautioned about the interruption or discontinuation of therapy; exacerbation of angina pectoris has occurred following the abrupt cessation of therapy and, when therapy is to be discontinued, the dosage should be gradually reduced over a period of several weeks.

Preparations: Tablets, 10, 20, 40, 60, and 90 mg. Long-acting capsules (Inderal LA), 60, 80, 120, and 160 mg. Oral solution, 4, 8, and 80 mg/ml. Ampules, 1 mg/ml.

PROPULSID®, see Cisapride

PROPYLENE GLYCOL

Solvent used as part of the vehicle in certain pharmaceutical formulations.

PROPYLHEXEDRINE—Benzedrex®

Nasal decongestant administered by inhalation.

Preparation: Inhaler, 250 mg.

PROPYLTHIOURACIL

Antithyroid agent used in the treatment of hyperthyroidism.

Preparation: Tablets, 50 mg.

PROSCAR®, see Finasteride

ProSom®, see Estazolam

PROSTACYCLIN®, see Epoprostenol

PROSTAGLANDIN E2, see Dinoprostone

PROSTAGLANDIN F2 ALPHA, see Dinoprost tromethamine

PROSTAGLANDIN 12® (PG 12), see Epoprostenol

PROSTAGLANDIN X® (PGX), see Epoprostenol

PROSTAPHLIN®, see Oxacillin sodium

ProStep®, see Nicotine

PROSTIGMIN®, see Neostigmine

PROSTIN E2, see Dinoprostone

PROSTIN F2 ALPHA, see Dinoprost tromethamine

PROSTIN VR PEDIATRIC®, see Alprostadil

PROSTIN 15M®, former name for Carboprost tromethamine

PROTAMINE SULFATE

Heparin antagonist indicated for intravenous use in the treatment of heparin overdosage and to neutralize heparin received during dialysis, cardiopulmonary bypass, and other procedures.

Preparations: Ampules, 10 mg/ml.

PROTAMINE ZINC INSULIN, see Insulin

PROTIRELIN—Relefact TRH®, Thypinone®

Thyrotropin-releasing hormone used intravenously as an adjunctive agent in the diagnostic assessment of thyroid function.

Preparation: Ampules, 0.5 mg.

PROTOPAM®, see Pralidoxime

PROTRIPTYLINE HYDROCHLORIDE—Vivactil®

Tricyclic antidepressant indicated in the treatment of symptoms of depression.

Preparations: Tablets, 5 and 10 mg.

PROTROPIN®, see Somatrem

PROVENTIL®—Proventil HFA®, see Albuterol

PROVERA®, see Medroxyprogesterone

PROZAC®, see Fluoxetine

PSEUDOEPHEDRINE HYDROCHLORIDE—Efidac/24®, Novafed®, Sudafed®

PSEUDOEPHEDRINE SULFATE—Afrinol®

Decongestant.

Actions and Uses: A sympathomimetic agent indicated for the temporary relief of nasal congestion due to the common cold and allergic disorders.

Warnings: Should not be used concurrently with a monoamine oxidase inhibitor. Use is best avoided in patients with advanced arteriosclerosis, symptomatic cardiovascular disease, moderate to severe hypertension, hyperthyroidism, or diabetes. Adverse reactions include restlessness, dizziness, insomnia, palpitations, tachycardia, and blood pressure elevation.

Administration: Oral.

Preparations: Tablets, 30 and 60 mg. Controlled-release capsules and tablets, 120 and 240 mg. Liquid, 15 and 30 mg/5 ml. Drops, 7.5 mg/0.8 ml.

PSYLLIUM—Metamucil®

Bulk laxative used in the treatment and prevention of constipation. Used in the management of chronic watery diarrhea. Contraindicated with abdominal pain, nausea, or vomiting (especially when associated with fever), serious adhesions, and dysphagia. Diabetics and cardiacs should read product labels to see which manufacturers include sugar, aspartame, and sodium in their formulations.

Preparations: Powder, effervescent powder, granules, chewable dosage form.

PULMOZYME®, see Dornase alfa

PURINETHOL®, see Mercaptopurine

PYRANTEL PAMOATE—Antiminth®

Anthelmintic indicated for the treatment of pinworm and roundworm infections.

Preparation: Oral suspension, 50 mg/ml.

PYRAZINAMIDE

Antitubercular agent used in combination with other antitubercular agents in patients in whom therapy with the primary agents has not been satisfactory.

Preparation: Tablets, 500 mg.

PYRETHRINS—A-200 Pyrinate®, RID®

Pediculicide indicated for topical use in the treatment of head lice, body lice, and pubic (crab) lice infestations.

Preparations: Liquid, gel, and shampoo, 0.17%, 0.3%, 0.33%.

PYRIDIUM®, see Phenazopyridine

PYRIDOSTIGMINE BROMIDE—Mestinon®

Cholinesterase inhibitor used in the treatment of myasthenia gravis. Also used parenterally as a reversal agent or antagonist to nondepolarizing muscle relaxants such as the curariform drugs.

Preparations: Tablets, 60 mg. Controlled-release tablets, 180 mg. Syrup, 60 mg/5 ml. Ampules, 5 mg/ml.

PYRIDOXINE—Vitamin B_6

Vitamin indicated for the treatment and prevention of pyridoxine deficiency resulting from inadequate diet, or use of drugs (e.g., isoniazid) that deplete pyridoxine. May also be useful in certain seizure disorders and anemias which are related to pyridoxine deficiency.

Preparations: Tablets, 10, 25, 50, 100, 200, 250, and 500 mg. Extended-release tablets, 100, 200, and 500 mg. Vials, 100 mg/ml.

PYRILAMINE MALEATE

Antihistamine: used in the management of allergic and related disorders, and also as an aid in the relief of insomnia.

Preparations: Tablets and capsules, 25 mg.

PYRIMETHAMINE—Daraprim®

Antimalarial agent indicated for the prophylaxis of malaria and in treating infections caused by chloroquine-resistant plasmodia. Also used as an adjunct to sulfonamide in the treatment of toxoplasmosis.

Preparation: Tablets, 25 mg.

Q

QUAZEPAM—Doral®

Benzodiazepine hypnotic.

Actions and Uses: Indicated for the treatment of insomnia characterized by difficulty in falling asleep, frequent nocturnal awakenings, and/or early morning awakenings. Due to accumulation, may give larger doses for 1–2 nights, then decrease.

Warnings: Contraindicated in pregnancy. Adverse reactions include daytime sedation, headache, fatigue, dizziness, dry mouth, and dyspepsia. Patients should be cautioned regarding activities such as driving and operating machinery, as well as interactions with other CNS-acting drugs including alcohol. Can cause dependence and is included in Schedule IV.

Administration: Oral.

Preparations: Tablets, 7.5 and 15 mg.

QUELICIN®, see Succinylcholine

QUESTRAN®, see Cholestyramine

QUESTRAN LIGHT®, see Cholestyramine

QUINACRINE HYDROCHLORIDE

Antimalarial agent that has been used in the prevention and treatment of malaria. Acts as suppressive agent and controls clinical attacks of malaria, but is not a true prophylactic agent and does not produce a radical cure. Use as an antimalarial has been largely superseded by more effective and less toxic drugs. Also used in the treatment of giardiasis and tapeworm infections. Has been utilized via intrapleural administration in patients who experience recurrent pneumothorax.

Preparation: Tablets, 100 mg.

QUINAGLUTE®, see Quinidine gluconate

QUINAMM®, see Quinine sulfate

QUINAPRIL HYDROCHLORIDE—Accupril®

Antihypertensive agent.

Actions and Uses: An angiotensin-converting enzyme (ACE) inhibitor that is a prodrug. Following oral administration, is converted to its active metabolite, quinaprilat. Indicated for the treatment of hypertension and may be used alone or in combination with a thiazide diuretic. Also indicated as adjunctive therapy in the management of congestive heart failure when added to conventional therapy including a diuretic or digitalis.

Warnings: Contraindicated in patients who are hypersensitive to the drug and in patients with a history of angioedema related to previous treatment with an ACE inhibitor. Adverse reactions include headache, dizziness, fatigue, cough, nausea and abdominal pain. May cause an elevation in serum potassium levels; the risk of hyperkalemia is increased in patients also taking a potassium-sparing diuretic, a potassium supplement, and/or a potassium-containing salt substitute. May cause symptomatic postural hypotension. There have been infrequent reports of angioedema of the face, extremities, lips, tongue, glottis, and larynx, especially following the first dose. Patients should be told to report immediately any symptoms suggesting angioedema and to stop taking the drug. When used during the second and third trimesters of pregnancy, ACE inhibitors have been reported to be associated with the development of neonatal hypertension, renal failure, and skull hypoplasia; use during pregnancy should be avoided. May increase serum lithium levels and concurrenttherapy should be closely monitored. Absorption is reduced when administered with a high-fat meal, and the drug is best administered apart from meals.

Administration: Oral.

Preparations: Tablets, 5, 10, 20, and 40 mg.

QUINESTROL—Estrovis®

Estrogen indicated in the treatment of moderate to severe vasomotor symptoms associated with the menopause, atrophic vaginitis, kraurosis vulvae, female hypogonadism, female castration, and primary ovarian failure.

Preparation: Tablets, 100μg.

QUINETHAZONE—Hydromox®

Diuretic indicated as adjunctive therapy in edema and in the management of hypertension.

Preparation: Tablets, 50 mg.

QUINIDINE GLUCONATE—Quinaglute®

Antiarrhythmic agent indicated in the prevention and treatment of a number of ventricular, atrial, and junctional (nodal) arrhythmias, and in the parenteral treatment of life-threatening *Plasmodium falciparum* malaria.

Preparations: Controlled-release tablets, 324 and 330 mg. Vials, 80 mg/ ml.

QUINIDINE POLYGALACTURONATE—Cardioquin®

Antiarrhythmic agent indicated in the prevention and treatment of a number of ventricular, atrial, and junctional (nodal) arrhythmias.

Preparation: Tablets, 275 mg.

QUINIDINE SULFATE

Antiarrhythmic agent indicated in the prevention and treatment of a number of ventricular, atrial, and junctional (nodal) arrhythmias.

Preparations: Capsules and tablets, 100, 200, and 300 mg. Controlled-release tablets, 300 mg. Ampules, 200 mg/ml.

QUININE SULFATE—Quinamm®

Antimalarial agent used in the treatment of chloroquine-resistant infections. Also used in the prevention and treatment of nocturnal leg cramps.

Preparations: Capsules and tablets, 130, 200, 260, 300, and 325 mg.

R

RAMIPRIL—Altace®

Antihypertensive agent.

Actions and Uses: An angiotensin-converting enzyme (ACE) inhibitor that is a prodrug. Following oral administration, is converted to its active metabolite, ramiprilat. Indicated for the treatment of hypertension and may be used alone or in combination with a thiazide diuretic. Treatment for CHF in stabilized patients post-MI has been found to reduce mortality.

Warnings: Adverse reactions include headache, dizziness, fatigue, and cough. May cause an elevation in serum potassium levels; the risk of hyperkalemia is increased in patients also taking a potassium-sparing diuretic, a potassium supplement, and/ or a potassium-containing salt substitute.

May cause symptomatic postural hypotension. There have been infrequent reports of angioedema of the face, extremities, lips, tongue, glottis, and larynx, especially following the first dose. Patients should be told to report immediately any symptoms suggesting angioedema and to stop taking the drug. When used during the second and third trimesters of pregnancy, ACE inhibitors have been reported to be associated with the development of neonatal hypertension, renal failure, and skull hypoplasia; use during pregnancy should be avoided. May increase serum lithium levels and concurrent therapy should be closely monitored.

Administration: Oral. If necessary, the capsules may be opened and the contents sprinkled on a small amount of applesauce or mixed in apple juice or water.

Preparations: Capsules, 1.25, 2.5, 5, and 10 mg.

RANITIDINE HYDROCHLORIDE—Zantac®

Antiulcer agent.

Actions and Uses: A histamine H2 receptor antagonist that inhibits gastric acid secretion. Indicated (1) in the short-term treatment of active duodenal ulcer; (2) for maintenance therapy for duodenal ulcer patients at reduced dosage after healing of acute ulcers; (3) for the treatment of pathological hypersecretory conditions (e.g., Zollinger-Ellison syndrome); (4) in the short-term treatment of active, benign gastric ulcer; (5) in the treatment of gastroesophageal reflux disease; and (6) in the treatment of erosive esophagitis, and in the maintenance treatment of healed erosive esophagitis.

Warnings: Adverse reactions include headache and GI effects.

Administration: Oral, intravenous, and intramuscular.

Preparations: Tablets, 150 and 300 mg. Geldose capsules, 150 and 300 mg. Efferdose tablets and granules, 150 mg. Syrup, 15 mg/ml. Vials, 25 mg/ml and 50 mg/100 ml containers.

RAUDIXIN®, see Rauwolfia serpentina

REGITINE®, see Phentolamine

REGLAN®, see Metoclopramide

RELA®, see Carisoprodol

RELAFEN®, see Nabumetone

REMERON®, see Mirtazapine

RENESE®, see Polythiazide

RENOVA®, see Tretinoin

REOPRO®, see Abciximab

RESCRIPTOR®, see Delvaviridine Mesylate

RESERPINE—Serpasil®

Rauwolfia alkaloid indicated in the treatment of hypertension and for the relief of symptoms in agitated psychotic states. Has been used parenterally in acute hypertensive and psychiatric conditions.

Preparations: Tablets, 0.1, 0.25, and 1 mg. Ampules, 2.5 mg/ml.

RESORCINOL

Antipruritic, anti-infective, and keratolytic agent used topically with other agents in the treatment of seborrheic dermatitis, acne, and other dermatologic conditions.

RESTORIL®, see Temazepam

RETEPLASE—Retavase®

Thrombolytic indicated to improve ventricular function post acute myocardial infarction (MI), to reduce the incidence of congestive heart failure.

Warnings: Contraindicated in patients with a history of cerebral vascular accident, active internal bleeding, intracranial or intraspinal surgery or trauma within the past two months, intracranial neoplasm, arteriovenous malformation or aneurysm, bleeding diathesis, severe uncontrolled hypertension and history of severe allergic reactions to altaplase, anistreplase or streptokinase. Use cautiously in patients with hypertension, recent major surgery, obstetrical delivery, organ biopsy, previous puncture of noncompressible vessel, GU or GI bleeding or trauma, high risk of left heart thrombus, subacute bacterial endocarditis, acute pericarditis, hemostatic defects, severe renal or hepatic dysfunction, cerebrovascular disease, hemorrhagic ophthalmic conditions, septic thrombophlebitis or occluded AV cannula at seriously infected sites, and patients above 75 years of age. Cholesterol embolization and/or reperfusion arrhythmias may occur. Avoid IM injections, noncompressible punctures, and unnecessary handling of patients. Minimize venipuncture. Check puncture sites.

Adverse reactions include bleeding (including intracranial hemorrhage) and reperfusion arrhythmias.

Administrations: 10 units IV over 2 minutes; then 30 minutes after initiation of first dose give a 2nd dose of 10 units IV over 2 minutes. Withhold 2nd dose if serious bleeding or anaphylaxis occurs.

Preparations: Powder for IV injection supplied with 2 ml diluent (preservative-free).

10.8 units/vial.

RETEVASE®, see Reteplase

RETIN-A®, see Tretinoin

RETINOIC ACID, see Tretinoin

RETROVIR®, see Zidovudine

REVERSOL®, see Edrophonium

REVEX®, see Nalmefene hydrochloride

RÉV-EYES®, see Dapiprazole hydrochloride

ReVia®, see Naltrexone hydrochloride

R-GENE®, see Arginine

REZULIN®, see Troglitazone

RHEOMACRODEX®, see Dextran

RHEUMATREX®, see Methotrexate

RHINOCORT®, see Budesonide

RHO(D) IMMUNE GLOBULIN—RhoGAM®

Immune globulin administered intramuscularly to prevent Rh immunization in Rh negative individuals exposed to Rh positive red blood cells. Indicated in pregnancy and other obstetric conditions when it is known or suspected that fetal red cells have entered the circulation of an Rh negative mother unless the fetus or the father can be shown conclusively to be Rh negative. Also indicated for any Rh negative female of childbearing age who receives a transfusion of Rh positive red blood cells or whole blood, or components prepared from Rh positive blood.

Preparations: Vials and syringes.

RHOGAM®, see Rh_o(D) immune globulin

RIBAVIRIN—Virazole®

Antiviral agent.

Actions and Uses: Indicated for the aerosol treatment of carefully selected hospitalized infants and young children with severe lower respiratory tract infections due to respiratory syncytial virus (RSV).

Warnings: Should not be used in infants requiring assisted ventilation because the drug may precipitate on the valves and tubing of the respirator and interfere with safe and effective ventilation. Is teratogenic in animals and, although presently indicated only in infants and young children, its potential value for viral infections in adults warrants recognition of the contraindication to its use during pregnancy.

Administration: Aerosol, delivered to an infant oxygen hood (or administered by face mask or oxygen tent if necessary). Is administered using a small-particle aerosol generator (model SPAG-2) and other aerosol-generating devices should not be used.

Preparations: Vials, 6 g.

RIBOFLAVIN—Vitamin B_2

Vitamin indicated in the prevention and treatment of riboflavin deficiency.

Preparations: Tablets, 10, 25, 50, and 100 mg.

RID®, see Pyrethrins

RIDAURA®, see Auranofin

RIFABUTIN—Mycobutin®

Antimycobacterial agent.

Actions and Uses: Is active against *Mycobacterium avium* and *Mycobacterium intracellulare* which comprise *Mycobacterium avium* complex (MAC). Indicated for the prevention of disseminated *Mycobacterium avium* complex (MAC) disease in patients with advanced human immunodeficiency virus (HIV) infection.

Warnings: Contraindicated in patients who are hypersensitive to rifampin. Adverse reactions include rash, gastrointestinal intolerance, neutropenia, flu-like syndrome, arthralgia, hepatitis, and a brown-orange discoloration of urine, feces, saliva, sputum, perspiration, tears, and skin, as well as permanent staining of soft contact lenses. May increase the activity of hepatic enzymes and reduce the effect of other therapeutic agents that are metabolized by these enzyme systems. Patients using oral contraceptives should be advised to use nonhormonal or additional methods of birth control while taking rifabutin. Should not be administered to patients with active tuberculosis because of the possibility of the development of tuberculosis that is resistant both to rifabutin and rifampin.

Administration: Oral, once a day. For patients who experience GI intolerance, administering doses twice a day with food may avoid these effects.

Preparations: Capsules, 150 mg.

RIFADIN®, see Rifampin

RIFADIN IV®, see Rifampin

RIFAMPIN—Rifadin®, Rifadin IV®, Rimactane®

Antitubercular agent indicated in the treatment of tuberculosis. Also indicated for the treatment of asymptomatic carriers of *Neisseria meningitidis.* Has a broad spectrum of action and is also useful in the treatment of staphylococcal infections, Legionnaire's disease, leprosy, and other infections.

Preparations: Capsules, 150 and 300 mg. Vials, 600 mg.

RILUZOLE—Rilutek®

Actions and Uses: Used in the treatment of Amyotrophic Lateral Sclerosis (ALS) to extend survival or time to tracheostomy. The etiology and pathogenesis are not known, but it has been hypothesized that motor neurons, made vulnerable through either genetic predisposition or environmental factors, are injured by glutamate. Riluzole's pharmacologic properties include an inhibitory effect on glutamate release, among others, which may account for its effect on ALS.

Warnings: Neutropenia may develop, usually within the first 2 months of treatment. Warn patients to report febrile illnesses as a trigger for prompt checking of white blood cell counts. Use cautiously in patients with a history of abnormal liver function tests. Elevation of serial LFTs (especially bilirubin) should preclude use of Riluzole. Use cautiously in patients with impaired renal function. Adverse reactions include asthenia, nausea, dizziness, diarrhea, anorexia, vertigo, somnolence, circumoral paresthesia (dose-related), decreased lung function, abdominal pain, pneumonia, and vomiting.

Administration: 50 mg orally on an empty stomach every 12 hours. No increased benefit can be expected from higher doses, but adverse events are increased.

Preparations: Tablets, 50 mg.

RIMACTANE®, see Rifampin

RIMANTADINE HYDROCHLORIDE —Flumadine®

Antiviral agent.

Actions and Uses: Indicated for the prophylaxis and treatment of illness caused by various strains of influenza A virus in adults and for prophylaxis in children aged one year and above.

Warnings: Contraindicated in patients who are hypersensitive to the drug or to amantadine. Adverse reactions include insomnia, dizziness, nervousness, fatigue, headache, nausea, vomiting, anorexia, dry mouth, and abdominal pain.

Administration: Oral.

Preparations: Tablets, 100 mg. Syrup, 50 mg/5ml.

RIMEXOLONE—Vexol®

Actions and Uses: Ophthalmic preparation containing benzalkonium chloride used in the treatment of postoperative inflammation and anterior uveitis.

Warnings: Contraindicated in epithelial herpes simplex Keratitis and other viral or fungal infections, including vaccinia and varicella. Do not use in the presence of ocular mycobacterial, fungal, or untreated purident infections. Use cautiously with ocular hypertension/glaucoma, optic nerve damage, defects in visual acuity and visual fields. Posterior subcapsular cataract formation or fungal invasion may occur with prolonged use. May mask secondary ocular infections. Corneal or scleral thinning may occur. Monitor intraocular pressures. Adverse reactions include blurred vision, discharge, discomfort, ocular pain, increased intraocular pressure, foreign body sensation , hyperemia, and pruritus.

Administration: Start 1–2 drops into the conjuctival sac(s) 4 times a day 24 hours after surgery and continue through the first 2 weeks postoperatively. Uveitis: 1–2 drops in conjunctival sac(s) every hour while awake the first week and then 1 drop every 2 hours while awake for the second week, then taper until resolved.

Preparations: Ophthalmic suspension, 5 and 10 ml.

RIMSO 50®, see Dimethyl sulfoxide

RINGER'S INJECTION

Intravenous electrolyte replacement solution containing sodium, potassium, calcium, and chloride.

Preparations: Solution, 500 and 1000 ml.

RIOPAN®, see Magaldrate

RISPERDAL®, see Risperidone

RISPERIDONE—Risperdal®

Antipsychotic agent.

Actions and Uses: Indicated for the management of the manifestations of psychotic disorders.

Warnings: Adverse reactions include extrapyramidal symptoms, insomnia, agitation, anxiety, headache, constipation, abdominal pain, tachycardia, and rhinitis. Patients should be cautioned about driving or operating hazardous machinery until they are reasonaably certain that the drug does not affect them adversely. Caution should also be exercised in patients taking other centrally-acting drugs, and patients should be advised to avoid the consumption of alcoholic beverages. May cause orthostatic hypotension, especially during the initial dose-titration period, and the initial dose should not exceed 1 mg twice daily to reduce the risk. May lengthen the QT interval and caution should be exercised in patients with risk factors for this complication (e.g., bradytcardia, use of other drugs that prolong the QT interval). May antagonize the effects of levodopa.

Administration: Oral.

Preparations: Tablets, 1, 2, 3, and 4 mg. Oral solution 1 mg/ml.

RITALIN®, see Methylphenidate

RITALIN SR®, see Methylphenidate

RITODRINE HYDROCHLORIDE—Yutopar®

Uterine relaxant indicated in the management of preterm labor in suitable patients for the purpose of prolonging gestation. Continue IV for 12–24 hours after contractions cease and begin po 30 minutes before IV is stopped.

Preparations: Tablets, 10 mg. Ampules, vials, and syringes, 10 mg/ml and 15 mg/ml.

RITONOVIR—Norvir®

Antiviral /protease inhibitor

Actions and Uses: Used in treatment of H.I.V. infection, either as monotherapy or in combination with other nucleoside analogues, or protease inhibitors.

Warnings: Use cautiously in patients with impaired hepatic function. Adverse reactions include GI upset, asthenia, abdominal pain, headache, anorexia, paresthesias, taste perversion, fever, hyperlipidemia, dizziness, rash, throat irritation, malaise, somnolence, insomnia, and sweating. Due to increased plasma concentrations of various agents, and also large increases in concentrations of highly metabolized sedatives and hypnotics, the co-administration of Ritonovir with such agents is contraindicated and prescribers should verify a patient's full drug profile prior to prescribing this agent.

Administration: Oral with meals.

Preparations: Capsules, 100 mg; oral solution, 80 mg/ml.

RMS®, see Morphine

ROBAXIN®, see Methocarbamol

ROBIMYCIN®, see Erythromycin base

ROBINUL®, see Glycopyrrolate

ROBITUSSIN®, see Guaifenesin

ROCALTROL®, see Calcitriol

ROCEPHIN®, see Ceftriaxone

ROCURONIUM BROMIDE—Zemuron®

Nondepolarizing neuromuscular blocking agent.

Actions and Uses: Indicated for inpatients and outpatients as an adjunct to general anesthesia to facilitate both rapid sequence and routine tracheal intubation, and to provide skeletal muscle relaxation during surgery or mechanical ventilation.

Warnings: Must be used with caution in patients with neuromuscular disease (e.g., myasthenia gravis) and in patients receiving other medications that may increase or prolong neuromuscular block. Action may be enhanced by the prior administration of succinylcholine, and rocuronium should not be administered until recovery from succinylcholine has been observed.

Administration: Intravenous. Should not be mixed with alkaline solutions in the same syringe or administered simultaneously during intravenous infusion through the same needle.

Preparation: Vials, 10 mg/ml.

ROFERON-A®, see Interferon alfa-2a recombinant

ROGAINE®, see Minoxidil

ROMAZICON®, see Flumazenil

ROPIVACAINE HYDROCHLORIDE—Naropin®

Long-acting local anesthetic indicated in local or regional anesthesia or surgery and management of acute pain, including the pain of obstetrical procedures.

Warnings: Contraindicated in patients with known hypersensitivity to any local anesthetic of this type, i.e., bupivacaine, lidocaine, mepivacaine. Adverse reactions include hypotension, fetal bradycardia, nausea, bradycardia, vomiting, parasthesia, and back pain. Carefully monitor vital signs including cardiovascular and respiratory status, and level of consciousness after each injection. Oxygen and resuscitative equipment should be available. Use cautiously in patients with severe hepatic, renal impairment and impaired cardiovascular function.

Administrations: Administer the smallest dose and concentration required to produce desirable results. Avoid rapid administration of large volume and use fractional (incremental) doses. Administer as infiltrate, block or epidural or intermittent bolus.

Preparations: Injection, 2, 5, 7.5, and 10 mg/ml.

ROWASA®, see Mesalamine

ROXANOL®, see Morphine

ROXANOL SR®, see Morphine

ROXICODONE®, see Oxycodone

RUBEX®, see Doxorubicin

RUFEN®, see Ibuprofen

RYTHMOL®, see Propafenone

S

SAFFLOWER OIL

Nutritional supplement used in the management of patients requiring caloric supplementation.

Preparation: Emulsion.

SALFLEX®, see Salsalate

SALAGEN®, see Pilocarpine hydrochloride

SALICYLAMIDE

Analgesic used in the management of mild to moderate pain.

Preparations: Tablets, 325 and 667 mg.

SALICYLIC ACID

Keratolytic agent used topically as an aid in the removal of excessive keratin in hyperkeratotic skin disorders including warts. Also used in combination with other agents in a number of dermatologic conditions including acne.

Preparations: Cream, ointment, liquid, gel, and

plaster in concentrations ranging from 1% to 60%.

SALMETEROL XINAFOATE—Serevent®

Antiasthmatic agent.

Action and Uses: Is a selective $beta_2$-adrenergic receptor agonist that is administered by oral inhalation. Has a long duration of action that permits twice-daily administration. Indicated for long-term, twice-daily (morning and evening) administration in the maintenance treatment of asthma and in the prevention of bronchospasm in patients 12 years of age and older with reversible obstructive airway disease, including patients with symptoms of nocturnal asthma, who require regular treament with inhaled, short-acting $beta_2$ agonists. Is also indicated for the prevention of exercise-induced bronchospasm and marhtenance treatment of CAPB-associated bronchospasm (including emphysema and chronic bronchitis). Patients must also be provided with a short-acting inhaled $beta_2$ agonist (e.g., albuterol) for the treatment of symptoms that occur despite twice-daily use of salmeterol. Should not be used to treat acute symptoms.

Warnings: Adverse reactions include headache, tremor, cough, and dizziness. Should be used with caution in patients with coronary insufficiency, cardiac arrhythmias, and hypertension, and in patients being treated with a tricyclic antidepressant or a monoamine oxidase inhibitor. Should not be used to treat acute symptoms.

Administration: Oral inhalation. Is administered twice daily (morning and evening, approximately 12 hours apart). If symptoms arise in the period between doses, a short-acting inhaled $beta_2$ agonist should be taken for immediate relief, and the patient should not take higher doses of salmeterol.

Preparation: Metered-dose inhaler, 21 ug per actuation. Powder for inhalation, 50 µg/blister. Diskus provider for inhalation, 50 µg/inh.

SALSALATE—Disalcid®, Salflex®

Salicylate analgesic/anti-inflammatory agent indicated for the relief of the signs and symptoms of rheumatoid arthritis, osteoarthritis, and related disorders.

Preparations: Capsules and tablets, 500 and 750 mg.

SALT, see Sodium chloride

SALURON®, see Hydroflumethiazide

SANDIMMUNE®, see Cyclosporine

SANDOSTATIN®, see Octreotide

SANOREX®, see Mazindol

SANSERT®, see Methysergide

SANTYL®, see Collagenase

SAQUINAVIR—Fortouase®, Invirase

Actions and Uses: Antiviral (HIV protease inhibitor) indicated in the management of advanced HIV infection in combination with zidovudine, and/or other nucleoside analogs.

Warnings: Use cautiously in patients with hepatic impairment. Adverse reactions include diarrhea, abdominal discomfort, nausea, asthenia, and rash.

Administration: Oral with food.

Preparations: Capsules, 200 mg.

SARGRAMOSTIM—Leukine®, Prokine®

Colony stimulating factor.

Actions and Uses: A human granulocyte-macrophage colony stimulating factor (GM-CSF) produced by recombinant DNA technology. Accelerates bone marrow recovery after autologous bone marrow transplantation. Indicated for acceleration of myeloid recovery in patients with non-Hodgkin's lymphoma, acute lymphoblastic leukemia, and Hodgkin's disease undergoing autologous bone marrow transplantation. Also indicated for patients who have undergone allogeneic or autologous bone marrow transplantation in whom engraftment is delayed or has failed.

Warnings: Contraindicated in patients with excessive leukemic myeloid blasts in the bone marrow or peripheral blood (greater than 10%). Adverse reactions include diarrhea, asthenia, rash, malaise, transient supraventricular arrhythmias, peripheral edema, and pleural and/or pericardial effusion. May cause dyspnea and special attention should be given to respiratory symptoms during or immediately following infusion, especially in patients with preexisting lung disease. Caution must be exercised in patients with any malignancy with myeloid characteristics because of the possibility that the drug may act as a growth factor for the tumor.

Administration: Intravenous. Should be administered not less than 24 hours after the last dose of chemotherapy and 12 hours after the last dose of radiotherapy. A complete blood count with differential is recommended twice per week during therapy.

Preparations: Vials, 250 and 500 ug.

SCOPOLAMINE HYDROBROMIDE—Hyoscine, Transderm-Scojp®

Anticholinergic agent indicated for parenteral use for preanesthetic medication, for obstetric amnesia in conjunction with analgesics, and for calming delirium. Also used orally and transdermally for the prevention of nausea and vomiting associated with motion sickness. Also indicated for ophthalmic use to produce cycloplegia and mydriasis.

Preparations: Capsules, 0.25 mg. Transdermal therapeutic system, 1.5 mg (used over a period of 3 days). Ampules and vials, 0.3 mg/ml, 0.4 mg/ml, 1 mg/ml. Ophthalmic solution, 0.25%

SECOBARBITAL SODIUM—Seconal®

Barbiturate used parenterally as a preanesthetic and for the emergency control of certain acute convulsive episodes.

Preparations: Vials and syringes, 50 mg/ml.

SECONAL®, see Secobarbital

SECTRAL®, see Acebutolol

SELEGILINE HYDROCHLORIDE—Eldepryl®

Antiparkinson agent.

Actions and Uses: Also known as deprenyl, it acts as a selective inhibitor of monoamine oxidase type B. Indicated as an adjunct to levodopa/carbidopa in the management of Parkinson's disease.

Warnings: Adverse reactions include nausea, abdominal pain, dry mouth, dizziness, fainting, confusion, hallucinations, and vivid dreams. Does not inhibit monoamine oxidase type A at the recommended dosage level, and is not likely to interact with the sympathomimetic amines and tyramine-containing foods that can cause hypertensive reactions when used concurrently with a nonselective monoamine oxidase inhibitor; however, the recommended dosage level should not be exceeded as the selectivity of selegiline is reduced with increasing daily doses. Concomitant use of selegiline with meperidine should be avoided.

Administration: Oral. Administered in divided doses at breakfast and lunch.

Preparation: Capsules, 5 mg.

SELENIUM SULFIDE—Selsun®

Antiseborrheic agent indicated for topical use in the treatment of dandruff and seborrheic dermatitis of the scalp, and also in the management of tinea versicolor.

Preparations: Lotion shampoo, 1% and 2.5%.

SELSUN®, see Selenium sulfide

SEMI-LENTE INSULIN, see Insulin

SEMPREX-D®, see AcrivastinePseudoephedrine hydrochloride

SENNA CONCENTRATE—Senokot®

Laxative used in the prevention and treatment of constipation.

Preparations: Tablets, granules, syrup, liquid, and suppositories.

SENOKOT®, see Senna concentrate

SEPTRA®, see Trimethoprim-sulfamethoxazole

SERAX®, see Oxazepam

SERENTIL®, see Mesoridazine

SEREVENT®, see Salmeterol xinafoate

SEROMYCIN®, see Cycloserine

SEROPHENE®, see Clomiphene

SEROSTIM®, see Somatropin

SERPASIL®, see Reserpine

SERTRALINE HYDROCHLORIDE—Zoloft®

Antidepressant.

Actions and Uses: Is a serotonin reuptake inhibitor. Indicated for the treatment of depression, panic disordr, and obsessive compulsive disorder (OCD).

Warnings: Adverse reactions include nausea, diarrhea, dyspepsia, dizziness, tremor, insomnia, somnolence, dry mouth, increased sweating, and sexual dysfunction in male patients (primarily ejaculatory delay). May decrease appetite resulting in significant weight loss. Concomitant use with a monoamine oxidase inhibitor (MAOI), or use within 14 days of treatment with a MAOI may result in serious, potentially fatal reactions (hyperthermia, rigidity, myoclonus, autonomic instability, with fluctuating vital signs and extreme agitation, which may proceed to delirium and coma). Sertraline should be stopped at least 14 days prior to MAO inhibitor therapy.

Administration: Oral.

Preparations: Tablets, 25, 50 and 100 mg.

SERZONE®, see Nefazodone hydrochloride

SEVOFLURANE®—Ultane®

Actions and Uses: Halogenated volatile anesthetic that provides rapid induction and emergence from anesthesia in inpatient and outpatient surgery.

Warnings: May cause malignant hyperthermia and is contraindicated in patients who are hypersensitive to the drug or other halogenated agents. Adverse reactions include agitation, somnolence, cough, breathholding, laryngospasm, airway obstruction, tachy- cardia, bradycardia, hypotension, nausea, and vomiting.

Administration: Inhalation.

Preparations: Liquid, 250 ml.

SHOHL'S SOLUTION MODIFIED®, See Sodium citrate

SILVADENE®, see Silver sulfadiazine

SILVER NITRATE

Anti-infective agent and cauterizing and caustic agent. Indicated for ophthalmic use in the prevention of gonococcal ophthalmia neonatorum. Has been used topically in the treatment of burns. Also has been used topically for its caustic and cauterizing actions in the treatment of certain dermatologic problems (e.g., warts).

Preparations: Ophthalmic solution, 1%. Ointment and solutions for topical use.

SILVER SULFADIAZINE—Silvadene®

Anti-infective agent used topically as an adjunct for the prevention and treatment of wound sepsis in patients with second- and third-degree burns.

Preparation: Cream, 1%.

SIMETHICONE—Mylicon®, Phazyme®

Antiflatulent indicated for relief of the painful symptoms of excess gas in the digestive tract.

Preparations: Tablets, 40, 50, 60, 80 and 95 mg. Chewable tablets, 125 mg. Capsules, 125 mg. Drops 40 mg/0.6ml.

SIMVASTATIN—Zocor®

Agent for hypercholesterolemia.

Actions and Uses: Is a prodrug which is converted to its active form following administration. Produces a significant reduction in total and low-density lipoprotein (LDL) cholesterol concentrations, a modest reduction in triglyceride concentrations, and an increase in high-density lipoprotein (HDL) cholesterol concentrations. Indicated as an adjunct to diet for the reduction of elevated total and LDL cholesterol concentrations in patients with primary hypercholesterolemia (type IIa and IIb) when the response to a diet restricted in saturated fat and cholesterol and other nonpharmacological measures has not been adequate. Also indicated in patients with coronary heart disease and hypercholesterolemia to reduce the risk of total mortality by reducing coronary death; reduce the risk of nonfatal myocardial infarction; and reduce the risk for undergoing myocardial revascularization procedures.

Warnings: Contraindicated in patients with active liver disease or unexplained persistent elevations of serum transaminases. Is also contraindicated in pregnant women and nursing mothers. Increases in serum transaminases may occur and it is recommended that liver function tests be monitored before treatment begins, every 6 weeks for the first 3 months, every 8 weeks during the remainder of the first year, and periodically thereafter (at about 6-month intervals). Adverse reactions include constipation, flatulence, dyspepsia, myalgia, myopathy, and, rarely, rhabdomyolysis. Patients should be advised to promptly report unexplained muscle pain, tenderness, or weakness.

Administration: Oral. Should be administered at bedtime.

Preparations: Tablets, 5, 10, 20, and 40 mg.

SINEMET—Combination of levodopa and carbidopa.

SINEMET—CR, Combination of levodopa and carbidopa (controlled-release)

SINEQUAN, see Doxepin

SINUMIST SR CAPLETS, see Guaifenesin

SKELAXIN, see Metaxalone

SKELID®, see Tiludronate

SLO-BID, see Theophylline

SLO-NIACIN, see Nicotinic acid

SLO-PHYLLIN, see Theophylline

SLOW-FE®, see Ferrous sulfate, exsiccated

SLOW-K®, see Potassium chloride

SLOW-MAG®, see Magnesium chloride

SODIUM ASCORBATE, see Vitamin C

SODIUM BENZOATE AND SODIUM PHENYLACETATE—Ucephan®

Agents for hyperammonemia.

Actions and Uses: Are metabolically active compounds which decrease elevated blood ammonia concentrations in patients with inborn errors of ureagenesis. Indicated as adjunctive therapy [with dietary management (low protein diet) and amino acid supplementation] for the prevention and treatment of hyperammonemia in the chronic management of patients with urea cycle enzymopathies.

Warnings: Adverse reactions include nausea and vomiting. Because of the sodium content of the product, the possibility of hypernatremia exists and caution should be exercised in patients with congestive heart failure, severe renal insufficiency, and in clinical states in which there is sodium retention with edema.

Administration: Oral. Ucephan is a concentrated solution and must be diluted before use. Because sodium phenylacetate has a lingering odor, care should be taken in mixing and administering the drug to minimize contact with skin and clothing.

Preparation: Oral solution. 10% sodium benzoate and 10% sodium phenylacetate.

SODIUM BICARBONATE—Baking soda

Antacid and alkalinizer. Used orally as a gastric antacid and urinary alkalinizer. Administered intravenously in the management of metabolic acidosis and to alkalinize the urine in the treatment of certain drug intoxications.

Preparations: Tablets, 325 and 650 mg.

Vials and syringes, 4%, 4.2%, 5%, 7.5%, and 8.4%.

SODIUM BIPHOSPHATE

Laxative often used in combination with sodium phosphate. Has also been used as a urinary acidifier.

SODIUM BORATE—Collyrium

Antiseptic and buffer indicated for ophthalmic use for flushing or irrigating the eye to remove loose foreign material.

Preparation: Ophthalmic solution.

SODIUM CELLULOSE PHOSPHATE—Calcibind®

Indicated for absorptive hypercalciuria type I with recurrent calcium oxalate or calcium phosphate nephrolithiasis.

Preparation: Powder, 2.5g packets.

SODIUM CHLORIDE—Salt

Used intravenously to replace fluid and electrolytes, as a genitourinary irrigant, as an abortifacient, for ophthalmic use in the treatment and diagnosis of ocular conditions, and for intranasal use to restore moisture and alleviate discomfort in certain nasal conditions.

Preparations: Solutions for intravenous infusion,

0.45%, 0.9% (normal saline); 3%, 5%. Vials for intravenous admixtures, 50 mEq, 100 mEq, and 625 mEq. Solutions for genitourinary irrigation, 0.45% and 0.9%. Solutions for inducing abortion, 20%. Ophthalmic solution or ointment, 2% and 5%. Nose drops and spray, 0.4% and 0.65%.

SODIUM CITRATE—Bicitra®, Shohl's solution modified®

Alkalinizing agent useful in conditions in which the maintenance of an alkaline urine is desirable, and in the alleviation of chronic metabolic acidosis such as results from chronic renal insufficiency.

Preparations: Solution, 500 mg/5 ml with citric acid. Also available in formulations with potassium citrate and citric acid.

SODIUM FLUORIDE—Luride®

Indicated for prevention of dental caries and certain dental procedures. Has been investigated for possible value in the treatment of osteoporosis.

Preparations: Tablets, 0.25, 0.5, and 1 mg fluoride. Drops, rinse, and gel.

SODIUM HYPOCHLORITE

Anti-infective agent and bleaching agent.

Preparation: Solution.

SODIUM IODIDE

Used in thyroid disorders. May be used adjunctively with an antithyroid drug in certain hyperthyroid patients. Radioactive form (sodium iodide I 131) has been used in the management of hyperthyroidism and selected cases of thyroid carcinoma.

Preparation: Solution.

SODIUM LACTATE

Administered intravenously in the treatment of metabolic acidosis.

Preparations: Vials, 50 mEq. Solution (for IV use), 167 mEq/l (1/6 molar).

SODIUM LAURYL SULFATE

Surfactant which is used in the preparation of certain pharmaceutical formulations and to enhance the distribution/penetration of some topically applied drugs.

SODIUM MORRHUATE

Sclerosing agent used in the intravenous treatment of small uncomplicated varicose veins of the lower extremities. May be useful as a supplement to venous ligation to obliterate residual varicose veins.

Preparations: Ampules and vials, 50 mg/ml.

SODIUM NITROPRUSSIDE—Nitropress®

Antihypertensive agent indicated for intravenous use for the immediate reduction of blood pressure of patients in hypertensive crisis and in the treatment of cardiac pump failure or cardiogenic shock. Also used to produce controlled hypotension during anesthesia in order to reduce bleeding in surgical procedures.

Preparation: Vials, 50 mg.

SODIUM PERBORATE

Antiseptic and cleansing agent included in some dentifrices.

SODIUM PHOSPHATE

Laxative often used in combination with sodium biphosphate. Also administered intravenously as a source of phosphate.

Preparations: Vials, 3 mM phosphate.

SODIUM POLYSTYRENE SULFONATE—Kayexalate®

Cation-exchange resin indicated for the treatment of hyperkalemia.

Preparation: Powder and suspension.

SODIUM SALICYLATE

Salicylate analgesic indicated for the relief of mild to moderate pain and inflammation.

Preparations: Enteric-coated tablets, 325 and 650 mg. Ampules, 1 g/10 ml.

SODIUM SULFATE

Laxative sometimes used in combination with other agents.

SODIUM TETRADECYL SULFATE—Sotradecol®

Sclerosing agent administered intravenously in the treatment of small uncomplicated varicose veins of the lower extremities.

Preparations: Ampules, 1% and 3%.

SODIUM THIOSALICYLATE

Salicylate analgesic/anti-inflammatory agent used parenterally in the management of acute gout, musculoskeletal disorders, and rheumatic fever.

Preparations: Ampules and vials, 50 mg/ml.

SODIUM THIOSULFATE—Tinver®

Used in the topical treatment of tinea versicolor and other dermatologic conditions including acne. Has also been used parenterally as adjunctive therapy in the management of cyanide toxicity, and also in the treatment of arsenic poisoning.

Preparations: Lotion, 25%. Ampules, 1 g/10 ml.

SOLGANAL®, see Aurothioglucose

SOLU-CORTEF®, see Hydrocortisone (as the sodium succinate)

SOLU-MEDROL®, see Methylprednisolone sodium succinate

SOMA®, see Carisoprodol

SOMATREM—Protropin®

Growth hormone.

Actions and Uses: Indicated for the long-term treatment of children who have growth failure due to a lack of adequate endogenous growth hormone secretion.

Warnings: Contraindicated in patients with closed epiphyses or when there is evidence of any progression of underlying intracranial lesion. Patients may experience glucose intolerance. Concurrent use of a glucocorticoid may inhibit the effect of somatrem. Some patients develop persistent antibodies to growth hormone.

Administration: Intramuscular.

Preparation: Vials, 5 and 10 mg.

SOMATROPIN—Humatrope®, Genotropin®, Nutropin®, Serostim®

Growth hormone.

Actions and Uses: Indicated for the long-term treatment of children who have growth failure due to Turner's syndrome or an inadequate secretion of normal endogenous growth hormone and in adults who have a deficiecy in growth hormone. Indicated in AIDS wasting or cachexia (Serostim®) as somatropin has been shown to increase lean body mass and a significant increase in body weight. Also indicated in growth failure in children associated with chronic renal insufficiency up to the time of renal transplant.

Warnings: Contraindicated in patients with closed epiphyses or when there is evidence of growth of intracranial lesions. Patients may experience glucose intolerance. Concurrent use of a glucocorticoid may inhibit the effect of somatropin. Some patients develop antibodies to growth hormone. Reevaluate AIDS patient if weight loss persists after 2 weeks of therapy. Give concomitant antiviral therapy. Discontinue if carpal tunnel syndrome persists after dosage reduction. Perform periodic fundoscopic exams.

Administration: Intramuscular.

Preparation: Vials, 5 and 10 mg.

SOMINEX®, see Diphenhydramine

SORBITOL

Urologic irrigant indicated for use in transurethral prostatic resection or other transurethral surgical procedures.

Preparations: Solutions, 3% and 3.3%.

SORBITRATE®, see Isosorbide dinitrate

SORIATANE®, see Acitretin

SOTALOL HYDROCHLORIDE—Betapace®

Antiarrhythmic agent.

Actions and Uses: Exhibits noncardioselective beta-adrenergic blocking activity and prolongs cardiacrepolarization. Indicated for the treatment of documented life-threatening ventricular arrhythmias such as sustained ventricular tachycardia.

Warnings: Contraindicated in patients with bronchial asthma, sinus bradycardia, second and third degree AV block, unless a functioning pacemaker is present, congenital or acquired long QT syndromes, cardiogenic shock, and uncontrolled congestive heart failure. May cause proarrhythmic events (e.g., torsades de pointes), the risk of which may be increased by excessive prolongation of the QT interval, history of cardiomegaly or congestive heart failure, reduction in heart rate, and reduction in serum potassium and/or magnesium. Should not be used in patients with hypokalemia or hypomagnesemia prior to the correction of the imbalance. Concurrent use with other agents known to prolong the QT interval is best avoided. Because of its beta-blocking activity, should be used with caution in patients with diabetes, bronchospastic diseases, sick sinus syndrome associated with symptomatic arrhythmias, a history of anaphylactic reactions to a variety of allergens, and patients suspected of developing thyrotoxicosis. When sotalol is administered concurrently with a beta-2-receptor agonist (e.g., terbutaline), the dosage of the latter agent may have to be increased.

Administration: Oral.

Preparation: Tablets, 80, 160, and 240 mg.

SOTRADECOL®, see Sodium tetradecyl sulfate

SPARFLOXACIN—Zagam®

Quinolone antibiotic indicated in the treatment of susceptible infections including community acquired pneumonia and acute bacterial exacerbation of chronic bronchitis. Although cross-resistance with other fluoroquinolones may be observed , certain bacterial isolates resistant to fluoroquinolones may be susceptible to sparfloxacin.

Warnings: Contraindicated in patients with a history of hypersensitivity to quinolones, i.e., levofloxacin, of loxacin, ciprofloxacin, norfloxacin or photosensitivity. Instruct patients to refrain from exposure to sun or UV light (direct or indirect) during or 5 days after treatment. Concomitant use of several agents may contraindicate use of Sparfloxacin and prescribers should review the patient's full profile and adjust the medication regimen accordingly. Not recommended for use in patients with hypokalemia, significant bradycardia, CHF, myocardial ischemia, atrial fibrillation or other pro-arrhythmic conditions. Use cautiously in patients with renal insufficiency. Maintain adequate hydration. Cautious use is recommended in patients with severe cerebral arteriosclerosis, epilepsy and other conditions that predispose to seizures or that lower seizure threshold. Not recommened in children < 18 years of age due to arthropathy. Discontinue if phototoxicity, rash or tendon pain, inflammation or rupture occur. Adverse reactions include photosensitivity, GI upset, headache, dizziness, insomnia, pruritus, taste perversion, QTc interval prolongation, flatulence, vasodilation, and convulsions.

AdminIstrations: 400 mg on day 1 and then 200 mg every 24 hours on days 2–10 for a total of 10 days of therapy (11 tablets). Reduce dose as per manufacturer's guidelines for impaired renal function (CrCl < 50ml/min).

Preparations: Tablets, 200 mg.

SPARINE®, see Promazine

SPASMOJECT®, see Dicyclomine

SPECTAZOLE®, see Econazole

SPECTINOMYCIN HYDROCHLORIDE—Trobicin®

Antibiotic indicated for intramuscular use in the treatment of acute gonorrheal urethritis and proctitis in the male and acute gonorrheal cervicitis and proctitis in the female.

Preparations: Vials, 2 and 4g.

SPECTROBID®, see Bacampicillin

SPIRONOLACTONE—Aldactone®

Potassium-sparing diuretic that is an aldosterone antagonist. Indicated in the management of edematous conditions, hypertension, primary hyperaldosteronism, and hypokalemia.

Preparations: Tablets, 25, 50, and 100 mg.

SPORANOX®, see Itraconazole

SSKI®, see Potassium iodide

STADOL®, see Butorphanol

STADOL NS®, see Butorphanol

STANOZOLOL—Winstrol®

Anabolic steroid indicated prophylactically to decrease the frequency and severity of attacks of angioedema in patients with hereditary angioedema and in selected cases of aplastic anemia to increase hemoglobin.

Preparation: Tablets, 2 mg.

STAPHCILLIN®, see Methicillin

STATICIN®, see Erythromycin base

STAVUDINE—Zerit®

Antiviral agent.

Actions and Uses: Indicated in advanced HIV infection in patients who have had prolonged prior zidovudine therapy.

Warnings: May cause peripheral neuropathy and patients should be advised to report symptoms such as tingling, burning, pain, or numbness in the hands or feet. Other adverse reactions include pancreatitis, diarrhea, nausea, vomiting, abdominal pain, headache, chills/fever, asthenia, myalgia, and rash.

Administration: Oral.

Preparations: Capsules, 15, 20, 30, and 40 mg. Oral solution, 1 mg/ml after reconsititution.

STELAZINE®, see Trifluoperazine

STILPHOSTROL®, see Diethylstilbestrol diphosphate

STIMATE®, see Desmopressinacetate

STOXIL®, see Idoxuridine

STREPTASE®, see Streptokinase

STREPTOKINASE—Streptase®

Thrombolytic enzyme indicated for parenteral use for the lysis of thrombi in the management of pulmonary embolism, deep vein thrombosis, arterial thrombosis and embolism, arteriovenous cannulae occlusion, and coronary artery thrombosis. Also indicated for intravenous use for acute myocardial infarction.

Preparations: Vials, 250,000, 600,000, and 750,000 IU.

STREPTOMYCIN SULFATE

Aminoglycoside antibiotic indicated in the parenteral treatment of tuberculosis and selected other infections caused by susceptible organisms.

Preparations: Vials, 1 and 5 g.

STREPTOZOCIN—Zanosar®

Actions and Uses: Antineoplastic agent indicated in the management of metastatic islet cell carcinoma of the pancreas.

Warnings: Use cautiously in renal or hepatic disease, patients with active infections or bone marrow suppression. Adverse reactions include nausea, vomiting, nephrotoxicity, and phlebitis at the IV site.

Administration: Intravenous.

Preparation: Vials, 1 g.

STRONTIUM-89 CHLORIDE—Metastron®

Agent for metastatic bone pain.

Actions and Uses: Is a radiopharmaceutical that decays by beta emission. Selectively concentrates in bone mineral and greater concentrations accumulate in primary bone tumors and in areas of metastatic involvement than can accumulate in normal bone. Has a slow onset of action (7–20 days) and a long duration of action (6 months). Indicated for the relief of bone pain in patients with painful skeletal metastases.

Warnings: May suppress the bone marrow and peripheral blood cell counts should be monitored at least every two weeks. Patients should discontinue calcium medications for about two weeks prior to receiving the drug. May cause fetal harm and women of childbearing potential should be advised to avoid becoming pregnant. Because the drug is radioactive, caution must be observed in handling and administering the drug, and patients should be instructed to observe appropriate cautions during the first week after the treatment.

Administration: Intravenous. Is administered by slow intravenous injection over 1–2 minutes.

Preparations: Vials, 4 millicuries (mCi).

SUBLIMAZE®, see Fentanyl citrate

SUCCIMER—Chemet®

Agent for lead poisoning in children.

Actions and Uses: Is a chelating agent that binds with lead and increases the urinary excretion of lead. Indicated for the treatment of lead poisoning in children with blood lead levels above 45 mg/dl. Use should always be accompanied by identification and removal of the source of the lead exposure.

Warnings: Adverse reactions include gastrointestinal effects (e.g., nausea, vomiting, diarrhea), increases in serum transaminases, and rash. Should be used with caution in patients with compromised renal function. Patients should be adequately hydrated. Elevated blood lead levels and associated symptoms may return rapidly after discontinuation of the drug.

Administration: Oral. In young children who cannot swallow capsules, the drug can be administered by separating the capsule and sprinkling the medicated beads on a small amount of soft food or putting them in a spoon and following with fruit drink.

Preparation: Capsules, 100 mg.

SUCCINYLCHOLINE CHLORIDE—Anectine®, Quelicin®, Sucostrin®

Depolarizing skeletal muscle relaxant for intravenous use as an adjunct to general anesthesia, to facilitate endotracheal intubation, and to provide skeletal muscle relaxation during surgery or mechanical ventilation.

Preparations: Ampules and vials, 20 mg/ml, 50 mg/ml, and 100 mg/ml. Vials, 500 mg and 1 g.

SUCOSTRIN®, see Succinylcholine

SUCRALFATE—Carafate®

Antiulcer agent.

Actions and Uses: Is an aluminum complex of sucrose sulfate indicated in the short-term treatment of duodenal ulcer and for maintenance therapy for duodenal ulcer.

Warnings: Adverse reactions include constipation. Simultaneous administration with other agents should be separated by an interval of at least 2 hours.

Administration: Oral. Should be administered on an empty stomach.

Preparation: Tablets, 1 g. Suspension, 1 g/10 ml.

SUDAFED®, see Pseudoephedrine

SUFENTA®, see Sufentanil

SUFENTANIL CITRATE—Sufenta®

Opioid analgesic/anesthetic indicated as an analgesic adjunct in the maintenance of balanced general anesthesia, and as a primary anesthetic agent for the induction and maintenance of anesthesia with 100% oxygen in patients undergoing major surgical procedures.

Preparations: Ampules, 50 μg/ml.

SULAMYD®, see Sulfacetamide

SULAR®, see Nisoldipine

SULCONAZOLE NITRATE—Exelderm®

Antifungal agent.

Actions and Uses: An imidazole antifungal agent indicated for the topical treatment of tinea pedis, tinea cruris, tinea corporis, and tinea versicolor.

Warnings: Adverse reactions include itching, burning, stinging, and redness.

Administration: Topical.

Preparations: Cream, 1%. Solution, 1%.

SULFABENZAMIDE

Sulfonamide anti-infective agent used in combination with other agents in the topical management of vaginal infections.

SULFACETAMIDE SODIUM—Sulamyd sodium®, Klaron®

Sulfonamide anti-infective agent indicated for ophthalmic use in the treatment of conjunctivitis, corneal ulcers, and other superficial ocular infections, and as adjunctive treatment in the management of trachoma. Also used topically in certain bacterial infections of the skin and seborrheic dermatitis, and in combination with other agents in the topical management of vaginal infections.

Preparations: Ophthalmic solution, 10%, 15%, and 30%. Ophthalmic ointment, 10%. Lotion, 10%.

SULFADIAZINE

Sulfonamide anti-infective agent indicated in the treatment of infections caused by susceptible organisms.

Preparation: Tablets, 500 mg.

SULFADOXINE

Sulfonamide anti-infective agent used in combination (Fansidar®) with pyrimethamine to achieve a synergistic effect in the prevention and treatment of malaria caused by chloroquine-resistant plasmodia.

Preparation: Tablets, 500 mg with 25 mg of pyrimethamine.

SULFAMERAZINE

Sulfonamide anti-infective agent used in combination with other sulfonamides.

SULFAMETHAZINE

Sulfonamide anti-infective agent used in combination with other sulfonamides.

SULFAMETHIZOLE—Thiosulfil Forte®

Sulfonamide anti-infective agent indicated for the treatment of urinary tract infections.

Preparation: Tablets, 500 mg.

SULFAMETHOXAZOLE—Gantanol®

Sulfonamide anti-infective agent indicated for the treatment of infections caused by susceptible organisms.

Preparations: Tablets, 500 mg and 1 g. Suspension, 500 mg/5 ml.

SULFAMYLON®, see Mafenide

SULFANILAMIDE—AVC®

Sulfonamide anti-infective agent used in the topical management of vaginal infections.

Preparations: Vaginal cream, 15%. Vaginal suppositories, 1.05 g.

SULFAPYRIDINE

Used in the treatment of dermatitis herpetiformis.

Preparation: Tablets, 500 mg.

SULFASALAZINE—Azulfidine®

Salicylate-sulfonamide.

Agent for ulcerative colitis indicated in the treatment of mild to moderate ulcerative colitis and as adjunctive therapy in severe ulcerative colitis, and for the prolongation of the remission period between acute attacks of ulcerative colitis. Also indicated in rheumatoid arthritis which has not responded adequately to salicylates or other NSAIDS.

Preparations: Tablets and enteric-coated tablets, 500 mg. Oral suspension, 250 mg/5 ml.

SULFATHIAZOLE

Sulfonamide anti-infective agent used in combination with other agents in the topical management of vaginal infections.

SULFINPYRAZONE—Anturane®

Uricosuric agent indicated in the treatment of chronic gouty arthritis and intermittent gouty arthritis.

Preparations: Tablets, 100 mg. Capsules, 200 mg.

SULFISOXAZOLE—Gantrisin®

SULFISOXAZOLE ACETYL

Sulfonamide anti-infective agent. Primarily used in the treatment of urinary tract infections, and is also useful in certain other infections.

Preparations: Tablets, 500 mg. Suspension (acetyl), 500 mg/5 ml.

SULFISOXAZOLE DIOLAMINE—Gantrisin®

Sulfonamide anti-infective agent used in the treatment of ocular infections.

Preparations: Ophthalmic solution and ointment, 4%.

SULFUR Used topically, usually in combination with other agents, in the treatment of acne, seborrheic dermatitis, and other dermatologic conditions.

SULFURATED LIME—Lime sulfur solution, Vlemasque®

Used topically in the treatment of acne and other dermatologic conditions.

Preparations: Cream, 6%. Topical solution.

SULINDAC—Clinoril®

Nonsteroidal anti-inflammatory drug.

Actions and Uses: Inhibits prostaglandin synthesis, and is indicated in the treatment of rheumatoid arthritis, osteoarthritis, ankylosing spondylitis, acute painful shoulder, and acute gouty arthritis.

Warnings: Should not be given to patients in whom aspirin or another NSAID causes asthma, rhinitis, urticaria, or other allergic-type reactions. May cause GI effects and use should be avoided in patients with active GI tract disease and closely monitored in patients with a previous history of such disorders. Other adverse reactions include dizziness, headache, edema, and rash. Should not be used concomitantly with dimethyl sulfoxide (DMSO).

Administration: Oral.

Preparations: Tablets, 150 and 200 mg.

SUMATRIPTAN SUCCINATE—Imitrex®

Agent for migraine.

Actions and Uses: Is a selective 5-hydroxytryptamine$_1$ (5-HT$_1$) receptor agonist that causes vasoconstriction of intracranial blood vessels. Indicated for the acute treatment of migraine attacks with or without aura and cluster headaches.

Warnings: Contraindicated in patients with ischemic heart disease (angina pectoris, history of myocardial infarction, or documented silent ischemia), Prinzmetal's angina, signs or symptoms consistent with ischemic heart disease, or uncontrolled hypertension. Should not be used concomitantly with ergotamine-containing preparations. Adverse reactions include pain or redness at the injection site, atypical sensations (e.g., sensations of warmth, tingling or paresthesia, pressure, burning, numbness, tightness), dizziness, weakness, neck pain/stiffness, jaw discomfort, flushing, chest discomfort, and transient increases in blood pressure. May cause vasospasm that may be additive to that caused by ergot-containing drugs, and it is recommended that the two agents not be administered within 24 hours of each other.

Administration: Subcutaneous, oral and nasal spray.

Preparations: Tablets, 25 and 50 mg. Vials, 6 mg. Unit-of-use syringes, 6 mg. Imitrex SELFdose system kit that contains two unit-of-use syringes containing 6 mg each and a SELFdose unit (a pushbutton autoinjector). Nasal spray, 5 and 20 mg/spray.

SUMYCIN®, see Tetracycline

SUPPRELIN®, see Histrelin acetate

SUPRANE®, see Desflurane

SUPRAX®, see Cefixime

SUPROFEN—Profenal®

Nonsteroidal anti-inflammatory drug for ophthalmic use.

Actions and Uses: Indicated for the inhibition of intraoperative miosis.

Warnings: Caution should be exercised in the treatment of patients having a history of sensitivity to aspirin or another nonsteroidal anti-inflammatory drug.

Administration: Ophthalmic.

Preparation: Ophthalmic solution, 1%.

SURMONTIL®, see Trimipramine

SURVANTA®, see Beractant

SUTILAINS—Travase®

Proteolytic enzymes applied topically as an adjunct for wound debridement of second- and third-degree burns, pressure ulcers, incisional, traumatic, and pyogenic wounds, and ulcers secondary to peripheral vascular disease.

Preparation: Ointment, 82,000 casein units/g.

SYMMETREL®, see Amantadine

SYNALAR®, see Fluocinolone

SYNALGOS-DC®, Combination of dihydrocodeine, aspirin, and caffeine

SYNAREL®, see Nafarelin acetate

SYNTHROID®, see Levothyroxine

SYNTOCINON®, see Oxytocin

SYPRINE®, see Trientine

T

TACARYL®, see Methdilazine

TACE®, see Chlorotrianisene

TACRINE HYDROCHLORIDE—Cognex®

Agent for Alzheimer's disease.

Actions and Uses: Also known as tetrahydroaminoacridine (THA). Is a reversible cholinesterase inhibitor that elevates acetylcholine concentrations in the cerebral cortex. Indicated for the treatment of mild to moderate dementia of the Alzheimer's type.

Warnings: Contraindicated in patients previously treated with tacrine who developed treatment-associated jaundice confirmed by elevated total bilirubin greater than 3 mg/dl. May increase serum transaminase levels (e.g., alanine aminotransferase [ALT]) and cause liver toxicity. Serum transaminase levels should be monitored every 2 weeks for the first 16 weeks, then monthly for 2 months, then every 3 months thereafter. Other adverse reactions include nausea, vomiting, diarrhea, dyspepsia, anorexia, myalgia, and ataxia.

Administration: Oral. Bioavailability is reduced by food by about 40–50% and doses are best administered at least one hour before meals. However, if gastrointestinal upset occurs, the drug may be taken with food to improve tolerability although a significant reduction in plasma concentrations should be expected.

Preparations: Capsules, 10, 20, 30, and 40 mg.

TACROLIMUS—Prograf®

Immunosuppressant.

Actions and Uses: Indicated for the prophylaxis of organ rejection in patients receiving allogeneic liver transplants. It is recommended that it be used concomitantly with adrenal corticosteroids.

Warnings: Contraindicated in patients who are hypersensitive to the drug, or to polyoxyl 60 hydrogenated castor oil (HCO-60) that is included in the parenteral formulation as a solubilizing agent. May cause nephrotoxicity; patients with impaired renal function should receive lower doses and caution should be exercised when it is used in patients who are also receiving other drugs that may cause nephrotoxicity (e.g., aminoglycosides). Should not be used concurrently with cyclosporine and it is recommended that tacrolimus or cyclosprine should be discontinued at least 24 hours prior to initiating the other. May cause hyperkalemia; serum potassium concentrations should be monitored, and the concurrent use of potassium-sparing diuretics should be avoided. Other adverse reactions include tremor, headache, hypertension, hyperglycemia, diarrhea, nausea, vomiting, abdominal pain, hypomagnesemia, anemia, pain, fever, and asthenia. Anaphylactic reactions have been experienced by some patients receiving the parenteral formulation, which may be due to the castor oil derivative used as the solubilizing agent. The parenteral formulation should be used only in patients who are unable to take the capsule formulation. Patients receiving the drug intravenously should be under continuous observation for at least the first 30 minutes following the start of the intravenous infusion and at frequent intervals thereafter.

Administration: Oral and intravenous infusion. Should be administered no sooner than 6 hours after transplantation. Patients should be converted from the intravenous to the oral formulation as soon as oral therapy can be tolerated. The parenteral formulation must be diluted and the diluted infusion solution should be stored in glass or polyethylene containers and should be discarded after 24 hours. It should not be stored in a polyvinyl chloride (PVC) container due to decreased stability and the potential for extraction of phthalates.

Preparations: Capsules, 1 and 5 mg. Ampules, 5 mg/ml.

TAGAMET®, see Cimetidine

TAGAMET HB®, see Cimetidine

TALWIN®, see Pentazocine

TAMBOCOR®, see Flecainide

TAMOXIFEN CITRATE—Nolvadex®

Antineoplastic agent indicated in the treatment of metastatic breast cancer in postmenopausal women, and in premenopausal women as an alternative to oophorectomy or ovarian radiation. Is also used in combination with cytotoxic agents following radical or modified radical mastectomy to delay recurrence of surgically curable breast cancer in postmenopausal women. Is also indicated for adjuvant treatment for axillary node-negative breast cancer. Is also indicated for advanced breast cancer in men.

Preparation: Tablets, 10 and 20 mg.

TAO®, see Troleandomycin

TAPAZOLE®, see Methimazole

TARKA®—Combination Ace Inhibitor (trandolapril) and calcium channel blocker (verapamil)

TAVIST®, see Clemastine

TAVIST-D®, Combination of clemastine and phenylpropanolamine

TAXOL®, see Paclitaxel

TAXOTERE®, see Docetaxel

TAZAROTENE—Tazorac®

Actions and Uses: Topical gel indicated for treatment of mild to moderate facial acne vulgaris or atable plaque psoriasis affecting up to 20% of the body surface area.

Warnings: Contraindicated in pregnancy (category X). Obtain a reliable negative pregnancy test within 2 weeks before starting therapy. Do not use on broken, eczematous, or sunburned skin. Warn patiens about sun sensitivity. Avoid sun and UV light, use adequate sun protection. Increased irritation may occur in extreme weather (e.g., wind, cold). Discontinue if excessive irritation occues. Adverse reactions include pruritus, burning, stinging, erythema, worsening of psoriasis, irritation, skin pain, desquamation, and other local reactions.

Administrations: Cleanse and dry skin. Apply thin film to lesions, once daily in the evening. Women of childbearing potential: begin therapy during normal menses.

Preparations: 0.05 and 0.1% aqueous gel.

TAZICEF®, see Ceftazidime

TAZIDIME®, see Ceftazidime

TAZORAC®, see Tazarotene

TECZEM®, Combination agent enalapril maleate and diltiazem maleate (ACE inhibitor and calcium channel blocker)

TEGOPEN®, see Cloxacillin

TEGRETOL®, see Carbamazepine

TELDRIN®, see Chlorpheniramine

TEMARIL®, see Trimeprazine

TEMAZEPAM—Restoril®

Benzodiazepine hypnotic.

Actions and Uses: A CNS depressant indicated for the management of insomnia.

Warnings: Contraindicated during pregnancy. Adverse reactions include residual sedation and other CNS effects upon awakening; patients should be cautioned regarding activities such as driving and operating machinery, as well as interactions with other CNS-acting drugs including alcohol. Can cause dependence and is included in Schedule IV.

Administration: Oral.

Preparations: Capsules and tablets, 7.5, 15 and 30 mg.

TEMOVATE®, see Clobetasol propionate

TEMPRA®, see Acetaminophen

TENEX®, see Guanfacine

TENIPOSIDE—Vumon®

Antineoplastic agent.

Actions and Uses: Is a derivative of podophyllotoxin, also known as VM-26. Indicated for use in combination with other anticancer agents for induction therapy in patients with refractory childhood acute lymphoblastic leukemia.

Warnings: Contraindicated in patients who are hypersensitive to etoposide or polyoxyethylated castor oil (Cremophor EL)—a solubilizing agent included in the formulation. Adverse reactions include myelosuppression (leukopenia, neutropenia, thrombocytopenia, anemia), mucositis, diarrhea, nausea, vomiting, infection, alopecia, and bleeding. Hypersensitivity reactions to the drug or to polyoxyethylated castor oil may occur and patients should be under continuous observation for at least 60 minutes following the start of the intravenous infusion and at frequent intervals thereafter. Transient hypotension has occurred following rapid intravenous administration and the drug should be administered only by slow intravenous infusion, lasting at least 30–60 minutes. Patients of childbearing potential should be advised to avoid becoming pregnant during treatment. Should not be used in nursing mothers.

Administration: Intravenous. Administered as an IV infusion over at least a 30- to 60-minute period; should not be given by rapid IV injection. The concentrated solution of teniposide may extract the plasticizer DEHP from plastic equipment or devices; thus, solutions of the concentrate should be prepared in non-DEHP containers such as glass or polyolefin plastic bags or containers, and teniposide solutions should be administered with non-DEHP-containing IV administration sets. Concentrated solution must be diluted with either 5% Dextrose Injection or 0.9% Sodium Chloride Injection. Gloves should be worn when handling and preparing the solutions.

Preparations: Ampules, 50 mg/ml (teniposide for injection concentrate).

TENORETIC®, Combination of atenolol and chlorthalidone

TENORMIN®, see Atenolol

TENSILON®, see Edrophonium

TENUATE®, see Diethylpropion

TEPANIL®, see Diethylpropion

TERAZOL 3®; TERAZOL 7®, see Terconazole

TERAZOSIN HYDROCHLORIDE —Hytrin®

Antihypertensive agent.

Actions and Uses: An alpha-1-selective adrenergic receptor blocking agent that causes vasodilatation and a reduction in blood pressure. Indicated in the treatment of hypertension and can be used alone or in combination with other antihypertensive agents. Also indicated for the treatment of benign prostatic hyperplasia.

Warnings: May cause orthostatic hypotension, resulting in symptoms such as dizziness, lightheadedness, palpitations and, in more severe cases, syncope. Syncope has occurred most often in association with the first dose or first few doses of therapy. To reduce the likelihood of syncope, treatment should be initiated with a 1-mg dose of terazosin, given at bedtime. Patients should be informed of the possibility of syncope and other orthostatic symptoms, and advised to avoid driving or other hazardous tasks for 12 hours after the first dose, after a dosage increase, and after interruption of therapy when treatment is resumed. They should also be advised to sit or lie down when symptoms associated with orthostatic hypotension occur, and to be cautious when rising from a sitting or lying position. Other adverse reactions include weakness, tiredness, fatigue, drowsiness, blurred vision, nasal congestion, nausea, peripheral edema, and weight gain.

Administration: Oral daily at bedtime.

Preparations: Tablets 1, 2, 5, and 10 mg.

TERBINAFINE HYDROCHLORIDE —Lamisil®

Topical antifungal agent.

Actions and Uses: An allylamine derivative that exhibits a fungicidal action by inhibiting squalene epoxidase, a key enzyme in sterol biosynthesis in fungi. Indicated for the topical treatment of interdigital tinea pedis, plantar tinea pedis (moccassin type) tinea cruris, and tinea corporis caused by *Epidermophyton floccosum, Trichophyton mentagrophytes,* or *Trichophyton rubrum.* Orally indicated in treatment of Onchomycosis of the toenail and fingernail due to tinea unguium.

Warnings: Adverse reactions include irritation and burning. Patients should be advised to avoid the use of occlusive dressings unless otherwise directed by the physician. Oral formulation contraindicated with preexisting hepatic disease or renal impairment (Cr Cl < 50 ml/min). Disontinue if hepatobiliary dysfunction or progressive skin rash or severe neutropenia occurs.

Monitor CBC and liver functions.

Administration: Oral and topical.

Preparations: Tablets, 250 mg. Cream and topical solution, 1%.

TERBUTALINE SULFATE— Brethaire®, Brethine®, Bricanyl®

Bronchodilator.

Actions and Uses: Stimulates beta-adrenergic receptors. Indicated for bronchial asthma and for reversible bronchospasm that may occur in association with bronchitis and emphysema. Also used in management of preterm labor (tocolytic).

Warnings: May cause increased heart rate and palpitations, and should be used cautiously in patients with cardiovascular disorders, especially those associated with arrhythmias. Other adverse reactions include nervousness, tremor, headache, nausea, vomiting, sweating, and muscle cramps. Other sympathomimetic agents should not be used concurrently. Beta-adrenergic blocking agents and terbutaline may inhibit the effect of each other.

Administration: Oral, oral inhalation, and subcutaneous.

Preparations: Tablets, 2.5 and 5 mg. Metered dose inhaler (Brethaire). Ampules, 1 mg/ml.

TERCONAZOLE—Terazol 3®; Terazol 7®

Antifungal agent.

Actions and Uses: Indicated for the local treatment of vulvovaginal candidiasis.

Warnings: Adverse reactions include headache, and vulvovaginal burning, itching, or irritation. Use during the first trimester of pregnancy should be avoided. Base contained in the vaginal suppository formulation may interact with certain rubber or latex products, such as those used in vaginal contraceptive diaphragms; therefore, concurrent use is not recommended.

Administration: Vaginal. Vaginal cream is administered for 7 consecutive days and the vaginal suppositories for 3 consecutive days.

Preparations: Vaginal cream (Terazol 7), 0.4%; vaginal suppository (Terazol 3), 80 mg.

TERPIN HYDRATE

Expectorant most frequently used with codeine in an elixir formulation indicated for respiratory symptoms.

TERRAMYCIN®, see Oxytetracycline

TESLAC®, see Testolactone

TESSALON®, see Benzonatate

TESTODERM®, see Testosterone

TESTOLACTONE—Teslac®

Antineoplastic agent indicated as adjunctive therapy in the treatment of advanced or disseminated breast cancer in postmenopausal women.

Preparation: Tablets, 50 mg.

TESTOSTERONE—Androderm®, Testoderm®

Androgen indicated for use in male patients for replacement therapy for conditions associated with a deficiency or absence of endogenous testosterone. Transdermal system is indicated for primary hypogonadism and hypogonadotropic hypogonadism.

Preparations: Transdermal systems (Androderm), 2.5 and 5 mg, (Testoderm), 10 and 15 mg.

TESTOSTERONE CYPIONATE—Depo-Testosterone®

Longer-acting ester of testosterone administered intramuscularly.

Preparations: Vials (in oil), 50 mg/ml 100 mg/ml, and 200 mg/ml.

TESTOSTERONE ENANTHATE—Delatestryl®

Longer acting ester of testosterone administered intramuscularly.

Preparations: Vials (in oil), 100 mg/ml, and 200 mg/ml.

TESTOSTERONE PROPIONATE

Androgen indicated for intramuscular use in male patients for replacement therapy in conditions associated with a deficiency or absence of endogenous testosterone—primary hypogonadism, hypogonadotropic hypogonadism, and delayed puberty. Also used in women with advancing inoperable metastatic mammary cancer who are 1 to 5 years postmenopausal.

Preparations: Vials, 25 mg/ml, 50 mg/ml, and 100 mg/ml.

TETRACAINE HYDROCHLORIDE—Pontocaine®

Local anesthetic indicated for spinal anesthesia, for anesthesia of the nose and throat, for ocular disorders, and skin conditions.

Preparations: Ampules (for spinal anesthesia), 0.2%, 0.3%, 1%, and powder. Solution (for anesthesia of the nose and throat), 2%. Ophthalmic solution and ointment (as base), 0.5%. Cream, 1%. Ointment (as base), 0.5%.

TETRACYCLINE HYDROCHLORIDE—Achromycin V®, Actisite®, Panmycin®, Sumycin®

Tetracycline antibiotic.

Actions and Uses: Active against many gram-positive and gram-negative bacteria, mycoplasmal, chlamydial, and rickettsial organisms, and certain spirochetes. Indicated in the treatment of respiratory and urinary tract infections and a number of other types of infections. Is useful as adjunctive therapy in the management of severe acne. Also indicated (for use as a periodontal fiber) as an adjunct to scaling and root planing for reduction of pocket depth and bleeding on probing in patients with adult periodontitis.

Warnings: Use is best avoided during the last half of pregnancy and in childhood to the age of 8 years because of the risk of discoloration of the teeth. Adverse reactions include nausea, vomiting, diarrhea, rash, and fungal superinfections. May cause photosensitivity reactions and patients should be cautioned to limit their exposure to sunlight and ultraviolet light. Must be used with caution in patients with impaired renal function. Absorption may be reduced by antacids, iron, calcium, and zinc salts, and other metal-containing formulations and foods; the administration of tetracycline and one of these agents should be separated by an interval of at least 1 hour.

Administration: Oral and topical.

Preparations: Capsules and tablets, 250 and 500 mg. Oral suspension, 125 mg/5 ml. Ointment, 3%. Topical solution. Periodontal fiber (Actisite), 12.7 mg.

TETRAHYDROZOLINE HYDROCHLORIDE—Tyzine®, Visine®

Decongestant: Indicated for nasal use and for ophthalmic use to provide temporary relief of burning, irritation, and discomfort associated with certain ocular conditions.

Preparations: Nasal solution, 0.05% and 0.1%. Ophthalmic solution, 0.05%.

THAM®, see Tromethamine with electrolytes

THEELIN®, see Estrone

THEO-DUR®, see Theophylline

THEO-24®, see Theophylline

THEOPHYLLINE (see list of preparations below for trade names)

Bronchodilator.

Actions and Uses: A xanthine derivative

indicated for the relief and/or prevention of symptoms of bronchial asthma and for reversible bronchospasm associated with chronic bronchitis and emphysema.

Warnings: Adverse reactions include nausea, vomiting, diarrhea, headaches, irritability, restlessness, insomnia, palpitation, tachycardia, flushing, and hypotension.

Administration: Oral. Controlled-release formulations should not be chewed or crushed. A high-fat content meal may increase the rate and extent of absorption of theophylline from certain formulations (e.g., Theo-24); the labeling for individual formulations should be consulted for guidelines regarding administration in relationship to meals.

Preparations: Capsules and tablets (Elixophyllin®, Slo-Phyllin®), 50, 100, 125, 200, 225, 250, and 300 mg. Controlled-release capsules and tablets (Elixophyllin SR®, Slo-bid gyrocaps®, Theo-24®, Theo-Dur®, Theovent®, Uni-Dur®, Uniphyl®), 50, 100, 125, 200, 250, 300, 400, 450, 500, and 600 mg. Liquid(Elixophyllin®, Slo-Phyllin®), 80, 112.5, and 150 mg/15 ml.

THEOPHYLLINE CALCIUM SALICYLATE

Bronchodilator used in combination with other agents in the treatment of asthma and other respiratory conditions.

THEOPHYLLINE ETHYLENEDIAMINE, see Aminophylline

THEOPHYLLINE SODIUM GLYCINATE

Bronchodilator indicated for the relief of bronchial asthma and for reversible bronchospasm associated with chronic bronchitis and emphysema.

THEOVENT®, see Theophylline

THIABENDAZOLE—Mintezol®

Anthelmintic indicated for the treatment of trichinosis, cutaneous larva migrans, visceral larva migrans, strongyloidiasis. Is also effective in numerous other helmintic infestations.

Preparations: Chewable tablets, 500 mg. Suspension, 500 mg/5 ml.

THIAMINE HYDROCHLORIDE—Vitamin B_1

Vitamin indicated for the treatment and prevention of thiamine deficiency and prevention of Wernicke's encephalopathy.

Preparations: Tablets, 5, 10, 25, 50, 100, 250, and 500 mg. Ampules and vials, 100 mg/ml and 200 mg/ml.

THIAMYLAL SODIUM

Barbiturate anesthetic administered intravenously for induction of anesthesia, for supplementing other anesthetic agents, as anesthesia for short surgical procedures, and for inducing hypnotic states.

Preparations: Vials, 1, 5, and 10 g.

THIETHYLPERAZINE MALEATE—Norzine®, Torecan®

Phenothiazine antiemetic indicated for the relief of nausea and vomiting.

Preparations: Tablets, 10 mg. Suppositories, 10 mg. Ampules, 10 mg/2 ml.

THIMEROSAL—Merthiolate®

Antiseptic used for antisepsis of intact skin, treatment of contaminated wounds, and for preoperative and postoperative use.

Preparations: Solution and tincture, 1:1000. Aeropump tincture, 1:1000.

THIOGUANINE

Antineoplastic agent indicated for the

treatment of acute nonlymphocytic leukemias and chronic myelogenous leukemia.

Preparation: Tablets, 40 mg.

THIOLA®, see Tiopronin

THIOPENTAL SODIUM—Pentothal®

Barbiturate anesthetic administered intravenously for induction of anesthesia, for supplementing other anesthetic agents, as anesthesia for short surgical procedures, for inducing hypnotic states, for control of convulsive seizures, in certain neurosurgical patients with increased intracranial pressure, and for narcoanalysis and narcosynthesis in psychiatric disorders. Has also been used in the form of a rectal suspension when preanesthetic sedation or basal narcosis by the rectal route is desired.

Preparations: Vials and syringes, 250, 400, and 500 mg, 1, 2.5, and 5 g. Rectal suspension, 400 mg/g.

THIOPLEX®, see Thiotepa

THIORIDAZINE HYDROCHLORIDE—Mellaril®

Phenothiazine antipsychotic agent.

Actions and Uses: Indicated for (1) the management of manifestations of psychotic disorders, (2) the short-term treatment of moderate to marked depression with variable degrees of anxiety, (3) the treatment of multiple symptoms such as agitation and anxiety in geriatric patients, (4) the treatment of severe behavioral problems in children marked by combativeness and/or explosive hyperexcitable behavior, and (5) the short-term treatment of hyperactive children who show excessive motor activity with accompanying conduct disorders.

Warnings: Adverse reactions include drowsiness and other CNS effects; patients should be cautioned regarding activities such as driving and operating machinery, as well as interactions with other CNS-acting drugs including alcohol. Other adverse reactions include extrapyramidal symptoms, tardive dyskinesia, dry mouth, blurred vision, and dermatitis.

Administration: Oral.

Preparations: Tablets, 10, 15, 25, 50, 100, 150, and 200 mg. Oral solution (concentrate), 30 and 100 mg/ml. Oral suspension (as the base), 25 and 100 mg/5 ml.

THIOSULFIL FORTE®, see Sulfamethizole

THIOTEPA—Triethylenethiophosphoramide, Thioplex®

Antineoplastic agent administered parenterally in the palliative treatment of adenocarcinoma of the breast, adenocarcinoma of the ovary, and for controlling intracavitary effusions secondary to diffuse or localized neoplastic disease of various serosal cavities, superficial papillary carcinoma of the bladder, lymphosarcoma, and Hodgkin's disease.

Preparation: Vials, 15 mg.

THIOTHIXENE—Navane®

Antipsychotic agent indicated in the management of the manifestations of psychotic disorders.

Preparations: Capsules, 1, 2, 5, 10, and 20 mg. Concentrate (as the hydrochloride), 5 mg/ml.

THORAZINE®, see Chlorpromazine

3TC®, see Lamivudine

THROMBIN—Thrombinar®, Thrombostat®

Hemostatic agent indicated for topical use whenever oozing blood and minor bleeding from capillaries and small venules is accessible. Also used in conjunction with absorbable gelatin sponge for hemostasis in various types of surgery.

Preparations: Vials, 1,000, 5,000, 10,000, 20,000, and 50,000 units.

THROMBINAR®, see Thrombin

THROMBOSTAT®, see Thrombin

THYLLINE®, see dyphylline

THYMOL

Anti-infective included in combination with other agents in certain topical formulations. Has also been included in mouthwash formulations for its aromatic and antiseptic properties.

THYROID

Agent for thyroid replacement.

Actions and Uses: Thyroid hormone and is indicated as replacement therapy in patients with hypothyroidism, and as a pituitary thyroid stimulating hormone (TSH) suppressant in the treatment or prevention of various types of goiters.

Warnings: Must be used cautiously in patients with cardiovascular disorders and endocrine disorders such as diabetes. Adverse reactions include headache, nervousness, palpitations, tachycardia, and nausea.

Administration: Oral.

Preparations: Tablets, 15, 30, 60, 90, 120, 180, 240, and 300 mg.

THYROTROPIN—Thyroid stimulating hormone, TSH, Thytropar®

Used for diagnostic purposes

Preparations: Vials, 10 IU of thyrotropic activity.

THYROXINE, see Levothyroxine

THYTROPAR®, see Thyrotropin

TIAZAC®, see Diltiazem

TICAR®, see Ticarcillin

TICARCILLIN DISODIUM—Ticar®

Penicillin antibiotic.

Actions and Uses: Is bactericidal and is active against many gram-positive and gram-negative bacteria, including *Pseudomonas aeruginosa.* Is usually used in conjunction with an amino-glycoside antibiotic in the treatment of *Pseudomonas* infections.

Warnings: Contraindicated in patients with a history of allergic reaction to any of the penicillins. Adverse reactions include hypersensitivity reactions, gastrointestinal effects, bleeding manifestations, and hypokalemia. Disodium salt is utilized and the administration of high doses may cause problems in patients in whom sodium intake must be closely monitored.

Administration: Intravenous and intramuscular.

Preparations: Vials, 1, 3, 6, 20, and 30 g.

TICARCILLIN DISODIUM/CLAVULANATE POTASSIUM—Timentin®

Penicillin antibiotic with beta-lactamase inhibitor. Clavulanic acid inhibits beta-lactamase enzymes and protects ticarcillin from degradation by these enzymes; the spectrum of action of ticarcillin is extended to include additional bacteria.

Preparations: Vials, 3.1 and 3.2 g (representing 3 g of ticarcillin and 0.1 and 0.2 g of clavulanic acid, respectively).

TICLID®, see Ticlopidine

TICLOPIDINE HYDROCHLORIDE—Ticlid®

Antiplatelet agent.

Actions and Uses: Is a platelet aggregation inhibitor that is thought to act primarily by inhibiting the adenosine diphosphate (ADP) pathway for platelet aggregation. Indicated to reduce the risk of thrombotic stroke in patients who have experienced stroke warning signs [e.g., transient ischemic attacks (TIAs)], and in patients who have had a completed thrombotic stroke. Use should be reserved for patients who are intolerant to aspirin therapy, or in situations in which there is a risk of stroke but aspirin is not indicated.

Warnings: Contraindicated in the presence of hematopoietic disorders such as neutropenia or thrombocytopenia. Contraindicated in the presence of a hemostatic disorder or active pathologic bleeding, and in patients with severe hepatic disease. May cause neutropenia with a resultant increased risk of infection; complete blood counts and white cell differentials should be performed every 2 weeks starting from the second week to at least the end of the third month of therapy. Causes a prolongation of bleeding time and its use has been associated with bleeding complications (e.g., ecchymosis, epistaxis, hematuria, gastrointestinal bleeding); should be used with caution in patients who may be at risk of increased bleeding from trauma, surgery, or pathological conditions, and in patients who have lesions with a propensity to bleed (e.g., ulcers). Medication may be discontinued 10–14 days prior to elective surgery. Patients should be advised that it may take them longer than usual to stop bleeding. The concomitant use of aspirin, an anticoagulant, or fibrinolyt-ic agent with ticlopidine is best avoided. Other adverse reactions include diarrhea, nausea, dyspepsia, gastrointestinal pain, and rash. Signs and symptoms of jaundice have occurred infrequently and patients should be advised to inform their physicians if they observe yellowing of the skin or whites of the eyes, or consistent darkening in the color of the urine or lightening in the color of the stools.

Administration: Oral. Should be administered with food.

Preparation: Tablets, 250 mg.

TIGAN®, see Trimethobenzamide

TILADE®, see Nedocromil sodium

TILUDRONATE—Skelid®

Actions and Uses: Indicated in the treatment of Paget's disease. In vitro studies indicated that tiludronate acts primarily on bone through a mechanism involving inhibition of osteoclastic activity, probably through a reduction in the enzymatic and transport process that leads to resorption of the mineralized matrix. Use in patients with severe renal failure (CrCl < 30 ml/min) not recommended. Maintain adequae calcium and vitamin D intake. Use cautiously in patients with upper GI disease.

Warnings: Adverse reactions include GI disorders (e.g., nausea, diarrhea, dyspepsia), chest pain, edema, paresthesia, hyperparathyroidism, arthrosis, rhinitis, sinusitis, cataract, conjunctivitis, and glaucoma.

Administrations: Take with 6–8 oz. of plain (not mineral) water at least 2 hours before or after any other beverages, food, or medication. 400 mg once daily for 3 months. May retreat after a 3-month posttreatment evaluation period.

Preparations: Tablets, 240 mg (equivalent to 200 mg tiludronic acid).

TIMENTIN®, see Ticarcillin disodium/clavulanate potassium

TIMOLOL MALEATE—Betimol®, Blocadren®, Timoptic®, Timoptic-XE®

Antihypertensive agent and agent for glaucoma.

Actions and Uses: A nonselective beta-adrenergic blocking agent indicated in the treatment of hypertension, and to reduce cardiovascular mortality and the risk of reinfarction in patients who have survived the acute phase of a myocardial infarction. Also indicated for migraine headache prophylaxis. Also indicated for ophthalmic administration in the treatment of chronic open-angle glaucoma, aphakic glaucoma, and secondary glaucoma.

Warnings: Contraindicated in patients with bronchial asthma or severe chronic obstructive pulmonary disease, sinus bradycardia, second- and third-degree AV block, overt cardiac failure, and cardiogenic shock. Adverse reactions include fatigue, dizziness, bradycardia, cold hands and feet, and, when administered in the ophthalmic dosage form, ocular irritation. Use is best avoided in patients with bronchospastic diseases, and therapy in diabetic patients must be closely monitored.

Administration: Oral and ophthalmic. Patients should be cautioned about the interruption or discontinuation of therapy; exacerbation of angina pectoris has occurred following the abrupt cessation of therapy and, when therapy is to be discontinued, the dosage should be gradually reduced over a period of 1 to 2 weeks.

Preparations: Tablets, 5, 10, and 20 mg. Ophthalmic solution, 0.25% and 0.5%. Ophthalmic gel (Timoptic-XE®), 0.25% and 0.5%.

TIMOPTIC®, see Timolol maleate

TIMOPTIC-XE®, see Timolol maleate

TINACTIN®, see Tolnaftate

TINDAL®, see Acetophenazine

TINVER®, see Sodium thiosulfate

TIOCONAZOLE—Vagistat®

Antifungal agent.

Actions and Uses: An imidazole antifungal agent indicated for use as a local single-dose treatment of vulvovaginal

candidiasis.

Warnings: Adverse reactions include burning and itching.

Administration: Vaginal

Preparations: Vaginal ointment, 6.5%.

TIOPRONIN—Thiola®

Agent for kidney stones.

Actions and Uses: Indicated for the prevention of cystine (kidney) stone formation in patients with severe homozygous cystinuria with urinary cystine greater than 500 mg/day, who are resistant to treatment with conservative measures of high fluid intake, alkali and diet modification, or who have had adverse reactions to penicillamine.

Warnings: Contraindicated during pregnancy. Adverse reactions include rash, pruritus, drug fever, lupus erythematosus-like effects, reduction in taste perception, and wrinkling and friability of the skin. May cause gastrointestinal, pulmonary, neurologic, renal, and hematologic reactions.

Administration: Oral. Should be given in divided doses 3 times a day at least one hour before or 2 hours after meals.

Preparation: Tablets, 100 mg.

TISSUE PLASMINOGEN ACTIVATOR, see Alteplase, recombinant

TITANIUM DIOXIDE

Sunscreen used topically in cream, lotion, and ointment formulations.

TIZANIDINE—Zanaflex®

Reduces muscle apasticity and is indicated in acute and intermittent management of increased skeletal muscle tone associated with spasticity.

Warnings: Use cautiously in impaired hepatic or renal function, in cardiovascular disease, and the elderly. Monitor ophthalmic and liver function (aminotransferases at baseline, 1, 3, 6 months and periodically thereafter). Adverse reactions include sedation, dry mouth, somnolence, asthenia, dizziness, constipation, elevated liver enzymes, vomiting, speech disorders, blurred vision, dyskinesia, nervousness, pharyngitis, hypotension (including orthostatic), hallucinations, and psychosis.

Administrations: Recommended dosage: 2–4 mg 3 times/day. Usual intial dose is 4 mg. May increase by 2–4 mg as needed every 6–8 hours to a maximum of 3 doses in 24 hours. Maximum dose is 36 mg/day. Reduce dose in renal impairment (CrCl < 25 ml/min).

Preparations: Tablets, 4 mg (scored).

TMP-SMX, see Trimethoprim-sulfamethoxazole

TOBRAMYCIN SULFATE—Nebcin®, Tobrex®

Aminoglycoside antibiotic.

Actions and Uses: Indicated for the parenteral treatment of serious infections caused by gram-negative bacteria including *Pseudomonas aeruginosa.* Is also effective in the treatment of staphylococcal infections. Has also been used topically in the treatment of ocular infections.

Warnings: May cause nephrotoxicity, ototoxicity, and neurotoxicity, and the concurrent or serial use of other nephrotoxic or ototoxic agents should be avoided.

Administration: Intravenous, intramuscular, and ophthalmic.

Preparations: Vials and syringes, 20 mg/2 ml, 60 mg/1.5 ml, 80 mg/2 ml., and 1.2 g. Ophthalmic solution and ointment, 0.3%.

TOBREX®, see Tobramycin

TOCAINIDE HYDROCHLORIDE—Tonocard®

Antiarrhythmic agent indicated for the suppression of symptomatic ventricular arrhythmias, including frequent premature ventricular contractions, unifocal or multifocal, couplets, and ventricular tachycardia.

Preparations: Tablets, 400 and 600 mg.

TOFRANIL®, see Imipramine

TOLAZAMIDE—Tolinase®

Sulfonylurea hypoglycemic agent.

Actions and Uses: Indicated as an adjunct to diet to lower the blood glucose in patients with non-insulin-dependent diabetes mellitus whose hyperglycemia cannot be controlled by diet alone.

Warnings: May cause hypoglycemia, and patients should be advised to contact their physician if symptoms of hypoglycemia develop. Adverse reactions include nausea, heartburn, pruritus, and erythema. Oral hypoglycemic agents have been suggested to be associated with increased cardiovascular mortality as compared with treatment by diet alone or diet plus insulin.

Administration: Oral.

Preparations: Tablets, 100, 250, and 500 mg.

TOLAZOLINE HYDROCHLORIDE—Priscoline®

Peripheral vasodilator indicated for intravenous use in the treatment of persistent pulmonary hypertension of the newborn when systemic arterial oxygenation cannot be satisfactorily maintained by usual supportive care.

Preparation: Ampules, 25 mg/ml.

TOLBUTAMIDE—Orinase®

Sulfonylurea hypoglycemic agent indicated as an adjunct to diet to lower the blood glucose in patients with non-insulin-dependent diabetes whose hyperglycemia cannot be satisfactorily controlled by diet alone.

Preparations: Tablets, 250 and 500 mg.

TOLECTIN®, see Tolmetin

TOLINASE®, see Tolazamide

TOLMETIN SODIUM—Tolectin®, Tolectin DS®

Nonsteroidal anti-inflammatory drug.

Actions and Uses: Inhibits prostaglandin synthesis and is indicated for the treatment of rheumatoid arthritis, juvenile rheumatoid arthritis, and osteoarthritis.

Warnings: Should not be given to patients in whom aspirin or another NSAID causes asthma, rhinitis, urticaria, or other allergic-type reactions. May cause GI effects, and use should be avoided in patients with active GI tract disease and closely monitored in patients with a previous history of such disorders. Other adverse reactions include headache, weakness, edema, elevated blood pressure, weight changes, and skin irritation. Effect may be reduced by sodium bicarbonate.

Administration: Oral. Bioavailability is reduced by food or milk and is best administered apart from meals.

Preparations: Tablets and capsules, 200, 400, and 600 mg.

TOLNAFTATE—Tinactin®

Antifungal agent used topically in the treatment of superficial fungal infections of the skin.

Preparations: Cream, powder, solution, gel, aerosol powder, and aerosol liquid, 1%.

TONOCARD®, see Tocainide

TOPAMAX®, see Topiramate

TOPICORT®, see Desoximetasone

TOPIRAMATE—Topamax®

Anticonvulsant indicated as adjunctive therapy for partial onset seizures in adults.

Warnings: Avoid abrupt cessation as this may precipitate seizures. Use cautiously in patients with hepatic or renal impairment. The risk of kidney stone formation is about 2–4 times that of untreated population. This may be reduced by increasing fluid intake. Adverse reactions include somnolence, dizziness, ataxia, speech disorders, psychomotor slowing, nervousness, paresthesia, nystagmus, tremor, fatigue, confusion, decreased weight, language or mood problems, anorexia, and anxiety.

Administrations: Initially 50 mg/day, titrate by 50 mg/day at 1 week intervals to target dose of 200 mg twice daily. Usual maximimum dose is 1.6 g/day. Halve dose in renal impairment (CrCl < 70 ml/min) and assess for slower titration.

Preparations: Tablets 25, 100, and 200 mg.

TOPOTECAN HYDROCHLORIDE—Hycamtin®

Antineoplastic.

Actions and Uses: Used in the treatment of patients with metastatic ovarian cancer after failure of initial or subsequent chemotherapy.

Warnings: Bone marrow suppression (primarily neutropenia) is the dose-limiting toxicity of topotecan. Administer only to patients with adequate bone marrow reserves (baseline neutrophil counts of at least 1500 cells/mm^3 and platelet count of 100,000 mm^3). Adverse effects include neutropenia, thrombocytopenia, and anemia.

Administration: IV infusion over 30 minutes daily for 5 consecutive days, starting on day 1 of a 21-day course. A minimum of 4 courses is recommended because median response time in clinical trials is 9–12 weeks. Usual dose: metastatic ovalian cancer: 1.5 $mg/m^2/day$ for 5 days.

Preparations: Powder for injection, 4 mg.

TOPROL XL®, see Metoprolol succinate

TORADOL®, see Ketorolac tromethamine

TORECAN®, see Thiethylperazine

TORNALATE®, see Bitolterol

TORSEMIDE—Demadex®

Diuretic.

Actions and Uses: Is a loop diuretic that is indicated for the treatment of edema associated with congestive heart failure, renal disease, or hepatic disease. Is also indicated for the treatment of hypertension and may be used alone or in combination with other antihypertensive agents.

Warnings: Contraindicated in patients who are hypersensitive to any sulfonylurea derivative. Is also contraindicated in patients who are anuric. Adverse reactions include excessive urination, headache, dizziness, and rhinitis. May cause electrolyte imbalance and periodic monitoring of serum potassium and other electrolytes is advised.

Administration: Oral and intravenous. When given intravenously, should be administered slowly over a period of two minutes.

Preparations: Tablets, 5, 10, 20, and 100 mg. Ampules, 20 and 50 mg.

TOTACILLIN®, see Ampicillin

TPA, see Alteplase, recombinant

TRACRIUM®, see Atracurium besylate

TRAMADOL HYDROCHLORIDE—Ultram®

Actions and Uses: Analgesic indicated for the management of moderate to moderately severe pain.

Warnings: Contraindicated in patients with alcohol, hypnotics, centrally acting analgesics, opioids, or psychotropic drugs. Adverse reactions include constipation, nausea, vomiting, dizziness, somnolence, central nervous system (CNS) stimulation, asthenia, and headache. Patients should be cautioned about driving or operating machinery. May increase the risk of seizures in patients with epilepsy. Unlikely to produce dependence and is not classified as a controlled substance.

Administration: Oral.

Preparations: Tablets, 50 mg.

TRANCOPAL®, see Chlormezanone

TRANDATE®, see Labetalol

TRANDOLAPRIL—Mavik®

Ace Inhibitor.

Actions and Uses: Inhibits angiotension converting enzyme (ACE). Used in treatment of hypertension as monotherapy or as an adjunct to other antihypertensive agents. Also indicated in stabilized patients after M.I. who have LV systolic dysfunction or DHF symptoms

Warnings: Do not use in patients with a history of Ace inhibitor - associated angioedema. Monitor for neutropenia in collagen, vascular, and/or renal disease. Monitor for hyperkalemia in diabetes. Use cautiously in patients with renal impairment, cardiovascular or cerebrovascular disease, or salt/ volume depletion. Adverse reactions include cough, dizziness, and diarrhea. Discontinue if laryngeal edema, angioedema, or jaundice occurs. (Black patients may have a higher risk of angioedema than non-Black patients.)

Administration: Usual range is 2–4 mg once daily to a maximum of 8 mg/day which may be given in two divided doses. Follow manufacturer's dosaging guidelines.

Preparations: Tablets, 1 mg (scored), 2 and 4 mg.

TRANEXAMIC ACID—Cyklokapron®

Antifibrinolytic agent.

Actions and Uses: Indicated in patients with hemophilia for short-term use (2 to 8 days) to reduce or prevent hemorrhage and to reduce the need for replacement therapy during and following tooth extraction.

Warnings: Contraindicated in (1) patients with acquired defective color vision, because this prohibits measuring one endpoint that should be followed as a measure of toxicity; and (2) patients with subarachnoid hemorrhage. Visual abnormalities have been experienced by some patients and, for patients who are to be treated continually for longer than several days, an ophthalmological examination is advised before commencing and at regular intervals during the course of treatment. Other adverse reactions include nausea, vomiting, diarrhea, and giddiness. Hypotension has been observed when intravenous injection is too rapid, and the solution should not be injected more rapidly than 1 ml per minute.

Administration: Oral and intravenous.

Preparations: Tablets, 500 mg. Ampules, 100 mg/ml.

TRANSDERM-NITRO®, see Nitroglycerin

TRANSDERM-SCOjP®, see Scopolamine

TRANXENE®, see Clorazepate

TRANYLCYPROMINE SULFATE—Parnate®

Monoamine oxidase inhibitor antidepressant indicated for the treatment of major depressive episode without melancholia.

Warnings: Hypertension or hypotension, coma, convulsions and death may occur with opioids (avoid use of meperidine within 14–21 days of MAO inhibitor therapy–decrease initial dose of other agents to 25% of usual dose). Serious potentially fatal adverse reactions may occur with concurrent use of other antidepressants. Avoid using within two weeks of each other (wait 5 weeks from end of fluoxetine therapy).

Preparation: Tablets, 10 mg.

TRASYLOL®, see Aprotinin

TRAVASE®, see Sutilains

TRAVERT®, see Invert sugar

TRAZODONE HYDROCHLORIDE—Desyrel®

Antidepressant.

Actions and Uses: Indicated for the treatment of depression.

Warnings: Is not recommended for use during the initial recovery phase of myocardial infarction. Adverse reactions include drowsiness and other CNS effects; patients should be cautioned regarding activities such as driving and operating machinery, as well as interactions with other CNS-acting drugs including alcohol. May cause priapism, and patients with prolonged or inappropriate penile erection should discontinue the drug and consult with the physician. Other adverse reactions include dry mouth, blurred vision, hypotension, nausea, and vomiting.

Administration: Oral.

Preparations: Tablets, 50, 100, 150, and 300 mg.

TRECATOR-SC®, see Ethionamide

TRENTAL®, see Pentoxifylline

TRETINOIN—Retinoic acid, vitamin A acid, Avita®, Renova®, Retin-A®

Agent for acne.

Actions and Uses: A vitamin A analog indicated for topical application in the treatment of acne.

Warnings: Skin may become excessively red, edematous, blistered, or crusted in some patients. May increase susceptibility to sunlight and patients should be advised to minimize exposure to sunlight, including sunlamps.

Administration: Topical.

Preparations: Cream, 0.025%, 0.05%, and 0.1%. Solution, 0.05%. Gel, 0.01% and 0.025%. Microspheres aqueous gel, 0.1%. Capsule, 10 and 25 mg.

TREXAN®, trade name formerly used for naltrexone

TRIACETIN—Glyceryl triacetate

Antifungal agent indicated for topical use in the treatment of athlete's foot and other superficial fungal infections.

Preparation: Cream, 25%.

TRIAMCINOLONE—Aristocort®, Kenacort®

Corticosteroid indicated in a wide range of endocrine, rheumatic, allergic, dermatologic, respiratory, hematologic, neoplastic, and other disorders.

Preparations: Tablets, 1, 2, 4, and 8 mg.

TRIAMCINOLONE ACETONIDE—Aristocort®, Azmacort®, Kenalog®, Nasacort®, Nasacort AQ®

Preparations: Vials (for intramuscular, intra-articular, intrabursal, and intradermal injection), 10 mg/ml and 40 mg/ml. Aerosol (for inhalation), 100 μg/actuation (Azmacort®). Cream and ointment, 0.025%, 0.1%, and 0.5%. Lotion, 0.025% and 0.1%. Aerosol (for topical use). Nasal spray, 55 μg/actuation (Nasacort®).

TRIAMCINOLONE DIACETATE—Aristocort®, Kenacort®

Preparations: Syrup, 2 mg/5 ml and 4 mg/5 ml. Vials (for intramuscular, intra-articular, intrasynovial, and intralesional injection), 25 mg/ml and 40 mg/ml.

TRIAMCINOLONE HEXACETONIDE—Aristospan®

Preparations: Vials (for intra-articular, intralesional, and sublesional injection), 5 mg/ml and 20 mg/ml.

TRIAMTERENE—Dyrenium®

Diuretic.

Actions and Uses: A potassium-sparing diuretic indicated in the treatment of edema associated with congestive heart failure, cirrhosis of the liver, and the nephrotic syndrome; also used in steroid-induced edema, idiopathic edema, and edema due to secondary hyperaldosteronism.

Warnings: Contraindicated in patients with anuria, severe hepatic or renal disease, or preexisting elevated serum potassium levels. Should not be used in patients receiving another potassium-sparing diuretic or potassium salts or supplements.

Administration: Oral.

Preparations: Capsules, 50 and 100 mg.

TRIAVIL®, Combination of amitriptyline and perphenazine

TRIAZOLAM—Halcion®

Benzodiazepine hypnotic.

Actions and Uses: A CNS depressant indicated in the management of insomnia.

Warnings: Contraindicated during pregnancy. Adverse reactions include residual sedation, amnesic effects, and other CNS effects upon awakening; patients should be cautioned regarding activities such as driving and operating machinery, as well as interactions with other CNS-acting drugs including alcohol. Can cause dependence and is included in Schedule IV.

Administration: Oral.

Preparations: Tablets, 0.125 and 0.25 mg.

TRICHLOROACETIC ACID

Cauterizing agent applied topically to warts and to debride callus tissue.

TRICHLORMETHIAZIDE—Metahydrin®, Naqua®

Thiazide diuretic indicated as adjunctive therapy in edema and in the management of hypertension.

Preparations: Tablets, 2 and 4 mg.

TRIDESILON®, see Desonide

TRIDIL®, see Nitroglycerin

TRIDIONE®, see Trimethadione

TRIENTINE HYDROCHLORIDE—Syprine®

Agent for Wilson's disease.

Actions and Uses: A chelating agent indicated in the treatment of patients with Wilson's disease who are intolerant of penicillamine.

Warnings: Adverse reactions include fever, skin eruption, and iron deficiency anemia. Mineral supplements should usually not be administered concurrently because they may reduce the absorption of trientine. Should be administered at least 1 hour before or 2 hours after meals and at least 1 hour apart from any other drug, food, or milk.

Administration: Oral.

Preparation: Capsules, 250 mg.

TRIETHYLENETHIOPHOSPHORAMIDE, see Thiotepa

TRIFLUOPERAZINE HYDROCHLORIDE—Stelazine®

Phenothiazine antipsychotic agent indicated for the manifestations of psychotic disorders.

Preparations: Tablets, 1, 2, 5, and 10

mg. Oral concentrate, 10 mg/ml. Vials, 2 mg/ml.

TRIFLUPROMAZINE HYDROCHLORIDE—Vesprin®

Phenothiazine antipsychotic agent and antiemetic indicated for parenteral use for the manifestations of psychotic disorders, and for the control of severe nausea and vomiting.

Preparations: Vials, 10 mg/ml and 20 mg/ml.

TRIFLURIDINE—Viroptic®

Antiviral agent indicated for ophthalmic use for the treatment of primary keratoconjunctivitis and recurrent epithelial keratitis due to *Herpes simplex* virus, types 1 and 2.

Preparation: Ophthalmic solution, 1%.

TRIHEXYPHENIDYL HYDROCHLORIDE—Artane®

Antiparkinson agent indicated for the treatment of parkinsonism and the management of drug-induced extrapyramidal reactions.

Preparations: Tablets, 2 and 5 mg. Controlled-release capsules, 5 mg. Elixir, 2 mg/5 ml.

TRIIODOTHYRONINE, see Liothyronine

TRILAFON®, see Perphenazine

TRILISATE®, see Choline magnesium trisalicylate

TRIMEPRAZINE TARTRATE—Temaril®

Phenothiazine antihistamine indicated for the treatment of pruritic symptoms in a number of allergic and nonallergic conditions.

Preparations: Tablets, 2.5 mg. Controlled-release capsules, 5 mg. Syrup, 2.5 mg/5 ml.

TRIMETHADIONE—Tridione®

Anticonvulsant indicated for the control of petit mal seizures that are refractory to treatment with other drugs.

Preparations: Tablets, 150 mg. Capsules, 300 mg.

TRIMETHOBENZAMIDE HYDROCHLORIDE—Tigan®

Antiemetic indicated for the control of nausea and vomiting.

Preparations: Capsules, 100 and 250 mg. Suppositories, 200 mg. Vials and syringes, 100mg/ml.

TRIMETHOPRIM—Proloprim®, Trimpex®

Antibacterial indicated in the treatment of urinary tract infections.

Preparations: Tablets, 100 and 200 mg.

TRIMETHOPRIM—SULFAMETHOX-AZOLE—TMP-SMX, Cotrimoxazole, Bactrim®, Septra®

Anti-infective agent.

Actions and Uses: Combined actions of the 2 agents result in a synergistic action against many microorganisms. Is active against many gram-positive and gram-negative bacteria as well as certain other organisms. Indications include urinary tract infections, acute otitis media, acute exacerbations of chronic bronchitis, shigellosis, treatment and prophylaxis of *Pneumocystis carinii* pneumonitis, and the treatment of travelers' diarrhea in adults due to susceptible strains of enterotoxigenic *E. coli.* Is also useful in a number of other infections including prostatic infections.

Warnings: Should not be used in

pregnancy at term or during the nursing period. Adverse reactions include nausea, vomiting, rash, and urticaria. Since serious reactions such as the Stevens-Johnson syndrome have occurred in some individuals, therapy should be discontinued at the first appearance of skin rash or other adverse effects.

Administration: Oral and intravenous.

Preparations: Tablets, 80/400 and 160/800 mg. Suspension, 40/200 mg/5 ml. Ampules and vials, 16/80 mg/ml.

TRIMETREXATE GLUCURONATE—NeuTrexin®

Anti-infective agent.

Actions and Uses: Is a structural analog of folic acid. Exhibits a folic acid antagonist (antifolate) action that leads to cell death of certain microorganisms such as *Pneumocystis carinii* that require folate metabolism for continued cell viability. Indicated with concurrent leucovorin administration (leucovorin protection) as alternative therapy for the treatment of moderate-to-severe *Pneumocystis carinii* pneumonia in immunocompromised patients, including patients with AIDS, who are intolerant of, or are refractory to tri- methoprim/ sulfamethoxazole (TMP/ SMX) therapy or for whom TMP/SMX is contraindicated.

Warnings: Contraindicated in patients who are hypersensitive to the drug, methotrexate, or leucovorin. It is essential that leucovorin be used concurrently to reduce the risk of bone marrow suppression, oral and gastrointestinal mucosal ulceration, and renal and hepatic dysfunction. It is recommended that blood tests be performed at least twice a week to assess absolute neutrophil counts and platelets, as well as renal function (serum creatinine) and hepatic function (AST, ALT, alkaline phosphatase). Adverse reactions include neutropenia, thrombocytopenia, anemia, increased AST and ALT, fever, rash, pruritus, nausea, and vomiting. It is recommended that zidovudine not be used during the period of trimetrexate therapy. May cause fetal harm if administered during pregnancy.

Administration: Intravenous. Administered once daily by IV infusion over 60–90 minutes. Leucovorin must be administered daily (every 6 hours) during treatment with trimetrexate and for 72 hours past the last dose of trimetrexate. The recommended course of treatment is 21 days of trimetrexate and 24 days of leucovorin. Trimetrexate must not be reconstituted or mixed with solutions containing either chloride ion or leucovorin because precipitation occurs instantly. The intravenous line must be flushed thoroughly with at least 10 ml of 5% Dextrose Injection before and after administering trimetrexate.

Prepartion: Vials, 25 mg trimetrexate.

TRIMIPRAMINE MALEATE—Surmontil®

Tricyclic antidepressant indicated for the relief of symptoms of depression.

Preparations: Capsules, 25, 50, and 100 mg.

TRIMOX®, see Amoxicillin

TRIMPEX®, see Trimethoprim

TRINALIN®, Combination of azatidine and pseudoephedrine

TRIOSTAT®, see Liothyronine

TRIOXSALEN—Trisoralen®

Photoactive agent indicated for repigmentation of idiopathic vitiligo, enhancing pigmentation, and increasing tolerance to sunlight in blond persons and those with fair complexions who suffer painful reactions when exposed to sunlight.

Preparation: Tablets, 5 mg.

TRIPELENNAMINE—PBZ®

Antihistamine indicated for the management of allergic disorders.

Preparations: Tablets (as the hydrochloride), 25 and 50 mg. Controlled-release tablets (as the hydrochloride), 100 mg. Elixir (as the citrate), equivalent to 25 mg of the hydrochloride/5 ml.

TRIPLE SULFAS, see Trisulfapyrimidines

TRIPROLIDINE HYDROCHLORIDE

Antihistamine used in combination with pseudoephedrine

TRISORALEN®, see Trioxsalen

TRISULFAPYRIMIDINES—Triple sulfas

Anti-infective agents (sulfadiazine, sulfamerazine, sulfamethazine) indicated in the treatment of infections caused by susceptible organisms.

Preparations: Tablets, 500 mg. Suspension, 500 mg/5 ml.

TRITEC®—Combination of ranitidine and bismuth citrate.

TROBICIN®, see Spectinomycin

TROGLITAZONE—Rezulin®

Antidiabetic (insulin resistance reducer) *agent* indicated in NIDDM patients on insulin whose hyperglycemia is inadequately controlled despite insulin therapy over 30 units/day given as multiple injections. Troglitazone lowers blood glucose by improving target cell response to insulin.

Warnings: Not for treating IDDM or diabetic ketoacidosis. May increase risk of hypoglycemia. Monitor glucose and reduce insulin dose if needed. Adverse reactions include asthenia, dizziness, GI disturbances, and reversible increases in serum transaminases.

Administrations: Initially 200 mg once daily with food. May increase after 2–4 weeks to usual dose of 400 mg once daily . Maximum dose is 600 mg/day. Reduce insulin dose by 10–25% when fasting blood glucose decreases to less than 120 mg/dl. Adjust insulin dosing further if needed.

Preparations: Tablets, 200 mg and 400 mg.

TROLAMINE SALICYLATE—Aspercreme®, Myoflex®

Salicylate analgesic indicated for topical use for the temporary relief of minor aches and pains of muscles and joints. Also used as a topical adjunct in arthritis.

Preparation: Cream, 10%.

TROLEANDOMYCIN—Tao®

Antibiotic indicated for infections caused by susceptible gram-positive bacteria.

Preparation: Capsules, 250 mg.

TROMETHAMINE—Tham®

Alkalinizing agent indicated for parenteral use for the prevention and correction of systemic acidosis in selected patients.

Preparation: Bottles, 18 g/500 ml.

TRONOLANE®, see Pramoxine

TRONOTHANE®, see Pramoxine

TROPICAMIDE—Mydriacyl®

Anticholinergic agent indicated for ophthalmic use to provide mydriasis and cycloplegia for diagnostic purposes.

Preparations: Ophthalmic solutions, 0.5% and 1%.

TRUSOPT®, see Dorzolamide hydrochloride

TRYPSIN

Proteolytic enzyme used in combination with other agents for enzymatic debridement and to promote normal healing.

TUBOCURARINE CHLORIDE—Curare

Nondepolarizing neuromuscular blocking agent indicated as an adjunct to anesthesia to induce skeletal muscle relaxation.

Preparation: Vials, 3 mg/ml.

TUMS®, see Calcium carbonate

TUSSI-ORGANIDIN®, Combination of codeine and iodinated glycerol

TYLENOL®, see Acetaminophen

TYLOX®, Combination of oxycodone and acetaminophen

TYZINE®, see Tetrahydrozoline

U

UCEPHAN®, see Sodium benzoate and sodium phenylacetate

ULTANE®, see Sevoflurane

ULTRA-LENTE INSULIN, see Insulin

ULTRAM®, see Tramadol hydrochloride

ULTRAVATE®, see Halobetasol propionate

UNASYN®, see Ampicillin sodium/sulbactam sodium

UNDECYLENIC ACID AND SALTS—Desenex®

Antifungal agent applied topically in the management of superficial fungal infections.

Preparations: Powder, cream, ointment, liquid, foam, and soap.

UNI-DUR® , see Theophylline

UNIPEN®, see Nafcillin

UNIPHYL®, see Theophylline

UNIRETIC®, Combination agent of morxipril hel and hydrochlorothiazide (ACE inhibitor and diuretic)

UNISOM®, see Doxylamine

UNIVASC®, see Moexipril hydrochloride

URACIL MUSTARD

Antineoplastic agent indicated for the treatment of chronic lymphocytic leukemia, non-Hodgkin's lymphomas, chronic myelogenous leukemia, polycythemia vera, and mycosis fungoides.

Preparation: Capsules, 1 mg.

UREA—Carbamide, Aquacare®,Ureaphil®

Osmotic agent administered intravenously to reduce intraocular pressure, and to reduce intracranial pressure in the control of cerebral edema. Also used topically to promote hydration and removal of excess keratin in dry skin and hyperkeratotic conditions.

Preparations: Bottles (for intravenous use), 40 g. Cream, 2%, 10%, 20%, 30%, and 40%. Lotion, 2%, 10%, 15%, and 25%.

UREA PEROXIDE, see Carbamide peroxide

UREAPHIL®, see Urea

URECHOLINE®, see Bethanechol

URISPAS®, see Flavoxate

UROCIT-K®, see Potassium citrate

UROFOLLITROPIN—Metrodin®

Gonadotropin administered intramuscularly and given sequentially with human chorionic gonadotropin for the induction of ovulation in selected patients with polycystic ovarian disease.

Preparation: Ampules, 0.83 mg.

UROKINASE—Abbokinase®

Thrombolytic enzyme indicated for parenteral use in the management of pulmonary embolism and coronary artery thrombosis. Also used for the restoration of patency to intravenous catheters.

Preparation: Vials, 250,000 IU.

URSODIOL—Actigall®

Gallstone solubilizing agent.

Actions and Uses: A bile acid that decreases hepatic synthesis and secretion of cholesterol. Used for dissolving gallstones and is indicated for patients with radiolucent, noncalcified gallbladder stones less than 20 mm in greatest diameter in whom elective cholecystectomy would be undertaken except for the presence of increased surgical risk due to systemic disease, advanced age, idiosyncratic reaction to general anesthesia, or for those patients who refuse surgery. Prevention of gallstone formation in obese patients experiencing rapid weight loss.

Warnings: Contraindicated in patients with a history of allergy to bile acids, chronic liver disease, or with gallstones of a type (e.g., calcified) against which ursodiol is not active. Adverse reactions include diarrhea. May cause hepatotoxicity and patients should have liver function tests performed. Choles-tyramine, colestipol, and aluminum-containing antacids may reduce the absorption and efficacy of ursodiol; therefore, doses should be separated from doses of these other medications by as long an interval as possible.

Administration: Oral. Therapy is usually continued for 6 to 24 months.

Preparation: Capsules, 300 mg.

UTICORT®, see Betamethasone benzoate

V

VAGISTAT®, see Tioconazole

VALACYCLOVIR—Valtrex®

Actions and Uses: Antiviral agent indicated for the treatment of herpes zoster (shingles) in immunocompetent adults. Also used for initial episodes and recurrent genital herpes.

Warnings: Thrombotic thrombocytopenic purpura (TTP)/hemolytic uremic syndrome (HUS) has been reported in patients with advanced human immunodeficiency virus (HIV) disease and also in bone marrow transplant and in renal transplant recipients; this reaction has not been reported in immunocompetent patients and valacyclovir is not indicated for the treatment of immunocompromised patients. Other adverse reactions include headache and nausea.

Administration: Oral.

Preparations: Capsules, 500 mg.

VALISONE®, see Betamethasone valerate

VALIUM®, see Diazepam

VALPROIC ACID—Depacon®, Depakene®
DIVALPROEX SODIUM—Depakote®

Anticonvulsant indicated for use in the treatment of simple (petit mal) and complex absence seizures. Also used adjunctively in patients with multiple seizure types which include absence seizures. Also indicated for the treatment of manic episodes associated with bipolar disorder and prophylaxis against migraine headaches.

Preparations: Capsules (as valproic acid), 250 mg. Syrup (as sodium valproate), 250 mg/5 ml. Enteric-coated tablets (divalproex sodium—representing a stable coordination compound comprised of sodium valproate and valproic acid in a 1:1 molar relationship), 125, 250, and 500 mg. Sprinkle capsules (divalproex sodium), 125 mg, 100 mg/ml solution for IV infusion.

VALRELEASE®, see Diazepam

VALSARTAN—Diovan®

Angiotension II receptor antagonist indicated in the treatment of hypertension as mono or combination therapy.

Warnings: Contraindicated in pregnancy, hyperaldosteronism, and biliary cirrhosis. Correct hypovolemia before beginning therapy or monitor closely. Use cautiously in severe CHF, renal artery stenosis, hepatic dysfunction or severe renal impairment. Adverse reactions include viral infection, fatigue, and abdominal pain. In clinical studies comparing valsartan to ACE inhibitors the incidence of dry cough was significantly greater in the ACE inhibitor group.

Administrations: Initially 80 mg once daily, after two to four weeks may increase to 160 mg or 320 mg once daily. Or, diuretic may be added (this has a greater effect than increasing dose above 80 mg). Clinical studies suggest valsartan's antihypertensive effects are independent of age, gender, and race.

Preparations: Capsules, 80 mg and 160 mg.

VALTREX®, see Valacyclovir

VANCENASE®, see Beclomethasone dipropionate

VANCENASE AQ®, see Beclomethasone dipropionate

VANCERIL®, see Beclomethasone dipropionate

VANCOCIN®, see Vancomycin

VANCOLED®, see Vancomycin

VANCOMYCIN HYDROCHLORIDE—Lyphocin®, Vancocin®, Vancoled®

Antibiotic used primarily for the intravenous treatment of staphylococcal infections. Also used orally for the treatment of staphylococcal enterocolitis and antibiotic-associated pseudomembranous colitis produced by *Clostridium difficile.*

Preparations: Vials, 500 mg. Capsules, 125 and 250 mg. Powder for oral solution, 1 and 10 g when reconstituted.

VANSIL®, see Oxamniquine

VANTIN®, see Cefpodoxime proxetil

VASCOR®, see Bepridil hydrochloride

VASERETIC®, Combination of enalapril and hydrochlorothiazide

VASODILAN®, see Isoxsuprine

VASOPRESSIN—Pitressin®

Hormone indicated for parenteral use in the prevention and treatment of postoperative abdominal distention, in abdominal roentgenography to dispel interfering gas shadows, and in diabetes insipidus.

Preparations: Ampules, 10 and 20 units.

VASOTEC®, see Enalapril

VASOXYL®, see Methoxamine

V-CILLIN K®, see Penicillin V potassium

VECURONIUM BROMIDE—Norcuron®

Nondepolarizing neuromuscular blocking agent indicated as an adjunct to general anesthesia, to facilitate endotracheal intubation and to provide skeletal muscle relaxation during surgery or mechanical ventilation.

Preparation: Vials, 10 mg.

VEETIDS®, see Penicillin V potassium

VELBAN®, see Vinblastine

VELOSEF®, see Cephradine

VELOSULIN®, see Insulin

VENLAFAXINE HYDROCHLORIDE—Effexor®, Effexor XR®

Antidepressant.

Actions and Uses: Is extensively metabolized and one of its metabolites, O-desmethylvenlafaxine (ODV), is also pharmacologically active. Inhibits the neuronal reuptake of both serotonin and norepinephrine. Indicated for the treatment of depression.

Warnings: Adverse reactions include somnolence, dizziness, insomnia, nervousness, anxiety, tremor, dry mouth, nausea, constipation, anorexia, weight loss, vomiting, asthenia, sweating, blurred vision, and, in men, abnormal ejaculation and impotence. Patients should be advised to avoid the consumption of alcoholic beverages, and cautioned about driving or operating machinery until they are certain that the drug does not adversely affect their ability to engage in such activities. May cause sustained increases in blood pressure and blood pressure should be monitored regularly. It is recommended that it not be used in combination with a monoamine oxidase inhibitor (MAOI), or within 14 days of discontinuing treatment with a MAOI. There should be at least a 7-day interval after stopping venlafaxine before starting therapy with a MAOI.

Administration: Oral. Administered with food for the purpose of reducing the occurrence of gastrointestinal side effects.

Preparations: Tablets, 25, 37.5, 50, 75, and 100 mg. Release capsules, 37.5, 75, and 150 mg.

VENTOLIN®, see Albuterol

VEPESID, see Etoposide

VERAPAMIL HYDROCHLORIDE—Calan®, Calan SR®, Covera HS®, Isoptin®, Isoptin SR®, Verelan®

Antianginal, antiarrhythmic, and antihypertensive agent.

Actions and Uses: Is a calcium channel blocking agent that is indicated in the treatment of (1) hypertension, (2) vasospastic and unstable angina, (3) chronic stable angina, (4) in association with digitalis for the control of ventricular rate at rest and during stress in patients with chronic atrial flutter and/or atrial fibrillation, and (5) prophylaxis of repetitive paroxysmal supraventricular tachycardia. Also indicated for intravenous use in the treatment of supraventricular tachycardia.

Warnings: Contraindicated in patients with hypotension or cardiogenic shock, sick sinus syndrome, second- or third-degree AV block and certain other cardiovascular disorders. Adverse reactions include constipation, dizziness, headache, and edema. May increase serum digoxin levels. Should not be administered IV to a patient also receiving a beta-adrenergic blocking agent IV; the concurrent oral administration of these agents may be beneficial in some patients but therapy must be closely monitored. Concomitant use with disopyramide is not recommended.

Administration: Oral and intravenous.

Preparations: Tablets, 80 and 120 mg. Controlled-release tablets, 120, 180, 240 and 360 mg. Ampules, vials, and syringes, 5 mg/2 ml.

VERCYTE®, see Pipobroman

VERELAN®, see Verapamil

VERMOX®, see Mebendazole

VERSED®, see Midazolam

VERSENATE CALCIUM DISODIUM®, see Edetate calcium disodium

VESPRIN®, see Triflupromazine

VIBRAMYCIN®, see Doxycycline

VIBRA-TABS®, see Doxycycline

VICODIN®, Combination of hydrocodone and acetaminophen

VICOPROFER®, Combination agent of hydrocodone bitartate and ibuprater (opiod and NSAID)

VIDARABINE—Vira-A®

Antiviral agent indicated for ophthalmic use for the treatment of acute keratoconjunctivitis and recurrent epithelial keratitis due to Herpes simplex virus types 1 and 2.

Preparations: Ophthalmic ointment, 3%.

VIDEX®, see Didanosine

VINBLASTINE SULFATE—Velban®

Antineoplastic agent administered intravenously in the treatment of Hodgkin's disease, lymphocytic lymphoma, histiocytic lymphoma, mycosis fungoides, advanced carcinoma of the testes, Kaposi's sarcoma, choriocarcinoma resistant to other agents, and carcinoma of the breast that is not responsive to other therapy.

Preparation: Vials, 10 mg.

VINCASAR PFS®, see Vincristine

VINCRISTINE SULFATE—Oncovin®, Vincasar PFS®

Antineoplastic agent administered intravenously in the treatment of acute leukemia, Hodgkin's disease, lymphosarcoma, reticulum-cell sarcoma, rhabdo- myosarcoma, neuroblastoma, and Wilm's tumor.

Preparations: Vials and syringes, 1, 2, and 5 mg.

VINORELBINE TARTRATE—Navelbine®

Actions and Uses: Antineoplastic agent indicated as monotherapy or in combination with cisplatin for the first line treatment of ambulatory patients with unresectable advanced non-small-cell lung cancer (NSCLC).

Warnings: Contraindicated in patients with pretreatment granulocyte counts of less than 1000 cells/mm_3. Cautious use is recommended in patients with previous irradiation or chemotherapy because of increased risk of myelosuppression. Granulocytopenia is the major dose limiting toxicity. Sepsis has occurred and patients should be taught to immediately report the occurrence of fever or chills. Adverse reactions include fatigue, peripheral neuropathy, alopecia, constipation, diarrhea, nausea and vomiting, chest pain, shortness of breath, and elevation of liver enzymes. Observe vesicant precautions.

Administration: Intravenous.

Preparations: Vials, 10 mg/ml.

VIOFORM®, see Clioquinol

VIOKASE®, see Pancrelipase

VIRA-A®, see Vidarabine

VIRACEPT®, see Nelfinavir

VIRAMUNE®, see Nevirapine

VIRAZOLE®, see Ribavirin

VIROPTIC®, see Trifluridine

VISINE®, see Tetrahydrozoline

VISKEN®, see Pindolol

VISTARIL®, see Hydroxyzine

VISTIDE®, see Cidofovir

VITACARN®, see L-Carnitine

VITAMIN A—Aquasol A®

Vitamin indicated for the treatment of vitamin A deficiency.

Preparations: Capsules, 10,000, 25,000, 50,000 IU. Drops, 5,000 IU/0.1 ml. Vials, 50,000 IU/ml.

VITAMIN A ACID, see Tretinoin

VITAMIN B1, see Thiamine

VITAMIN B2, see Riboflavin

VITAMIN B3, see Nicotinic acid

VITAMIN B6, see Pyridoxine

VITAMIN B12, see Cyanocobalamin

VITAMIN B COMPLEX

Vitamin mixture usually including thiamine, riboflavin, niacin, pantothenic acid, pyridoxine, and cyanocobalamin.

VITAMIN C—Ascorbic acid, sodium ascorbate, Cevalin®

Vitamin indicated in the prevention and treatment of scurvy. Has been suggested to be of benefit in high doses in the prevention and treatment of colds. Has been used as a urinary acidifier.

Preparations: Tablets, 25, 50, 100, 250, and 500 mg. Chewable, controlled-release, and effervescent tablets. Solution, syrup, powder, and crystals. Ampules and vials, 100 mg/ml, 250 mg/ml, and 500 mg/ml.

VITAMIN D, see Cholecalciferol and Ergocalciferol

VITAMIN D2, see Ergocalciferol

VITAMIN D3, see Cholecalciferol

VITAMIN E—Aquasol E®

Vitamin indicated for the treatment and prevention of vitamin E deficiency. Has been used in certain premature infants to reduce the toxic effects of oxygen therapy on the lung parenchyma, and to decrease the severity of hemolytic anemia in infants.

Preparations: Capsules, 50, 100, 200, 400, 500, 600, 1000 IU. Drops, 15 IU/0.3 ml.

VITAMIN K, see Menadiol sodium diphosphate

VITAMIN K1, see Phytonadione

VIVACTIL®, see Protriptyline

VIVELLE®, see Estradiol

VLEMASQUE®, see Sulfurated lime

VOLMAX®, see Albuterol sulfate

VOLTAREN®, see Diclofenac

VONTROL®, see Diphenidol

VOSOL®, see Acetic acid

VP-16®, see Etoposide

VUMON®, see Teniposide

W

WARFARIN SODIUM—Coumadin®

Coumarin anticoagulant.

Actions and Uses: Indicated for (1) the prophylaxis and treatment of venous thrombosis and its extension, (2) the treatment of atrial fibrillation with embolization, (3) the prophylaxis and treatment of pulmonary embolism, (4) as an adjunct in the treatment of coronary occlusion, (5) for the prevention and treatment of thromboembolic complications associated with cardiac valve replacements, and (6) to reduce the risk of death, recurrent myocardial infarction and thromboembolic events such as stroke or systemic embolization after myocardial infarction.

Warnings: Contraindicated during pregnancy, in patients with bleeding tendencies associated with active ulceration, hemorrhagic tendencies, or blood dyscrasias or in patients who have recently undergone or are to undergo surgery of the CNS or eye, or other surgery that has resulted in large open surfaces. Adverse reactions include hemorrhage and therapy must be closely monitored. Effect may be increased by the concurrent administration of allopurinol, antibiotics, cimetidine, erythromycin, monoamine oxidase inhibitors, phenylbutazone, quinidine, salicylates, sulfonylurea hypoglycemic agents, and trimethoprim-sulfamethoxazole, as well as other agents. Effect may be reduced by barbiturates, carbamazepine, griseofulvin, and other agents.

Administration: Oral, intravenous, and intramuscular.

Preparations: Scored tablets, 1, 2, 2.5, 3, 5, 7.5, and 10 mg. Vials, 2 mg/ml, 5 mg/ml.

WELLBUTRIN®, see Bupropion

WELLCOVORIN®, see Leucovorin

WHITFIELD'S OINTMENT, see Benzoic acid

WINSTROL®, see Stanozolol

WINTERGREEN OIL, see Methyl salicylate

WOOL FAT, see Lanolin

WYAMINE®, see Mephentermine

WYCILLIN®, see Procaine penicillin G

WYDASE®, see Hyaluronidase

WYMOX®, see Amoxicillin

WYTENSIN®, see Guanabenz

X

XALATAN®, see Latanoprost

XANAX®, see Alprazolam

XYLOCAINE®, see Lidocaine

XYLOMETAZOLINE HYDROCHLORIDE—Otrivin®

Decongestant used topically for the relief of nasal congestion.

Preparations: Nose drops, 0.05% and 0.1%. Nose spray, 0.1%.

Y

YODOXIN®, see Iodoquinol

YOHIMBINE HYDROCHLORIDE

Has been suggested to have an aphrodisiac effect

Preparation: Tablets, 5 mg.

YUTOPAR®, see Ritodrine

Z

ZAFIRLUKAST—Accolate®

Antiasthmatic (leukotriene receptor antagonist). Indicated in prophylaxis and chronic treatment of asthma.

Warnings: Not for primary treatment of acute asthma attacks. Use cautiously in cirrhosis. Adverse reactions include headache, infection (respiratory tract), and nausea. Remind patients that this drug should be taken regularly as prescribed and not to make changes in dosing on their own. This drug is not a bronchodilator. While it may be used during an acute episode, it is not indicated for the reversal of acute bronchospasm.

Administrations: Take twice daily on an empty stomach.

Preparations: Tablets, 20 mg

ZAGAM®, see Sparfloxacin

ZALCITABINE—Hivid®

Antiviral agent.

Actions and Uses: Also known as dideoxycytidine or ddC. Inhibits the replication of the human immunodeficiency virus (HIV). Is converted by cellular enzymes to the active antiviral metabolite that inhibits viral replication, in part, by interfering with reverse transcriptase. Indicated for use in combination with zidovudine for the treatment of adult patients (i.e., 13 years of age and older) with advanced HIV infection (CD4 cell count less than or equal to 300 cells/mm_3) who have demonstrated significant clinical or immunologic deterioration. Also indicated for second-line monotherapy in HIV-infected patients who experience disease progression with zidovudine or are intolerant to zidouvdine.

Warnings: May cause peripheral neuropathy which may become severe and potentially irreversible if the drug is not stopped promptly; patients should be advised to report symptoms such as tingling, burning, pain, or numbness in the hands or feet. Use should be avoided in patients with moderate or severe peripheral neuropathy, and the concurrent use with other drugs that have the potential to cause peripheral neuropathy (e.g., didanosine) should be avoided where possible. May cause pancreatitis and, if a patient develops abdominal pain and nausea, vomiting, or elevated amylase levels, the use of the drug should be interrupted until the possibility of pancreatitis is excluded. Other adverse reactions include esophageal ulcers, cardiomyopathy, congestive heart failure, anaphylactoid reactions, oral ulcers, nausea, dysphagia, anorexia, abdominal pain, vomiting, rash, pruritus, headache, dizziness, myalgia, fatigue, pharyngitis, anemia, leukopenia, and elevation of hepatic enzymes. May cause fetal harm and women of childbearing potential should not receive the drug unless they are using effective contraception.

Administration: Oral.

Preparations: Tablets, 0.375 and 0.75 mg.

ZANAFLEX®, see Tizanidine

ZANTAC®, see Ranitidine

ZARONTIN®, see Ethosuximide

ZAROXOLYN®, see Metolazone

ZEBETA®, see Bisoprolol fumarate

ZEMURON®, see Rocuronium bromide

ZEPHIRAN®, see Benzalkonium chloride

ZERIT®, see Stavudine

ZESTORETIC®, Combination of lisinopril and hydrochlorothiazide

ZESTRIL®, see Lisinopril

ZIAC®, Combination of bisoprolol and hydrochlorothiazide

ZIDOVUDINE—AZT, Retrovir®

Antiviral agent.

Actions and Uses: Also known as azidothymidine (AZT), it inhibits the replication of certain retroviruses including human immunodeficiency virus (HIV), which causes acquired immunodeficiency syndrome (AIDS). Indicated for the management of adult patients with symptomatic HIV infection [AIDS and advanced AIDS-related complex (ARC)] who have a history of cytologically confirmed pneumonia (PCP) or an absolute CD4 (T4 helper/inducer) lymphocyte count of less than 200/mm_3 in the peripheral blood before therapy is begun. Also indicated for the management of patients with HIV infection who have evidence of impaired immunity, and for HIV-infected children who have HIV-related symptoms or who are asymptomatic with abnormal laboratory values indicating significant HIV-related immunosuppression. Also indicated for the prevention of maternal-fetal HIV transmission.

Warnings: Hematologic toxicity (e.g., granulocytopenia, anemia) is the adverse event reported most frequently and may require dose adjustment, discontinuation of the drug and/or blood transfusions. Frequent (at least every 2 weeks) blood counts are strongly recommended in patients taking the medication. Other adverse reactions include headache, nausea, insomnia, and myalgia. Caution must be exercised in patients taking other medications that are nephrotoxic, cytotoxic, or that interfere with the number or function of red blood cells and/or white blood cells, because the risk of toxicity may be increased. Probenecid may increase the activity of zidovudine.

Administration: Oral and intravenous.

Preparations: Capsules, 100 mg. Tablets, 300 mg. Syrup, 50 mg/5 ml. Vials, 10 mg/ml.

ZILABRACE®, see Benzocaine

ZILADENT®, see Benzocaine

ZILEUTON—Zyflo®

Antiasthmatic indicated in the prophylaxis and chronic treatment of asthma.

Warnings: Contraindicated in acute liver disease. Do not administer if transaminase levels are greater than or equal to three times the upper limit of normal. Evaluate liver function before initiation of and during therapy (discontinue if signs of liver disease occur). Use cautiously in patients with a history of liver disease or alcohol consumption. Adverse reactions include dyspepsia, pain, nausea, asthenia, headache, and myalgia. Documented drug interactions require a full drug profile review and adjustment of the regimen accordingly.

Administrations: 600 mg, 4 times a day without regard to meals.

Preparations: Tablets, 600 mg (scored).

ZINACEF®, see Cefuroxime sodium

ZINC CHLORIDE

Trace metal supplement to intravenous solutions given for total parenteral nutrition.

ZINC GLUCONATE

Dietary supplement to prevent or treat deficiencies of zinc.

Preparations: Tablets, 35, 50, and 105 mg.

ZINC OXIDE

Protectant and antiseptic applied topically in

the treatment of various dermatologic conditions.

Preparations: Ointment, 25%. Paste, 25% with 25% starch.

ZINC SULFATE

Trace metal supplement to intravenous solutions given for total parenteral nutrition. Also used as a dietary supplement to prevent or treat deficiencies of zinc. Has been investigated in dermatologic and arthritic disorders, and also in situations in which there is delayed wound healing associated with zinc deficiency. Also used in an ophthalmic solution for the relief of minor eye irritation.

Preparations: Vials, 1 mg/ml and 5 mg/ml. Capsules and tablets, 110 and 220 mg. Ophthalmic solution, 0.25%.

ZINECARD® , see Dexrazoxane

ZITHROMAX®, see Azithromycin

ZOCOR®, see Simvastatin

ZOFRAN®, see Ondansetron

ZOLADEX®, see Goserelin acetate

ZOLICEF®, see Cefazolin

ZOLOFT®, see Sertraline

ZOLPIDEM TARTRATE—Ambien®

Hypnotic.

Actions and Uses: Is an imidazopyridine derivative that is indicated for the short-term treatment of insomnia.

Warnings: Adverse reactions include drowsiness, dizziness, drugged feelings, and diarrhea. Patients should be cautioned against engaging in activities requiring complete mental alertness or motor coordination, including potential impairment of the performance of such activities the following day. Patients should also be warned about the risk of additive depressant effects when other agents with central nervous system depressant activity (including alcohol) are used concurrently. Has a potential for causing problems of dependence and abuse, and is classified in Schedule IV.

Administration: Oral. For faster sleep onset, should not be administered with or immediately after a meal. Use should generally be limited to a period of 7 to 10 days.

Preparations: Tablets, 5 and 10 mg.

ZONALON®, see Doxepin hydrochloride

ZONASAR®, see Streptozocin

ZORPRIN®, see Aspirin

ZOSTRIX®, see Capsaicin

ZOSTRIX—HP®, see Capsaicin

ZOSYN®, see Piperacillin sodium/tazobactam sodium

ZOVIRAX®, see Acyclovir

Z-PAK®, see Azithromycin

ZYBAN®, see Bupropion

ZYFLO®, see Zileuton

ZYLOPRIM®, see Allopurinol

ZYMASE®, see Pancrelipase

ZYPREXA®, see Olanzapine

ZYRTEC®, see Cetirizine Hydrochloride

PART II
New Drugs

AMLEXANOX 5%

Aphthasol®

DESCRIPTION/ACTIONS

Anti-inflammatory adhesive oral paste indicated in the treatment of aphthous ulcers (canker sores). Amlexanox has been shown to accelerate the healing of canker sores. Mechanism of action not fully understood.

PRECAUTIONS/ADVERSE REACTIONS

Not for use in immunocompromised patients. Discontinue if rash or contact mucositis occurs. Pregnancy Cat B. Use cautiously in nursing mothers. Adverse reactions include transient local pain, burning and/or stinging. Instruct patients to consult physician or dentist if ulcer does not heal after 10 days.

ADMINISTRATION

Begin treatment at earliest onset of symptoms. Apply 1/4 inch to each ulcer four times daily (preferably following oral hygiene after meals and at bedtime). Wash hands after application. Continue until ulcer heals.

PREPARATIONS

5 g tubes of 5% adhesive oral paste.

ARDEPARIN

Normiflo®

DESCRIPTION/ACTIONS

Antithrombolic indicated in prevention of post-op DVT, which may lead to pulmonary embolism, in patients undergoing elective knee replacement surgery. Ardeparin is a low molecular weight (LMW) heparin whose activity results from its ability to prevent fibrin formation by the inhibition of thrombin generation by anti-X_a and anti II-a effects.

PRECAUTIONS/ADVERSE REACTIONS

Contraindicated in severe hemorrhagic diathesis, active major bleeding; Type II thrombocytopenia associated with a positive in vitro test for anti platelet antibody associated with ardeparin sodium, heparin, or pork allergy.

Use cautiously in neuraxial anesthesia and post-op indwelling epidural catheter or spinal puncture (risk of epidural or spinal hematoma), asthma, heparin-induced thrombocytopenia, bleeding disorders, severe renal dysfunction (monitor carefully if serum Cr≥2mg/dl), severe uncontrolled hypertension, acute bacterial endocarditis, acute ulceration and angiodysplastic GI disease, bleeding diathesis, nonhemorrhagic stroke, invasive procedures, recent brain, spinal, or eye surgery.

Adverse reactions include hemorrhage, hematoma, thrombocytopenia, local reactions (e.g., hematoma, pain), fever, allergic reaction, GI upset, constipation, rash, pruritus, edema, dizziness, insomnia, and anemia.

ADMINISTRATION

50 anti-X_a units/Kg every 12 hours by SC injection. Begin treatment the evening of the day of surgery or the following morning and continue for 14 days or until patient is fully ambulatory (whichever is shorter).

Administer by deep SC injection. Do not give by IM injection to avoid the potential for a hematoma at the injection site.

PREPARATIONS

5,000 anti-X_a units in 0.5 mL.

10,000 anti-X_a units in 0.5 mL.

BECAPLERMIN

Regranex®

DESCRIPTION/ACTIONS

Diabetic foot ulcers are among the most difficult types of wounds to heal and are associated with serious complications such as severe infections and amputations. Becaplermin has been shown to increase the incidence of complete healing of these ulcers when used as adjunct to good ulcer care. Good ulcer care is inclusive of complete initial sharp debridement, ongoing debridement as needed, non-weight bearing regimen, systemic treatment of infection if present (no topical antibiotics or antiseptics), maintenance of a moist wound environment, and assessment of oxygen perfusion.

Becaplermin is recombinant human platelet- derived growth factor with biological activity similar to that of endogenous platelet - derived growth factor. This activity includes promoting the chemotactic recruitment and proliferation of cells involved in wound repair and enhancing the formulation of granulation tissue.

Indicated as an adjunct in the treatment of lower extremity diabetic neuropathic ulcers that extend into the subcutaneous tissue or beyond and have an adequate blood supply.

PRECAUTIONS/ADVERSE REACTIONS

Contraindicated in neoplasia at the application site. Not for use in wounds that close by primary intention, in pregnancy (category C), and in nursing mothers.

Adverse reactions include erythematous rash.

ADMINISTRATION

Apply for 12 hour duration once daily until complete healing has occurred. Measure size of ulcers and adjust at 1–2 week intervals. Calculate amount of gel based on ulcer size and gel tube size as per manufacturer's guidelines. Squeeze calculated length of gel onto clean nonabsorbent measuring surface (e.g., wax paper). Spread gel over entire ulcer to thickness of about $^{1}/_{16}$ inch (size of the thickness of a dime). Cover with saline dressing for 12 hours. After 12 hours remove dressing, rinse, and replace with clean normal saline dressing.

PREPARATIONS

0.01% gel in 2, 7.5 and 15 g tubes.

BROMFENAC

Duract®

DESCRIPTION/ACTIONS

An NSAID indicated in short term (usually less than 10 days) management of pain. Not indicated for the treatment of conditions such as osteoarthritis or rheumatoid arthritis. A peripherally acting analgesic that belongs to the nonsteroidal inflammatory drug (NSAID) class. Unlike other NSAIDS is not indicated for conditions other than pain.

PRECAUTIONS/ADVERSE REACTIONS

Contraindicated in aspirin allergy, chronic hepatitis or other known severe liver disease, and late pregnancy. Pregnancy Category C.

Use cautiously in hepatic or renal impairment. Monitor liver function (esp ALT) if use for >4 weeks, asthma, fluid retention, hypertension, CHF, history of peptic ulcer disease and/or GI bleed or patients at risk of GI bleed. Monitor patients with coagulation disorders. Use not recommended in nursing mothers.

Adverse reactions include GI upset, liver enzyme elevations, headache, abdominal pain, dizziness, somnolence, constipation and asthenia.

ADMINISTRATION

25 mg every 6–8 hours as needed.

If taken with high fat food may need 50 mg dose.

Max 150 mg/day.

PREPARATIONS

Capsules, 25 mg.

BUDESONIDE

Pulmicort Turbuhaler®

DESCRIPTION/ACTIONS

Pulmicort is a potent adrenocortical steroid with locally acting anti-inflammatory and immune modifer properties. Use of aerosolized steroids may decrease the requirement for or avoid use of systemic glucocorticoids and delay pulmonary damage that occurs from chronic asthma. Inhaled steroids do not provide systemic effect and caution should be used when weaning systemic steroids to avoid adrenal insufficiency. Pulmicort is indicated in the maintenance and prophylactic treatment of asthma including patients who require systemic corticosteroids and those who may benefit from systemic dose reduction/elimination.

PRECAUTIONS/ADVERSE REACTIONS

Contraindicated in acute asthma/status asthmaticus. Use cautiously in active untreated infections, patients with diabetes, glaucoma, underlying immunosuppression, systemic glucocorticoid therapy, pregnancy, nursing mothers, and children <6.

Adverse reactions include headache, dysphonia, hoarseness, oropharyngeal fungal infections, bronchospasm, cough, wheezing, dry mouth, esophageal candidiasis, dyspepsia, gastroenteritis, back pain, and flu-like symptoms.

ADMINISTRATION

Adults: Previously controlled on bronchodilators alone: 1–2 sprays twice daily (up to 2 sprays twice daily)

Previously controlled on other inhaled glucocorticoids: 1–2 sprays twice daily (up to 4 sprays twice daily)

Previously controlled on oral glucocorticoids: 2–4 sprays twice daily (up to 4 sprays twice daily).

Children >6: 1 spray twice daily (up to 2 sprays twice daily).

PREPARATIONS

160 μg/actuation powder in a 200 dose turbuhaler.

CAPECITABINE

Xeloda®

DESCRIPTION/ACTIONS

Antineoplastic agent indicated in the treatment of patients with metastatic breast cancer resistant to both pacitaxel and an anthracycline - containing chemotherapy regimen or resistant to pacitaxel and for whom further anthracycline therapy is not indicated.

PRECAUTIONS/ADVERSE REACTIONS

Contraindicated in patients with hypersensitivity to 5-flurouracil. Use cautiously in patients with renal or hepatic impairment and carefully monitor function during therapy.

Adverse effects include diarrhea which can be severe. Provide supportive treatment to minimize dehydration and electrolyte imbalance. Other adverse effects are hand and foot syndrome (plantar erythrodyesthesia or chemotherapy induced acral erythema), cardiotoxicity (MI, angina, dysrhythmias, cardiogenic shock, sudden death, ECG changes), hyperbilirubinemia, anemia, neutropenia, thrombocytopenia, nausea, vomiting, stomatitis and others.

ADMINISTRATION

2,500 mg/m^2/day orally in two divided doses (~12 hours apart) at the end of a meal for 2 weeks followed by a 1-week rest period given as 3-week cycles.

PREPARATIONS

Tablets, 150 and 500 mg.

CARVEDILOL

Coreg®

DESCRIPTION/ACTIONS

A noncardioselective *B*-blocker/alpha-I blocker indicated in mild or moderate heart failure (NYHA class II or III) and hypertension.

PRECAUTIONS/ADVERSE REACTIONS

Contraindicated in decompensated class IV NYHA heart failure requiring intravenous inotropic therapy, asthma related bronchospastic conditions 2nd or 3rd degree AV block, sick sinus syndrome (unless paced), cardiogenic shock, severe bradycardia, hepatic impairment and history of carvedilol-associated hepatic injury.

Use cautiously in peripheral vascular disease, nonallergic bronchospasm, diabetes, hyperthyroidism, hepatic dysfunction, prinzemetal's angina, pheochromocytom, and anesthesia . Monitor renal function in ischemic heart disease, diffuse vascular disease, underlying renal insufficiency and/or if systolic BP <100mmHg. Avoid abrupt cessation. Pregnancy Category C. Use not recommended in nursing mothers.

Adverse reactions include bradycardia, orthostatic hypotension, edema, AV block, GI upset, hyperglycemia, increased weight, dizziness, and others.

ADMINISTRATION

Take with food

Adults:	>18 y/o: Initially 3.125 mg twice daily for 2 weeks.
	Only if tolerated, may increase to 6.25 mg twice daily.
	Continue to double dose at 2 week intervals as tolerated.
	Maximum (<85 kg) 25mg twice daily.
	Maximum (>85 kg) 50mg twice daily.
Children:	<18 years: Not recommended
	Dose increases must be physician monitored
	Reduce dose if pulse <55

PREPARATIONS

Tablets, 3.125, 6.25, 12.5, and 25 mg.

CERIVASTATIN

Baycol®

DESCRIPTION/ACTIONS

Cerivastatin is a competitive inhibitor of HMG-CoA reductase, an enzyme which is responsible for an early, rate limiting step in biosynthesis of cholesterol (C). Cholesterol biosynthesis inhibition reduces the level of cholesterol in hepatic cells, which stimulates the synthesis of LDL receptors, thereby increasing the uptake of cellular LDL particles. The result of these processes is a reduction in the level of plasma cholesterol concentration. In hypercholesterolemia cerivastatin has been shown to reduce plasma total-C, LDL-C, Apoβ, and triglycerides (TG) and to increase plasma HDL-C.

Maximal effect is seen within 4 weeks of initiation of treatment and this is when repeat lipid determinations should be made.

Indicated as an adjunct to diet in primary hypercholesterolemia and mixed dyslipidemia (Types IIa and IIb) for the reduction of elevated total cholesterol (total C) and LDL-cholesterol (LDL-C) levels when response to dietary therapy is inadequate.

PRECAUTIONS/ADVERSE REACTIONS

Contraindicated in active liver disease, unexplained persistent elevated serum transaminases, pregnancy (category C), and nursing mothers.

Use cautiously in alcoholics (start at low dose and monitor closely), homozygous familial hypercholesterolemia, and severe renal insufficiency.

Monitor liver function before and during therapy. Discontinue if AST or ALT levels of >3 × upper limit of normal (ULN). Monitor for endocrine dysfunction. Discontinue if myopathy, elevated CPK levels develop or if pregnancy occurs. Suspend treatment if a predisposition to the development of renal failure secondary to rhabdomyolysis develops.

Adverse reactions include rhinitis, pharyngitis, headache, myalgia, elevated serum transaminases or creatininekinase. Instruct patients to promptly report symptoms of myopathy especially if fever or malaise is present.

ADMINISTRATION

0.3 mg once daily in the PM.

0.2 mg once daily in the PM if significant renal impairment (CrCl , 60 ml/min)

PREPARATIONS

Tablets, 0.2 and 0.3 mg.

CLOPIDOGREL

Plavix®

DESCRIPTION/ACTIONS

An inhibitor of platelet aggregation indicated in the reduction of atherosclerotic events (MI, stroke, and vascular death) in patients with altherosclerosis documented by recent stroke or MI or established peripheral arterial disease. Inhibiting platelet function has been shown to decrease morbidity in patients with established atherosclerotic cardiovascular disease, as evidenced by stroke, myocardial infarction, or the need for bypass surgery or angioplasty. This indicates platelets participate in the initiation and/or evolution of these events and it follows that inhibiting platelets could reduce their incidence.

Clopidogrel is a direct inhibitor of adenosine diphosphate (ADP) induced platelet aggregation. The modification that occurs at the ADP receptor is irreversible. Consequently, platelets exposed to clopidogrel are affected for the remainder of their lifespan.

PRECAUTIONS/ADVERSE REACTIONS

Contraindicated in active pathologic bleeding (e.g., peptic ulcer, intracranial hemorrhage). Use cautiously in the presence of the risk of bleeding (e.g., surgery, ulcers, trauma, concomitant NSAIDS), and severe hepatic disease. Consider discontinuing 7 days prior to surgery. Not recommended for use in children. Pregnancy Category C.

Adverse reactions include diarrhea, rash, pruritus, purpura, other GI disturbances, GI ulcers, hemorrhage, neutropenia/agranulocytosis (rare).

Instruct patients to report unusual or prolonged bleeding or fever.

ADMINISTRATION

75 mg once daily for adults.

PREPARATIONS

Tablets, 75 mg.

DANAPAROID SODIUM

Orgaran®

DESCRIPTION/ACTIONS

Antithrombolic indicated in prevention of post-op DVT, which may lead to pulmonary embolism, in patients undergoing elective hip replacement surgery. Danaparoid is a low molecular weight (LMW) heparin whose activity results from its ability to prevent fibrin formation by the inhibition of thrombin generation by anti-X_a and anti II-a effects. The ratio of anti-X_a to anti IIA activity is greater than 22:1. Danaparoid only has minor effects on platelet function and aggregation.

Danaparoid's anti-X_a activity is not equivalent to heparin or other LMW heparins. Therefore, this product can not be interchanged on a unit for unit basis with either heparin or with any other LMW heparin products.

PRECAUTIONS/ADVERSE REACTIONS

Contraindicated in severe hemorrhagic diathesis, active major bleeding, Type II thrombocytopenia associated with a positive in vitro test for anitiplatelet antibody associated with danaparoid sodium, heparin, or pork allergy.

May cause bleeding or hematomas within the spinal column if used concurrently with spinal or epidural anesthesia.

Use cautiously in asthma, heparin-induced thrombocytopenia, bleeding disorders, severe renal dysfunction (monitor carefully if serum Cr≥2 mg/dl), severe uncontrolled hypertension, acute bacterial endocarditis, acute ulceration and angiodysplastic GI disease, bleeding diathesis, nonhemorrhagic stroke, invasive procedures, recent brain, spinal, or eye surgery.

Not interchangeable (unit for unit) with heparin or other low molecular weight heparin products. Pregnancy Category C.

Adverse reactions include hemorrhage, thrombocytopenia, local reactions (e.g., hematoma, pain), fever, GI upset, constipation, rash, pruritus, edema, dizziness, insomnia, and anemia.

ADMINISTRATION

Begin treatment 1–4 hours pre-op and then not sooner than 2 hours after surgery.

750 anti-Xa units SC twice daily. Rotate sites.

Treat 7–10 days, not to exceed a maximum of 14 days.

PREPARATIONS

750 units/0.6 mL solution for SC injection, contains sulfites.

DOLASETRON MESYLATE

Anzemet®

DESCRIPTION/ACTIONS

Selective 5-HT_3 receptor antagonist indicated in the prevention of nausea and vomiting associated with emetogenic cancer chemotherapy, including initial and repeat courses. Also indicated in the prevention and treatment of post-op nausea and vomiting.

Serotonin 5-HT_3 receptors are present on the nerve terminals of the vagus and in the CNS in the chemoreceptor trigger zone of the area postrema. It is postulated that cancer chemotherapeutic agents cause nausea and vomiting by releasing serotonin from the enterocromaffin cells of the small intestine, and that the released serotonin then activates 5-HT_3 receptors on the vagus nerve to initiate the vomiting reflex. By blocking the receptor sites, dolasetron can interfere with this cascade.

PRECAUTIONS/ADVERSE REACTIONS

Use cautiously in patients at risk of developing prolongation of cardiac conduction intervals, especially Qt_C (e.g., congential QT syndrome, hypokalemia, hypomagnesemia). Pregnancy Category B. Not recommended for use in nursing mothers.

Adverse reactions include headache, dizziness, pain, fatigue, diarrhea, tachycardia, and ECG changes.

ADMINISTRATION

Oral:

Adults ≥ 16 years : tablets-100 mg within 1 hour before chemotherapy or within 2 hours of surgery.

Injection:

1. IV 100 mg over 30 seconds or infuse over up to 15 minutes.
2. Chemotherapy induced nausea and vomiting:
   1.8 mg/kg about 30 minutes before chemotherapy or may give 100 mg IV.
3. Prevention of post-op nausea and vomiting:
   12.5 mg about 15 minutes before stopping anesthesia.
4. Treatment of post-op nausea and vomiting:
   12.5 mg as soon as needed.
   Children <2 years not recommended

5. Children 2–16 years.

Oral:

Tablets: 1.8 mg/kg (max 100 mg) within 1 hour of chemotherapy or
1.2 mg/kg (max 100 mg) within 2 hours before surgery.

Injection:

1. May be given by IV injection as an adult dose, or may be diluted in apple or apple-grape juice and taken orally.
2. Chemotherapy-induced nausea and vomiting: 1.8 mg/kg (max 100 mg) diluted in juice and taken orally within 1 hour of chemotherapy.
3. Prevention of post-op nausea and vomiting: .35mg/kg IV (max 12.5 mg) about 15 minutes before stopping anesthesia or 1.2 mg /kg (max 100 mg) diluted in apple or apple-grape juice and taken orally within 2 hours before surgery.
4. Treatment of post-op nausea and vomiting: .35 mg/kg IV as soon as needed.

PREPARATIONS

Tablets, 50 and 100 mg

Injection, single use ampules 12.5 mg/0.625mL.

Single use vials 100 mg/5 mL.

EPTIFIBATIDE

Integrilin®

DESCRIPTION/ACTIONS

Platelet aggregation inhibitors indicated in combination with heparin for treating acute coronary syndrome (unstable angina/non Q-wave myocardial infarction) including patients who are to be managed medically and those undergoing percutaneous transluminal angioplasty or artherectomy.

PRECAUTIONS/ADVERSE REACTIONS

Contraindicated in the following conditions within previous 30 days: active internal bleeding, bleeding diathesis, stroke, major surgery or severe trauma. Contraindicated with a history of intracranial hemmorrhage, intracranial neoplasm, arteriovenous malformation, aneurysm, hemorrhagic stroke, thrombocytopenia after previous Tirofiban therapy, symptoms or findings suggestive of aortic dissection, severe hypertension, acute pericarditis and concomitant parenteral GI 11b/111A inhibitor.

Use cautiously in patients with renal failure, platelet count <150,000/mm^3 or hemorrhagic retinopathy. Properly care for femerol artery access site to minimize bleeding. Minimize other arterial and venous punctures, IM injections, catheter use and other invasive procedures to minimize bleeding risk. Avoid use of noncompressible IV access sites. Do baseline platelet counts, hemoglobin, hematocrit, and monitor during therapy. Discontinue Tirofiban if confirmed thrombocytopenia occurs. Adjust heparin to maintain aPTT at two times control.

Adverse reactions include bleeding decreased hemoglobin and/or hematocrit, reduced platelet counts, edema, vasovagal reaction and others.

ADMINISTRATION

Acute coronary syndrome: 180 µg/Kg (max 22.6 mg) IV over 1–2 minutes (bolus) as soon as possible after diagnosis, then 2 µg/kg/min (max 15 mg/hr) by continuous IV infusion until discharge or coronary artery bypass surgery, up to 72 hours.

Percutaneous Coronary Intervention (PCI): reduce infusion rate to 0.5 µg/kg/min and continue for 20–24 hours post procedure, allowing for 96 hours of therapy.

PCI without acute coronary syndrome: 135 µg/Kg IV bolus immediately following procedure, then 0.5 µg/Kg/min by continuous infusion for 20–24 hours.

PREPARATIONS

Vials, 2 mg/mL (10 mL for bolus dose).

Vials, 0.75 mg/mL (100 mL for infusion).

FENOFIBRATE

Tricor®

DESCRIPTION/ACTIONS

Drug's mechanism of action has not been fully defined but apparently lowers plasma triglycerides by inhibiting triglyceride synthesis, resulting in a reduction of very low density lipoprotein (VLDL) released into circulation. The mechanism may also be related to its ability to stimulate the catabolism of triglyceride-rich lipoprotein (i.e., VLDL). Indicated as an adjunct to diet in treating adults with very high elevations of serum triglyerceride levels (Type IV and V hyperlipidemias) who are at risk of pancreatitis and who do not adequately respond to strict dietary measure of control.

Fenofibrate reduces serum uric acid levels in both hyperuricemic and normal individuals by increasing urinary excretion of uric acid.

PRECAUTIONS/ADVERSE REACTIONS

Contraindicated in hepatic dysfunction (including primary biliary cirrhosis and unexplained persistent liver function abnormality), severe renal dysfunction and gallbladder disease. Fenofibrate can cause dose related hepatoxicity. Liver function should be monitored at baseline and at regular intervals for the duration of treatment. Pancreatitis has been reported in patients taking fenofibrate but it is a secondary phenomenon through biliary tract stone or sludge formation and obstruction of the bile duct.

Use cautiously in patients with renal impairment. Monitor CBC for at least a year. Monitor liver function regularly and discontinue if ALT (SGPT) levels are >3 × upper limit of normal (ULN). Discontinue if myopathy or gallstones occur. Pregnancy category C. Not recommended in nursing mothers.

Adverse reactions include rash, flu-like symptoms, eye irritation, dizziness, eructation, myopathy, rhabdomyolysis, increased serum transaminases, hepatitis, cirrhosis, cholelithiasis, pancreatitis, increased BUN/Cr., transient moderate hematologic changes, thrombocytopenia, and agranulocytosis (rare).

ADMINISTRATION

Give with meals. Initially 67 mg once daily. May increase at 4–8 week intervals up to a maximum of 201 mg/day. Discontinue if significant improvement is not seen in 2 months.

PREPARATIONS

Capsules, 67 mg.

FINASTERIDE

Propecia®

DESCRIPTION/ACTIONS

Type II 5α-reductase specific inhibitor indicated in the treatment of male pattern hair loss (androgenetic alopecia) in men only.

In men with male pattern hair loss, the balding scalp contains miniaturized hair follicles and an increased amount of 5α-dihydratestosterone (DHT) compared with hair scalp. Finasteride decreases scalp and serum DHT levels in these men, apparently interrupting a key factor in the development of androgenetic alopecia in those who are genetically predisposed to this condition.

PRECAUTIONS/ADVERSE REACTIONS

Contraindicated in woman and children. Woman of childbearing potential must not handle crushed or broken tablets. Pregnancy category X.

Use cautiously in hepatic dysfunction. Consider doubling PSA in men ≥41 years of age without BPH who are undergoing PSA test.

Instruct patients that the benefits may not be seen for 3 months. Must continue to sustain effect. Reversal of effects seen within 12 months of discontinuation.

Adverse reactions include decreased libido, erectile dysfunction, ejaculation disorder (all rare).

ADMINISTRATION

1 mg once daily.

PREPARATIONS

Tablest, 1 mg.

GREPAFLOXACIN

Raxar®

DESCRIPTION/ACTIONS

Fluoroquinolone antibiotic indicated in the treatment of susceptible mild to moderate infections including acute bacterial exacerbation of chronic bronchitis, community acquired pneumonia, nongonococcal urethritis and cervicitis, and uncomplicated gonorrhea.

Grepafloxacin is a broad spectrum antibiotic against a wide range of aerobic gram-positive and gram-negative bacteria, as well as some atypical organisms.

PRECAUTIONS/ADVERSE REACTIONS

Contraindicated in hepatic failure, Qtc prolongation, concomitant drugs that can increase Qtc interval and/or cause torsades de pointes unless cardiac monitoring is assured (e.g., hospitalization).

Not recommended for use in hypokalemia, nursing mothers, significant bradycardia, CHF, myocardial ischemia, atrial fibrillation or other pro-arrhythmic condition. Discontinue if tendon pain, inflammation, or rupture occurs; if rash phototoxicity, signs of hypersensitivity or if other serious adverse reactions occur on treatment. Maintain adequate hydration. Use cautiously in severe cerebral atherosclerosis, epilepsy and other conditions that predispose to seizures or lower seizure threshold. Avoid exposure to sun or UV light. Pregnancy Category C.

Adverse reactions include nausea, taste perversion, headache, dizziness, diarrhea or other gastrointestinal disturbances, vaginitits, pruritus, leukopenia, asthenia, insomnia, rash, anorexia, somnolence, dry mouth, photosensitivity, pain, CNS stimulation, superinfection, possible fever, severe dermatologicial reactions, and others.

ADMINISTRATION

Children <18 years not recommended

>18 years:

- acute bacterial exacerbation of chronic bronchitis:
  400 or 600 mg once daily for 10 days.
- community acquired pneumonia: 600 mg once daily for 10 days,
- urethritis or cervicitis: 400 mg once daily for 7 days
- gonorrhea: 400 mg as single dose

PREPARATIONS

Tablets, 200 mg.

HYDROQUINONE

Lustra®

DESCRIPTION/ACTIONS

A depigmenting agent indicated in ultraviolet-induced dyschromia and discoloration of the skin due to pregnancy, oral contraceptives, hormone replacement therapy or skin trauma. Hydroguinone contains glycolic acid and an antioxidant complex. Does not contain any sunscreening or sunblocking agents. The topical application of hydroquinone produces a reversible depigmentation of skin by inhibition of enzymatic oxidation of tyrosine to 3-(3,4-dihydroxyphenyle) alanine (dopa) and suppression of other melanocyte metabolic processes.

PRECAUTIONS/ADVERSE REACTIONS

Do skin sensitivity test before use. If itching, vesicle formation, or excessive inflammation occurs, avoid further treatment. Avoid sun and UV light. Avoid contact with eyes. Pregnancy category C.

Adverse reactions include localized contact dermatitis (discontinue if occurs).

ADMINISTRATION

Apply to affected areas twice daily (am and PM).

Discontinue if lightening effect does not occur after 2 months.

PREPARATIONS

4% cream in 10 oz jar.

INTERFERON ALFACON-1

Intergen®

DESCRIPTION/ACTIONS

Interferon Alfacon-1 is a non-naturally occurring type-1 interferon that is produced by genetically engineered E. Coli cells. Two major types of interferon, Type1 and 2, have been identified. Type 1 interferon induces varied biologic responses which include antiviral, antiproliferative and immunomodulatory effects, regulation of cell surface major histocompatibility, antigen expression, and regulation of cytokine expression.

Indicated in treatment of chronic Hepatitis C virus (HCV) infection in patients with compensated liver disease who have anti-HCV serum antibodies and/or presence of HCV-RNA.

PRECAUTIONS/ADVERSE REACTIONS

Contraindicated in hypersensitivity to E. Coli derived products. Use only under the supervision of qualified MD's. Do not interchange brands. Exclude other causes of hepatitis (e.g., Hepatitis B, Autoimmune Hepatitis). Use cautiously in cardiac disease, endocrine disorders, autoimmune disorders, leukopenia (esp. granulocytopenia), thrombocytopenia, and other myelosuppressive conditions. Withhold treatment if absolute neutrophil count $<500 \times 10^6/L$ or if platelet count is$<50 \times 10^9/L$.

Not recommended for use in severe psychiatric disorders or decompensated liver disease. Discontinue if either occurs. Not for use in pregnancy (category C) or nursing mothers. Do pre-treatment eye exams in diabetics and hypertensives. Refer to opthlamologist if visual disturbances occur.

Monitor lab values (blood counts, TSH, and T_4 creatinine, albumin, triglycerides, bilirubin) before, two weeks after starting, and periodically thereafter.

Adverse reactions include flu like symptoms, pain, edema, psychiatric /CNS effects (e.g., depression, insomnia, dizziness), local reactions, GI upset, cardiac or upper respiratory effects, rash, alopecia, pruritis, visual or lab abnormalities.

Instruct patients in effective contraception (both males and females).

ADMINISTRATION

9 µg SC three times per week for 24 weeks. May withhold or reduce dose to 7.5 µg if intolerable adverse event(s) occur(s).

If tolerated and unresponsive or relapsed, may give 15 ug SC three times per week for 6 months.

PREPARATIONS

9 and 15 µg vials for SC inj., preservative free.

IRBESARTAN

Avapro®

DESCRIPTION/ACTIONS

Angiotensin II receptor antagonist indicated in the treatment of hypertension as mono or combination therapy.

Irbesartan blocks the vasoconstrictor and aldosterone-secreting effects of angiotensin II by selectively blocking the binding of angiotensin II to the At1 receptor in many tissues. This mechanism of action is independent of the pathways for angiotensin II synthesis, which differentiates irbesartan and other angiotensin II receptor antagonists from the angiotensin converting (ace) inhibitors.

PRECAUTIONS/ADVERSE REACTIONS

Correct salt/volume depletion (e.g., patients vigorously treated with diuretics or those on dialysis) before beginning therapy, or use a low initial dose. Use cautiously in renal impairment, severe CHF, renal artery stenosis. Pregnancy Category C in 1st trimester. Pregnancy Category D in 2nd and 3rd trimesters.

Adverse reactions include diarrhea, dyspepsia and fatigue.

ADMINISTRATION

Initially 150 mg once daily; may increase to 300 mg once daily. Or, may add a low dose of diuretic. Salt/volume depletion: initially 75 mg once daily

PREPARATIONS

Tablets, 75, 150, and 300 mg.

LEPIRUDAN

Refludan®

DESCRIPTION/ACTIONS

Heparin-induced Thrombocytopenia (HIT) is a serious allergy-like reaction to heparin. The clinical picture of HIT is characterized by thrombocytopenia alone or in combination with thromboembolic complications. Lepirudan is the 1st agent available to treat this condition.

Lepirudan is indicated to treat HIT and associated thromboembolic disease in order to prevent further thromboembolic complications.

PRECAUTIONS/ADVERSE REACTIONS

Carefully assess risk in patients with increased risk of bleeding (e.g., recent puncture of large vessels or organ biopsy, anomaly of vessels or organs, recent cerebrovascular accident, stroke, intercerebral surgery or other neuraxial procedures, severe uncontrolled hypertension, bacterial endocarditis, advanced renal impairment, hemorrhagic diathesis, recent major surgery, recent major bleeding). Obtain baseline aPTT ratio and continue to monitor closely during therapy. Use cautiously in renal insufficiency, liver injury, and reexposure.

Adverse reactions include hemorrhagic events, abnormal liver function, allergic skin reactions, infections, multiorgan failure, and ventricular fibrillation.

ADMINISTRATION

Initial dose: .4 mg/kg (max 44 mg) by Slow IV bolus (over 15–20 seconds) followed by 0.15 mg/kg per hour (max 16.5 mg/hr) as continuous infusion for 2–10 days or longer. Titrate dose as per manufacturer's guidelines to achieve target aPTT ratio. Reduce dose for renal impairment (CrCl <60 mL/min)

PREPARATIONS

50 mg Vials.

LETROZOLE

Femara®

DESCRIPTION/ACTIONS

Letrozole is a nonsteroid aromatase inhibitor indicated in advanced breast cancer in postmenopausal woman with disease progression following antiestrogen therapy.

In postmenopausal woman, estrogens are derived mainly from the action of aromatase, an enzyme which converts adrenal androgens to estrone and estradiol. Letrozole is a highly specific inhibitor of aromatase. The treatment of woman with letrozole significantly lowers serum estrone, estradiol and estrone sulfate.

PRECAUTIONS/ADVERSE REACTIONS

Adverse reactions include pain, nausea, headache, fatigue, arthralgia, GI upset, edema, hot flashes, hypercalcemia, alopecia, depression, elevated liver enzymes, thrombocytopenia (rare), and others.

Pregnancy Category D. Use cautiously in severe hepatic impairment.

ADMINISTRATION

2.5 mg once daily until tumor progression is evident

PREPARATIONS

Tablets, 2.5 mg.

MOMETASONE FUROATE

Nasonex®

DESCRIPTION/ACTIONS

Corticosteroid indicated in prophylaxis and treatment of seasonal allergic rhinitis symptoms and treatment of perennial allergic rhinitis symptoms.

PRECAUTIONS/ADVERSE REACTIONS

Use not recommended in tuberculosis, varicella, vaccinia, unhealed nasal wounds,untreated fungal, bacterial, and viral infections or ocular herpes simplex. Discontinue if nasopharyngeal candida infection occurs. If adrenal insufficiency exists following systemic corticosteroid therapy, replacement with topical corticosteroids may exacerbate symptoms of adrenal insufficiency (e.g., depression). Monitor for vision changes or if there is a history of glaucoma or cataracts. Pregnancy Category C. Cautious use in nursing mothers.

Adverse reactions include headache, viral infection, pharyngitis, epistaxis, cough, upper respiratory tract infections, pain, sinusitis, and others.

Instruct patients to adhere to dosing and interval recommendations. Advise patients to seek medical advice if exposed to chickenpox or measles.

ADMINISTRATION

Two sprays in each nostril once daily

Prophylaxis: Begin 2–4 weeks prior to anticipated pollen season

PREPARATIONS

50 μg/spray in 17 g (120 sprays) metered dose, manual pump spray.

MONTELUKAST

Singulair®

DESCRIPTION/ACTIONS

A leukotriene antagonist indicated in prophylaxis and chronic treatment of asthma. The cysteinyl leukotrienes are products of arachidonic acid metabolism and are released from various cells including mast cells and eosinophils. Cysteinyl leukotrienes and leukotriene receptor occupation have been correlated with the pathopbysiology of asthma. Montelukast inhibits physiological actions of LTD_4 (a specific cysteinyl leukotreine) at the Cys LT receptor without any agonist activity.

PRECAUTIONS/ADVERSE REACTIONS

Not for primary treatment of acute attack. Not for monotherapy in treatment and management of exercise induced bronchospasm. Monitor patients closely when withdrawing from oral steroids.

Adverse reactions include headache, asthenia/fatigue, fever, GI disturbances, laryngitis, and pharyngitis.

Instruct patients to report increased need for short acting bronchodilators. Have appropriate rescue meds available. Continue usual regimen for exercise-induced bronchospasm prophylaxis.

Pregnancy Category B.

ADMINISTRATION

6–14 years-5 mg chewable tablet once daily in the PM.

>15 years-10 mg once daily in the PM.

<6 years—not recommended.

PREPARATIONS

Chewable tabs in cherry flavor, 5 mg.

Tablets, 10 mg.

NARATRIPTAN

Amerge®

DESCRIPTION/ACTIONS

Selective 5-HT $_{IB/ID}$ receptor agonist indicated in acute treatment of migraine with or without aura, in adults. Effective in relieving the pain and other symptoms associated with migraine (e.g., nausea, photophobia). Due to its long half life relative to other "triptans" it may be an appropriate choice for patients who have longer lasting migraines.

PRECAUTIONS/ADVERSE REACTIONS

Confirm diagnosis. Exclude underlying cardiovascular disease, supervise 1st dose, and consider ECG monitoring in patients with likelihood of unrecognized coronary disease (e.g., postmenopausal woman, men over 40, hypertension hyerpcholestrolemia, obesity, diabetes, smokers, strong family history). Monitor cardiovascular function in long-term intermittent use. Use cautiously in hepatic or renal dysfunction. Not recommended for use in the elderly.

Contraindicated in ischemic cardiac disease (e.g., history of MI, angina pectoris, silent myocardial ischemia) cerebrovascular disease (e.g., stroke, TIA), or peripheral vascular disease (e.g., ischemic bowel disease), uncontrolled hypertension, severe renal or hepatic impairment, basilar or hemoplegic migraine, and within 24 hours of other 5-HT, agonist or ergot type drugs. Pregnancy category C.

Adverse reactions include paresthesia, dizziness, drowsiness, malaise/fatigue, throat/neck symptoms (pain, pressure tightness).

ADMINISTRATION

Adults >18 y/o: 1 mg or 2.5 mg with fluids, may repeat once every 4 hours to a maximum of 5 mg/24 hours

The safety of treating, on average, more than 4 headaches in a 30-day period has not been established.

In mild to moderate renal or hepatic impairment, consider lower initial dose and reduce maximum to 2.5 mg/24 hours

PREPARATIONS

Tablets, 1 and 2.5 mg.

QUETIAPINE

Seroquel®

DESCRIPTION/ACTIONS

The pathophysiology of schizophrenia is complex and not completely understood. While earlier theories focused on the dopaminergic system, newer theories address the interplay between the seratonergic pathways as well as the involvement of muscarinic, alpha adrenergic, and histamine systems. Symptoms are generally categorized into two groups, positive (delusions, disorganized speech, hallucinations and behavior disturbance) and negative (avolition, flattened affect, anhedonia, and social withdrawal). Pharmacotherapy is aimed at improving these target symptoms while maintaining the most tolerable side effect profile at the lowest possible dose.

Quetiapine is a dibenzepine indicated in the management of the symptoms of psychotic disorders including schizophrenia. Studies indicate that some drugs in the dibenzepine class are effective in patients resistant to antipsychotic therapy and may be more effective in relieving negative symptoms than conventional agents.

PRECAUTIONS/ADVERSE REACTIONS

Contraindicated in hypersentitivity or lactation. Use cautiously in cardiovascular disease, cerebrovascular disease, dehydration or hypovolemia (increased risk of hypotension), history of siezures, Alzheimer's dementia, ≥ 65 y/o, hepatic impairment, hypothryroidism, history of suicide attempt, pregnancy Category C and children (safety not established). Hepatic enzyme elevations usually occurred within the first 3 weeks of treatment and promptly returned to pre-study levels with ongoing treatment. In hepatic impairment adjust dosing downwards.

Adverse reactions include dizziness, weight gain, leukopenia, flu-like syndrome, anorexia, constipation, dry mouth, dyspepsia, palpitations, peripheral edema, postural hypotension, cough, dypsnea, pharyngitis, ear pain, rhinitis, cognitive impairment, extrapyramidal symptoms, sedation, and tardive dyskinesia,

ADMINISTRATION

Initial dose of 25 mg twice daily.

Increase in increments of 25–50 mg twice daily or 3 times daily on second and third day, as tolerated, to a target dose range of 300–400 mg/day by the 4th day, given in 2 or 3 divided doses. Dose increments/decrements are recommended at 25–50 mg twice daily at intervals ≥ 2 days. Maximum dose-800 mg/day.

Antipsychotic efficacy was demonstrated at 150–750 mg/day. When restarting patients off quetiapine for <1 week dose titratration is not necessary and the maintenance dose may be reinitiated. After 1 week off quetiapine follow the initial titration schedule.

PREPARATIONS

Tablets, 25, 100, and 200 mg.

RALOXIFENE HCL

Evista®

DESCRIPTION/ACTIONS

Following menopause or oophorectomy, estrogen levels decrease, leading to increase in bone resorption and bone loss. The compensatory increase in bone formation that occurs is inadequate to offset resorptive losses. This imbalance between resumption and formation is related to a loss in estrogen, and may also involve age-related impairment of osteoblasts or their precursors. Raloxifene reduces bone resorption and decreases overall bone turnover. The relationship between the increase in bone mineral density (BMD) that is seen with Raloxifene and skeletal fracture rates has not been established.

Raloxifene is a selective estrogen receptor modulator (SERM) indicated in the prevention of osteoporosis in postmenopausal women. Data suggests drugs in this class may have the ability to act like estrogen in some tissues but not in others. Clinical data indicate that raloxifene has estrogen-like effects on bone (increase BMD) and on lipid (decrease in total and LDL-Cholesterol levels) metabolism. Preclinical data demonstrate that raloxifene is an estrogen antagonist in uterine and breast tissue.

PRECAUTIONS/ADVERSE REACTIONS

Contraindicated in pregnancy (Category X) or in women who may become pregnant and in woman with active or a history of venous thrombophlebitis. Not for use in premenopausal women. Not recommended with concomitant systemic estrogen therapy. Use cautiously in hepatic dysfunction.

Discontinue 72 hours before and during prolonged immobilization and resume when fully ambulatory.

Adverse reactions include hot flashes, leg cramps, and venous thromboembolic events (rare).

Instruct patients in calcium and Vitamin D rich diet and supplement if inadequate. Add weight-bearing exercise and modify other risk factors as appropriate. Inform patients to avoid prolonged restrictions of movement during travel.

ADMINISTRATION

60 mg once daily

PREPARATIONS

Tablets, 60 mg.

REPAGLINIDE

Prandin®

DESCRIPTION/ACTIONS

Antidiabetic agent chemically unrelated to the sulfonylureas. It lowers glucose by stimulating the release of insulin from the pancreas. Its action is dependent upon functioning β cells in the pancreatic islets. Compared to other oral antidiabetic agents, repaglinide has a quick onset of action and a short duration of action. Following oral administration, peak plasma levels occur within 1 hour, and it is rapidly eliminated from the blood with a half life of about 1 hour.

It is indicated as an adjunct to diet and exercise in Type 2 diabetes, as monotherapy or in combination with metformin.

PRECAUTIONS/ADVERSE REACTIONS

Contraindicated in Type 1 diabetes and diabetic ketoacidosis. Titrate carefully in renal or hepatic dysfunction. Use cautiously in elderly, debilitated, malnourished, stressed, adrenal or pituitary insufficiency. Increases the risk of hypoglycemia. Monitor for initial effect and for secondary failure. Pregnancy category C. Not recommended for use in nursing mothers.

Adverse reactions include hypoglycemia, upper respiratory infection, headache, diarrhea, constipation, arthralgia, back or chest pain. Oral antidiabetics may increase the risk of cardiovascular mortality.

Instruct patients to adhere to diet and exercise programs. Test blood glucose and HbA_{1C} regularly. Inform patients about management of hypoglycemia and explain primary vs. secondary failure.

ADMINISTRATION

Take within 30 minutes before meals. Treatment—naive of HbA1c <8%: initially 0.5 mg with 2–4 meals daily. Previously treated with antidiabetic agents and HbA1 ≥8%: initially 1–2 mg with 2–4 meals daily. For both, titrate by doubling dose at intervals of at least 1 week. Range: 0.5 mg–4 mg with 2–4 meals daily. Maximum dose of 16 mg/day. Should not be taken without meals.

PREPARATIONS

Tablets, 0.5, 1, and 2 mg.

RISEDRONATE

Actonel®

DESCRIPTION/ACTIONS

For treatment of patients with Paget's disease of the bone having alkaline phosphatase at least 2 times the upper limit of normal or those who are symptomatic or at risk for future complications from their disease. The major pharmacologic action is inhibition of normal and abnormal bone resorption.

PRECAUTIONS/ADVERSE REACTIONS

ium and vitamin D if dietary intake is inadequate. Take calcium, aluminum, and magnesium-containing agents at a different time of day to prevent interference with risedronate absorption.

Correct hypocalcemia before initiating treatment with risedronate. Not recommended for use in patients with severe renal failure(CrCl <30 mL/min). Small, asymptomatic decreases in serum calcium and phosphate may occur.

Adverse reactions include rash, influenzalike symptoms, edema, asthenia, sinusitis, amblyopia, dry eye, bronchitis, tinnitus, and neoplasm.

ADMINISTRATION

30 mg once daily ≥30 minutes before first food or drink (except water) of the day for 2 months.

Avoid lying down for 30 minutes after taking to reduce possibility of GI side effects.

Retreatment may be considered (following a posttreatment observation period ≥ 2 mos) if relapse occurs or treatment fails to normalize serum alkaline phosphatase.

PREPARATIONS

Tablets, 30 mg.

SIBUTRAMINE HYDROCHLORIDE

Meridia®

DESCRIPTION/ACTIONS

Antiobesity agent indicated as an adjunct to a reduced calorie diet in the management of obesity including weight loss and the maintenance of weight loss. Recommended for obese patients with an initial body mass index ≥30 kg/m^2 or >27 kg/m^2 in the presence of other risk factors such as hypertension, diabetes, and/or dyslipidemia.

PRECAUTIONS/ADVERSE REACTIONS

Contraindicated in arteriosclerosis, cardiovascular disease, hypertension, hyperthyroidism, glaucoma, agitation, drug or alcohol abuse, or during or within 14 days of MAOI's.

Discontinue if dyspnea, angina pectoris, syncope, lower extremity edema or other symptoms of primary pulmonary hypertension occur. Discontinue after a few weeks as tolerance to anorectic effect occurs. Use cautiously in diabetes. Prescribe a limited total amount to prevent overdose. Pregnancy Category C. Not recommended for use in nursing mothers.

Adverse reactions include CNS overstimulation, dizziness, palpitations, arrhythmias, hypertension, psychosis, dry mouth, GI disturbances, urticaria, impotence, primary pulmonary hypertension/and or regurgitant cardiac valvular disease.

ADMINISTRATION

10 mg once daily.

After 4 weeks may titrate to 15 mg once daily, if tolerated.

PREPARATIONS

Capsules, 5 mg, 10mg, 15 mg.

SILDENAFIL CITRATE

Viagra®

DESCRIPTION/ACTIONS

An oral tablet indicated for the treatment of erectile dysfunction (ED). The physiologic mechanism of penile erection involves the release of nitric oxide into the corpus cavernovsum during sexual stimulation. Nitric oxide activates the enzyme guanylate cyclase, resulting in an increase in cGMP levels. This increase in cGMP in the corpus cavernosum causes smooth muscle relaxation, allowing blood to flow into the erectile tissue. Sildenafil enhances the effect of nitric oxide by inhibiting PDE5, an enzyme responsible for the degradation of cGMP in the corpus cavernosum. Sildenafil has no direct relaxant effect on the corpus cavernosum, nor does it have any activity in the absence of sexual stimulation.

PRECAUTIONS/ADVERSE REACTIONS

Contraindicated with concomitant organic nitrates or nitric oxide donors. Use cautiously in anatomical penile deformation, predisposition to priapism, or in patients for whom sexual activity is inadvisable or contraindicated. Avoid use in bleeding disorders, active peptic ulceration, concomitant erectile dysfunction treatment, or retinosis pigmentosa. Not indicated for use in woman, children, or newborns.

Adverse reactions include headache, flushing, dyspepsia, nasal congestion, UTI, abnormal vision (color tinge to vision, increased light sensitivity, blurred vision), diarrhea, dizziness, and rash.

ADMINISTRATION

Take 1 dose as needed about 1 hour (0.5–4 hours) before sexual activity at a frequency of up to once daily. Use initial dose of 50 mg. May decrease dose to 25 mg or increase dose to a maximum of 100 mg. In elderly, hepatic impairment, severe renal impairment, or concomitant CYP3A4 inhibitors consider an initial dose of 25 mg.

PREPARATIONS

Tablets, 25, 50, and 100 mg.

TAMSULOSIN HYDROCHLORIDE

Flomax®

DESCRIPTION/ACTION

An A_{Ia} Adrenergic antagonist indicated in benign prostatic hyperplasia. Obstruction of bladder output is responsible for most of the symptoms of BPH. The urethral obstruction is partially a result of increased smooth muscle tone in the prostate and bladder neck leading to constriction of the bladder outlet. Tamsulosin blocks receptors causing smooth muscle relaxation in the bladder neck and prostate, resulting in an improvement in urine flow and a reduction in the symptoms of BPH.

PRECAUTIONS/ADVERSE REACTIONS

Rule out prostate cancer. Use cautiously in patient syncope. Adverse reactions include abnormal ejaculation, postural hypotension, dizziness, rhinitis, cough, somnolence, sinusitis, amblyopia, decreased libido, insomnia, and syncope.

ADMINISTRATION

Do not crush, chew, or open caps.

Take 1/2 hour after the same meal each day.

Initially 0.4 mg once daily, may increase to 0.8 mg once daily after 2–4 weeks if response is inadequate.

If therapy is interrupted resume at 0.4 mg once daily and retitrate.

PREPARATIONS

Capsules, 0.4 mg.

TIAGABINE HYDROCHLORIDE

Gabitril®

DESCRIPTION/ACTION

Antiepileptic agent indicated as an adjunct in partial seizures. In vitro studies suggest that the antiseizure effect of Tiagabine may be due to its ability to enhance the activity of GABA, the major inhibitory neurotransmitter in the CNS. These studies have shown that Tiagabine blocks GABA intake into the presynaptic neurons, leaving more GABA to be available for receptor binding on the surfaces of post synaptic cells.

PRECAUTIONS/ADVERSE REACTIONS

Avoid abrupt cessation. Use cautiously in nursing mothers, hepatic impairment, and the elderly. Pregnancy Category C.

Adverse reactions include dizziness, asthenia, somnolence, GI upset/pain, nervousness, tremor, abdominal pain, concentration difficulties, other CNS effects, serious rash, and possible long term opthalmologic effects.

ADMINISTRATION

Take with food. Use lower doses and titrate slower if not on concomitant enzyme -inducing drugs (e.g. phenytoin, phenobarbital, carbamezepine)

Children:	Not recommended
12–18 years:	4 mg once daily for 1 week
	May increase to 8 mg/day in 2 divided doses for 1 week
	May then increase by 4–8 mg weekly to clinical response or up to 32 mg/day in 2–4 divided doses.
>18 years:	4mg once daily for 1 week may increase by 4–8 mg weekly to clinical response or up to 56 mg/day in 2–4 divided doses.

PREPARATIONS

Tablets, 4, 12, 16, and 20 mg.

TIROFIBAN

Aggrastat®

DESCRIPTION/ACTIONS

Platelet aggregation inhibitor indicated in combination with heparin for treating acute coronary syndrome (unstable angina/non Q-wave myocardial infarction) including patients who are to be managed medically and those undergoing percutaneous transluminal angioplasty or atherectomy.

PRECAUTIONS/ADVERSE REACTIONS

Contraindicated in the following conditions within previous 30 days: active internal bleeding, bleeding diathesis, stroke, major surgery or severe trauma. Contraindicated with a history of intracranial hemorrhage, intracranial neoplasm, arteriovenous malformation, aneurysm, hemorrhagic stroke, thrombocytopenia after previous Tirofiban therapy, symptoms or findings suggestive of aortic dissection, severe hypertension, acute pericarditis and concomitant parenteral GI 11b/111A inhibitor.

Use cautiously in patients with renal failure, platelet count ≤150,000/mm^3 or hemorrhagic retinopathy. Properly care for femerol artery access site to minimize bleeding. Minimize other arterial and venous punctures, IM injections, catheter use and other invasive procedures to minimize bleeding risk. Avoid use of non-compressible IV access sites. Do baseline platelet counts, hemoglobin, hematocrit and monitor during therapy. Discontinue tirofiban if confirmed thrombocytopenia occurs. Adjust heparin to maintain aPTT at two times control.

Adverse reactions include bleeding, decreased hemoglobin and/or hematocrit, reduced platelet counts, edema, vasovagal reaction, and others.

ADMINISTRATION

Initial rate of 0.4 µg/kg per minute for 30 minutes then 0.1 µg/kg per minute. In severe renal insufficiency (Cr Cl <30mL/min) reduce both the loading and maintenance rate by half. Stop infusion if bleeding cannot be controlled by pressure. Pregnancy Cat B, Nursing mothers, and children <18 not recommended.

PREPARATIONS

Premixed 50 µg/mL vials.

Concentrate, 250 µg/mL.

TOLCAPONE

Tasmar®

DESCRIPTION/ACTION

Anti-Parkinson agent indicated as an adjunct to Carbidopa/Levodopa in idiopathic Parkinson's disease.

Tolcapone is a COMT (catechol-0-methyltransferase) inhibitor that improves a patients ability to function and perform basic daily activities. It can be used for both "non-fluctuating" patient's (those whose response to levodopa is relatively stable) and "fluctuating" patients (those with "wearing-off" and "on-off" phenomena and dyskinesias.) Tolcapone has been shown to enhance and extend the actions and benefits of Carbidopa/Levodopa.

COMT is one of two main enzymes that break down Levodopa before it reaches the brain. By inhibiting COMT, Tolcapone produces plasma levels of Levadopa that are more sustained than those seen with Carbidopa/Levadopa alone. This results in more sustained dopaminergic stimulation in the brain, which may allow for a reduction in the dose of levodopa.

PRECAUTIONS/ADVERSE REACTIONS

Contraindicated in concomitant non-selective MAOI's (e.g., phenelzine). Use cautiously in orthostatic hypertension/syncope, severe renal impairment (CrCl ≤25 mL/min), severe hepatic impairment. Monitor transaminases every month for the first 3 months, then every 6 weeks for the next 3 months (more frequently if elevation occurs). Discontinue if enzyme elevations ≥5 times the upper limit of normal or jaundice occurs. Pregnancy Category C.

Adverse reactions include dyskinesias, nausea, sleep disorders, dystonia, excessive dreaming, anorexia, muscle cramps, orthostatic complaints, somnolence, diarrhea, confusion, dizziness, headache, hallucinations, vomiting, constipation, fatigue, upper respiratory or urinary tract infection, falling, increased sweating, syncope, xerostomia, urine discoloration, and others.

ADMINISTRATION

100 or 200 mg three times daily to a maximum of 600 mg /day.

Moderate to severe hepatic cirrhosis use lower dose range.

PREPARATIONS

Tablets, 100 and 200 mg.

TOLTERODINE TARTRATE

Detrol®

DESCRIPTION/ACTIONS

A competitive muscarinic receptor antagonist indicated in treatment of patients with symptoms of urinary frequency, urgency, or urge incontinence. The main effects are an increase in residual urine and a decrease in detrusor pressure.

PRECAUTIONS/ADVERSE REACTIONS

Contraindicated in urinary retention, gastric retention, and uncontrolled narrow-angle glaucoma. Use cautiously in patients with bladder outflow obstruction, obstructive GI disease (e.g., pyloric stenosis), narrow-angle glaucoma, renal impairment, and hepatic dysfunction. Pregnancy Category C. Not recommended in nursing mothers.

Adverse reactions include dry mouth, dyspepsia, headache, constipation, xerophthalmia, hypertension, dizziness, and other anticholinergic effects. May cause blurred vision.

ADMINISTRATION

2 mg twice daily, may decrease to 1 mg twice daily. Significant hepatic dysfunction or CYP3A4 inhibitors, administer 1 mg twice daily.

PREPARATIONS

Tablets, 1 and 2 mg.

TOREMIFENE

Fareston®

DESCRIPTION/ACTIONS

Toremifene is a nonsteroidal antiestrogenic drug that binds to estrogen receptors. The antitumor effect of toremifene is thought to be due to its antiestrogenic effects, thereby blocking the growth stimulating effect of estrogen in the tumor. Its antiestrogen effect is evidenced by decreases in serum concentrations of luteinizing hormone and follicle stimulating hormone.

Indicated in metastatic breast cancer in postmenopausal women with estrogen-receptor positive or unknown tumors.

PRECAUTIONS/ADVERSE REACTIONS

Contraindicated in pregnancy (Category D) and nursing mothers.

Use not recommended in history of thromboembolic disorders and long-term treatment not recommended in patients with pre-existing endometrial hyperplasia. If bone metastases present, monitor for hypercalcemia for first few weeks. Discontinue if severe hypercalcemia occurs. Use cautiously with leukopenia and thrombocytopenia. Monitor blood counts, calcium levels and liver, function.

Adverse reactions include hot flashes, sweating, GI upset, vaginal discharge/bleed, dizziness, edema, tumor flare, hypercalcemia, elevated liver tests; cardiac, ocular, and thrombotic events.

Instruct patients to report vaginal bleeding and symptoms of hypercalcemia.

ADMINISTRATION

60 mg once daily until disease progression slows.

PREPARATIONS

Tablets, 60 mg.

TROVAFLOXACIN

ALATROFLOXACIN

Trovan®

DESCRIPTION/ACTIONS

Quinolone broad-spectrum antibiotic indicated in the treatment of susceptible infections.

PRECAUTIONS/ADVERSE REACTIONS

Discontinue if tendon pain, inflammation, or rupture occurs; if rash phototoxicity or other hypersensitivity occurs; or if CNS stimulation, psychosis, or increased intracranial pressure occur, severe atherosclerosis, epilepsy, or other conditions that predispose to seizures. Monitor liver function. Maintain adequate hydration. Avoid excessive sun and UV light. Pregnancy Category C. Not recommended for use in nursing mothers.

Adverse reactions include dizziness, lightheadedness, nausea, headache, vomiting, diarrhea, injection site reaction (IV), and pseudomembranous colitis.

ADMINISTRATION

Give each dose once daily. Avoid rapid IV Administration—infuse over 60 minutes, 100–300 mg as per manufacturer's guidelines for specific infectious organism being treated.

PREPARATIONS

Tablets, 100 and 200 mg.

Injection, 5 mg/mL concentrate for IV infusion after dilution in 40 and 60 mL single use vials

ZOLMITRIPTAN

Zomig®

DESCRIPTION/ACTIONS

Acts as an agonist at specific 5-hydroxytryptamine receptor sites in intracranial blood vessels and sensory trigeminal nerves. Exerts cranial vessel vasoconstriction with resultant decrease in migraine headache.

Indicated in the acute treatment of migraine headache with or without auras.

PRECAUTIONS/ADVERSE REACTIONS

Use not recommended in children. Contraindicated in ischemic heart disease (history of MI, angina pectoris, documented silent ischemia), coronary artery vasospasm (e.g., Prinzmetal's angina), uncontrolled hypertension, other significant cardiovascular disease, basilar or hemiplegic migraine, within 24 hours of other 5-HT1 agonists or ergot-type drugs, during or within 2 weeks after discontinuing MAOI's.

Confirm diagnosis and exclude underlying cardiovascuar disease. Supervise 1st dose and consider monitoring ECG in patients with likelihood of unrecognized coronary disease (e.g., postmenopausal women, men over age 40), hypertension, hydrocholesterolemia, obesity, diabetes, smokers, strong family history). Monitor cardiovascular function in longer-term intermittent use. Use not recommended in Wolff-Parkinson-White Syndrome or arrhythmias associated with other cardiac accessory conduction pathway disorders. Use cautiously in hepatic dysfunction, elderly, and nursing mothers. Pregnancy Category C.

Adverse reactions include paresthesia, asthenia, nausea, dizziness, pain, chest or neck tightness/heaviness, somnolence, and warm feeling.

ADMINISTRATION

INITIALLY 2.5 mg or lower (may break 2.5 mg tab by hand).

If headache returns may repeat after 2 hours; max 10 mg/day. Reevaluate if no response.

The safety of treating more than 3 headaches in a 30-day period has not been established.

Use low dose in hepatic impairment.

PREPARATIONS

Tablets, 2.5 mg and 5 mg.